OXFORD MEDICAL PUBLICATIONS

Optic neuritis and its differential diagnosis

Optic neuritis and its differential diagnosis

G. D. Perkin
Consultant Neurologist, Charing Cross Hospital

F. Clifford Rose
Consultant Neurologist, Charing Cross Hospital

Consultant Neurologist, Medical Ophthalmology Unit, St. Thomas's Hospital

Oxford New York Toronto
OXFORD UNIVERSITY PRESS
1979

Oxford University Press, Walton Street, Oxford OX2 6DP

Oxford London Glasgow New York
Toronto Melbourne Wellington Cape Town
Ibadan Nairobi Dar es Salaam Lusaka Addis Ababa
Kuala Lumpur Singapore Jakarta Hong Kong Tokyo
Delhi Bombay Calcutta Madras Karachi

© G. D. Perkin and F. Clifford Rose, 1979

British Library Cataloguing in Publication Data
Perkin, G. D.
  Optic neuritis and its differential diagnosis.
  – (Oxford medical publications).
  1. Optic neuritis – Diagnosis 2. Diagnosis, Differential
  I. Title II. Rose, Frank Clifford III. Series
  617.7'3   RE728.0/   78–40806

ISBN 0–19–261156–9

Set, printed and bound in Great Britain by Fakenham Press Limited, Fakenham, Norfolk

Preface

With the opening of the Royal Eye Medical Ophthalmology Unit in 1963, it became possible to make a close in-patient study of optic neuritis. In all, 172 cases were collected and the majority reviewed 6 years later. The results form the basis of this monograph, which in addition considers the literature of the subject and the problems of differential diagnosis.

A study devoted to demyelination of a tiny part of the central nervous system may be considered an esoteric exercise. There are, however, cogent reasons for paying so much attention to the optic nerve in multiple sclerosis. Pathological evidence indicates that areas of demyelination in the nerve are almost inevitable in cases of long standing. Furthermore its accessibility both for clinical and physiological analysis allows a more ready assessment of its function than is possible for other parts of the central nervous system. The introduction of visual evoked responses and other techniques has enabled identification of optic nerve lesions which hitherto have remained undetected. It does not seem over-optimistic to assume that the greater understanding of the behaviour of multiple sclerosis which they provide can lead in turn to a clearer idea of the factors determining the progression and clinical declaration of the disease.

Department of Neurology,   G.D.P.
Charing Cross Hospital,   F.C.R.
London, 1978

Acknowledgements

The study on which this book is based progressed through the particular interest of Dr. P. M. A. Bowden, at present Consultant in Forensic Psychiatry at St. George's Hospital, London, to whom we wish to express our grateful thanks.

We are indebted to the surgeons at the Royal Eye Hospital, and in particular Mr. A. I. Friedmann, for referring cases and for their encouragement. The ophthalmological assessments at the follow-up examination in 1969 were kindly performed by Mr. P. I. Condon, F.R.C.S., Mr. P. Eustace, F.R.C.S., and Mr. J. C. McGrand, F.R.C.S.

The illustrations for this book have been prepared by the staff of the Medical Illustration Department, Charing Cross Hospital, under the guidance of Miss P. M. Turnbull.

We are indebted to Miss B. Laatz for her secretarial work during the preparation of the manuscript, and to Dr. K. D. MacRae, Senior Lecturer in Statistics, Charing Cross Hospital, for the statistical analyses.

Figures

Figs. 0.1 and 0.2 are reproduced by permission of the *Journal of Neurophysiology* and Dr. C. R. Michael; Figs. 4.23, 4.24, 4.25, and 4.26 by permission of the Ophthalmological Society of the United Kingdom; Figs. 4.27 and 4.28 by permission of Dr. Max Chamlin (from Figs. 1 and 2 in *Archives of Ophthalmology*, Vol. 50, pp. 699–713, 1953, © 1953, American Medical Association). Fig. 4.30 is by permission of the Ophthalmological Society of the United Kingdom. Figs. 5.2, (a), (b), and (c) are reproduced by permission of Professor W. F. Hoyt from Fig. 1 in *Archives of Ophthalmology*, Vol. 87, pp. 1–11, 1972, © 1972, American Medical Association. Fig. 5.3 is reproduced by permission of the editor of the *American Journal of Ophthalmology*, Figs. 5.4, 5.5 (a) and (b) were kindly loaned by Dr. G. A. S. Lloyd, Consultant Radiologist, and have been reproduced by permission of the editors of the *British Journal of Radiology*, having previously been published as Figs. 6, 7, and 7b in *British Journal of Radiology*, Vol. 44, pp. 405–11, 1971. Fig. 5.6 is reproduced by permission of Dr. J. Lawton Smith and the editor of the *American Journal of Ophthalmology*. Fig. 5.7 is reproduced by permission of Dr. M. K. Rubinstein from Fig. 1 in *Archives of Ophthalmology*, Vol. 80, pp. 42–4, 1968, © 1968, American Medical Association. Figs. 6.1, 6.2, and 6.3 are reproduced from Figs. 2,6 (A and B) and 13 (E and F) in *Archives of Ophthalmology* Vol. 20, pp. 201–54, 1938, © 1938, American Medical Association. Fig. 6.4 is reproduced by permission of Dr. B. W. Miller and the editor of the *American Journal of Ophthalmology*. Fig. 7.1 is reproduced by permission of Dr. A. L. Feldmahn from Fig. 1 in *Archives of Ophthalmology*, Vol. 65, pp. 381–5, 1961, © 1961, American Medical Association. Fig. 7.2 is reproduced from Fig. 142 in Traquair's *Clinical perimetry* (7th edn), 1957 by permission of the publishers, Henry Kimpton Ltd., London. Fig. 7.3 is reproduced by

viii *Acknowledgements*

permission of the Ophthalmological Society of the United Kingdom. Fig. 7.4 is reproduced by permission of Mr. A. D. Mackenzie and the editor of *Brain*. Fig. 8.1 is reproduced by permission of the Ophthalmological Society of the United Kingdom. Fig. 8.2 is reproduced by permission of Mr. M. D. Sanders and the editor of the *British Journal of Ophthalmology*. Fig. 8.3 is reproduced by permission of Dr. J. W. Goldzieher, from the *Archives of Neurology*, Vol. 65, p. 190, 1951, © 1951, American Medical Association. Fig. 10.1 is reproduced by permission of Dr. F. A. Davis and the editor, the *Journal of Neurology, Neurosurgery and Psychiatry*. Fig. 10.2 is reproduced by permission of Dr. F. A. Davis and the editor of *Neurology*. Fig. 11.3 is reproduced by permission of Dr. F. A. Davis and the editor, *Acta Neurologica Scandinavica*. Figs. 11.4 and 11.5 are reproduced by permission of Dr. C. L. Schauf and the editor of the *Journal of Neurology, Neurosurgery and Psychiatry*. Figs. 12.5 and 12.6 are reproduced by permission of Dr. H. S. Thompson and the editor of the *American Journal of Ophthalmology*. Fig. 12.9 is reproduced by permission of Dr. Lars Frisén from Fig. 3 in *Archives of Ophthalmology*, Vol. 92, pp. 91–7, 1974, © 1974, American Medical Association. Figs. 14.2 and 14.3 are reproduced by permission of Dr. A. M. Halliday and the Ophthalmological Society of the United Kingdom.

Contents

Introduction
The optic nerve—some basic aspects

A central or paracentral scotoma is the characteristic finding since the macular fibres are those commonly affected by demyelination (McAlpine 1972).

Optic nerve anatomy

The optic nerve, between 35 and 55 mm in length, is divided into four sections—intra-ocular (1 mm), orbital (20–30 mm), canalicular (4–10 mm), and intra-cranial (3–16 mm). The intra-orbital length considerably exceeds the distance from the pole of the eye to the optic foramen (18 mm) determining the S shape of the nerve in the resting position, though this disappears when the eye is fully abducted. The diameter of the nerve increases from 1 mm at the intra-ocular point, through 3–4 mm in the orbit, to 4–7 mm within the cranial cavity.

Relationships

The optic disc is some 3·5 mm medial to the fovea centralis. The central retinal artery and vein enter the nerve infero-medially 5 to 15 mm behind the globe, as it runs postero-medially along the orbital axis to the optic foramen. The ciliary ganglion lies lateral to the nerve, between it and the lateral rectus muscle. At the optic foramen the ophthalmic artery lies below and laterally, with medially the inferior division of the third nerve, the sixth nerve, and the naso-ciliary artery. At the apex of the orbit the nerve is surrounded by the recti, of which the superior and medial rectus arise partly from its nerve sheath. Despite this, in our experience, abduction of the eye is more likely to be painful than adduction in cases of optic neuritis. In the optic canal the nerve lies lateral to the sphenoidal sinus and sometimes the posterior ethmoidal sinus, a relationship discussed in more detail in Chapter 6.

The nerve sheath

The retrolaminar part of the nerve is enclosed in a sheath composed of dura, arachnoid, and pia. The dura lining the optic canal splits at the orbital opening one part continuing over the orbital bone, the other forming the outer layer of the optic nerve sheath and eventually blending with the outer scleral fibres. Externally a layer of fascia separates it from the remaining orbital contents. The arachnoid sheath clothes the nerve as it leaves the basal cisterns and finally fuses with the sclera. The pia is closely applied to the nerve and is continuous with the various septa which traverse it.

The nerve fibres

Approximately 130 million rods and 7 million cones transmit information to the 1·1–1·3 million fibres in the optic nerve (Potts, Hodges, Shelman, Fritz, Levy, and Mangnall, 1972a). In the prelaminar region, the nerve fibres are arranged in 800–1200 fascicles surrounded by tube-like glial channels formed by astrocytes. Histograms of axis cylinder size show a unimodal distribution peaking at 0·25–0·5 μm (Potts *et al.* 1972b), the corresponding figure for fibre diameter in the primate being 1·2 μm. At the lamina cribrosa a bridge of dense connective tissue crosses the scleral canal, perforated by numerous openings for the transmission of nerve fibre bundles lined by astrocytes. The myelin sheath stops shortly behind the lamina cribrosa, but on occasions extends along the retinal fibres. Here it is visible on fundoscopy, and may disappear following a demyelinating episode (Gartner 1953).

The septa of connective tissue composed of collagen and elastic fibres, separate the individual fascicles and are continuous with the pial sheath. Between the septa a neuroglial framework separates individual fibres, comprising fibrous astrocytes and oligodendrocytes. The latter are arranged in columns between the fibres with projections surrounding the myelin sheaths (Duke-Elder and Wybar 1961). Infrequent microglial cells are also found. It has been suggested that the intercellular clefts of 10–20 nm between the glial cells and nerve fibres permit rapid transport of ions and molecules.

In the distal optic nerve, the disposition of fibres reflects the retinal pattern. Upper retinal fibres lie dorsal to lower and temporal fibres lateral to nasal fibres, with the macular pathway occupying a superficial sector-shaped area laterally. More proximally, the macular fibres occupy a central position. Foveal destruction in the rhesus monkey leads to degeneration of up to one quarter of all optic nerve fibres, virtually confined to those less than 0·75 μm in diameter (Potts *et al.* 1972c). Arcuate fibres lie in the superior and inferior temporal optic nerve and maintain this distribution throughout its course (Hoyt 1962).

Blood supply

Arterial

Prelaminar. Supply of this part has been attributed to centripetal branches from the peripapillary choroidal vessels (Hayreh 1969) or to scleral branches of the short posterior ciliary artery entering through the border tissue of Elschnig (Ernest, 1976; Lieberman, Maumenee, and Green 1976).

Lamina cribrosa. This portion of the optic nerve receives centripetal branches from the short posterior ciliary arteries and occasionally from the circle of Zinn.

Retro-laminar nerve. This part of the nerve has both centripetal and longitudinal vessels of pial origin. The longitudinal system, which extends to the retinal surface, anastomoses with three transverse systems—arterioles from the short posterior ciliary artery, choroidal capillaries or short posterior ciliary branches at the prelaminar level, and branches from the central retinal artery in the region of the disc (Lieberman *et al.* 1976).

Orbital nerve. The periphery is supplied by vessels of the pial sheath derived from branches of the internal carotid artery. The axial portion receives branches from the central retinal artery, the central retinal collateral arteries, and the central artery of the optic nerve.

Intracanalicular and intracranial. These parts of the optic nerve are supplied by peripheral branches from the pial plexus.

Venous

The venous pattern of the anterior optic nerve is relatively uniform, predominantly draining to the central retinal vein, with smaller vessels passing to the choroid and pia mater.

Optic nerve physiology (Arden 1976; Holden 1976)

The concept of the division of the retina into temporal and nasal halves with completely distinct visual projections has had to be modified. In the cat, a central strip of some 0·2 mm, corresponding to a visual angle of 1°, contains ganglion cells which project to either optic tract. In addition, though all fibres nasal to this strip project contralaterally, only 75 per cent of the cells temporal to the strip project ipsilaterally the remainder giving rise to decussating fibres. A similar arrangement exists in the monkey.

Each ganglion cell, though projecting to a single nerve fibre, transmits impulses from a large number of receptor cells. The receptive field of a cell in the visual system is defined as that area of the retina, or of the visual field, within which illumination will influence (excite or inhibit) the discharge of that particular cell (Michael 1968*a*). In the cat, many of the receptive fields are roughly circular with a centre and surround zone. The central zone may be excited by increased illumination (an on-centre cell) or decreased illumination (an off-centre cell), the surround having the reverse response to the centre. A similar arrangement is found in the ground-squirrel (Fig. 0.1). In some cases the field centre has to be light adapted or the background luminance increased before a consistent surround response is elicited. In the cat, with dark adaptation, the surround response tends to disappear. Other ganglion cells have a more complex receptive field organization, with on- and off-zones overlapping. Such cells may respond to particular directions of movement (Fig. 0.2) or to the orientation of the object (Michael 1968*b*). The ganglion cells are more concentrated near the fovea and of smaller size. Such cells have a smaller receptive field (0·5° in the cat) compared to the peripheral cells (8°) and are subject to a greater degree of surround inhibition.

Three types of ganglion cell are distinguished (X, Y, and W) according to differing morphological and physiological characteristics (Table 0.1). The proportion of Y cells decreases towards the central area in both the cat and the monkey, where X cells predominate. The higher resolution with central vision has been attributed to the smaller receptive field and intense surround inhibition of the X cell. The sensitivity of the peripheral retina to movement can be equated with the properties of Y cells; in particular their responsiveness to target velocity.

The very small W ganglion cells, which connect to correspondingly small

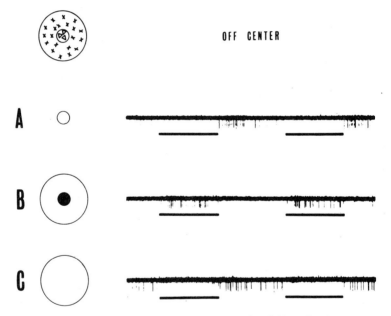

Fig. 0.1. Responses of an off-centre unit. Receptive field outlined in upper left-hand corner of figure. Crosses designate on-responses; triangles, off-discharges. Diameter of field 0·5°. In each example black bars indicate the 1-s periods of illumination. A: spot covering field centre (0·5°) completely suppressed the resting activity and evoked a strong off-response. B: annulus, 0·5° inner diameter — 4° outer diameter, elicited an on-response. C: 4° spot caused complete inhibition of resting activity followed by resumption of spontaneous rate. Intensity of stimuli, $1 \cdot 9 \log_{10}$ cd/m²; background illumination $0 \log_{10}$ cd/m². cd = candela (from Michael 1968*a*).

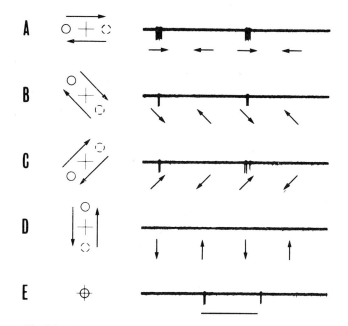

Fig. 0.2. Responses of a directionally selective unit to a white spot moving through the field centre in different directions. Geometrical centre of receptive field indicated by a cross in each example. Size of stimulus, 10 min; field centre 1°. In A the preferred direction of motion evokes the strongest response; the reverse or null direction has no effect. In B and C intermediate directions evoke weaker responses. In D, movement at right angles to the preferred—null axis evokes no response. The on-off response to the centered stationary stimulus is shown in E. Intensity of stimulus $2\cdot0$ $\log_{10}$ cd/m²; background, 0 $\log_{10}$ cd/m². (cd = candela). Rate of movement, 10°/s. Black bar indicates 1 s (from Michael 1968*b*).

axons, appear particularly responsive to a specific orientation or direction of movement. These cells do not however appear to be a homogeneous group and their exact function remains uncertain.

In the cat, three types of optic nerve fibre have been identified, differing in receptive field characteristics, conduction velocity, and central connections. The compound action potential of the cat's optic nerve and tract contains three components, T_1, T_2, and T_3, thought to correspond to the X, Y, and W ganglion cells. Conduction velocities in the axons connected to these cells are highest for the Y group and lowest for the W group. Differing values have been obtained but usually lie between $5\cdot5$ and 14 m/s for W axons, 9–14 m/s for X axons, and 29–39 m/s for the Y axons. In the cat, X and Y cells project to the lateral geniculate nucleus, whilst W and Y cells project to the tectum.

Table 0.1 Characteristics of ganglion cells in the retina

	X	Y
Size	Small	Large
Position	Mainly central	Mainly peripheral
Connecting axons	Small	Large
Axonal conduction velocity (CAT)	9–14 m/s	29–39 m/s
Destination (CAT)	Lateral geniculate nucleus	Lateral geniculate nucleus and optic tectum
Receptive field (CAT)	0.5°	8°
Response to sustained light	Sustained	Transient
Response to brief light pulses	More delayed and sustained	More rapid and transient
Flicker-fusion rate (at which individual light flashes not signalled by individual spikes)	Slower	More rapid
Discharge rate altered by stimulus remote from receptive field	No	Yes
Response to grating stimulus	Can be abolished by altering phase angle of stimulus	Never completely abolished whatever phase of grating
Response to rapid movement	No	Yes

Centrifugal fibres

In addition to pupillary and visual afferent fibres, the optic nerve contains efferent fibres destined for the retina, passing through the inner plexiform layer to terminate in association with the amacrine cells. There is some evidence that stimulation of these fibres modifies ERG responses. In pigeons, removal of the efferent system increases the inhibitory surround of the retinal ganglion cell receptive field (Pearlman and Hughes 1973).

The pathological changes in optic neuritis

Berliner (1935) found the pathological changes in optic neuritis predominated in the perivascular zones, particularly between the papilla and the entrance of the central retinal artery. Gartner (1953) examined 14 eyes from 10 patients in whom the diagnosis of multiple sclerosis had been confirmed at post-mortem examination. All had involvement of the visual pathways, though an attack of optic neuritis had been diagnosed in life in only two of them. Optic nerve atrophy was almost always found, and though usually including a considerable portion of the papillomacular bundle was never confined to it, extending to adjacent fibres and sometimes the periphery. The nerves contained an increased number of glial cells with fibroblasts and lymphocytes seldom showing a perivascular distribution. The optic nerve head showed extensive gliosis with sclerosis of the blood-vessel walls. Atrophy of retinal nerve fibres with their associated ganglion cell bodies was particularly prominent at the macula. All the cases examined by Gartner (1953) were in an advanced state of the disease by the time of their admission. The ultra-structure of the optic nerve in a patient with multiple sclerosis has been recently described (de Preux and Mair 1974). Both optic nerves had areas of partial and complete demyelination on light microscopy, the completely demyelinated zones being denuded of oligodendrocytes. The naked axons showed swollen, vacuolated mitochondria. In the partially demyelinated nerve oligodendrocytes persisted and in all areas there was an excess of fibrous astrocytes. Some phagocytes contained nuclear inclusion bodies, though of a type differing from those described in nerve cells and astrocytes of multiple sclerosis patients.

Pathophysiology of optic nerve demyelination

Demyelination of nerve fibres, whatever their function, may lead to complete conduction block, slowing of conduction, or a failure to transmit a rapid train of impulses (Davis and Schauf 1975). Though demyelination could account for the rapid onset of vision loss in optic neuritis, alternative mechanisms for the equally rapid recovery have been sought, including the concept of optic nerve oedema (Halliday and McDonald 1977). The amplitude of the visual evoked response (Chapter 14) recovers in line with visual acuity, but delay, established at the time of the attack, seldom does so, suggesting it reflects—at least in part—continuing demyelination. The degree of conduction block in experimental peripheral nerve demyelination depends on local electrolyte concentration. With a fall in ionized calcium concentration, conduction is restored in some previously blocked fibres. With increasing myelin loss, conduction fails at progressively lower temperatures in peripheral nerve fibres, a finding probably also applicable to the central nervous system. For a given degree of demyelination, blocking temperature falls as axonal diameter decreases (Schauf and Davis 1974).

Peripheral field defects may be more common than is normally appreciated in multiple sclerosis, their subtle quality failing to attract the attention of the patient or his physician. In most published series however, and in our own experience, central scotomata have predominated. Post-mortem studies of the optic nerve in multiple sclerosis patients indicate that plaques tend to extend outside the limits of the papillomacular bundle, though admittedly in many of these cases multiple episodes of optic nerve demyelination might have occurred prior to examination. It seems unlikely that morphological factors alone explain the predominance of central defects.

Optic nerve oedema has been suggested as a possible factor in the pathogenesis of conduction failure in acute optic neuritis. A compressive effect, with consequent demyelination, would be an unlikely explanation since, using as a model the effect of compression on peripheral nerve fibres (Neary and Eames 1975), larger myelinated axons would be more affected than the small diameter fibres subserving foveal function. The greater concentration of fibres in the papillo-macular bundle may render them more susceptible to the metabolic disturbances likely to be present in an area of acute demyelination. The smaller axonal diameter of foveal fibres might also be relevant, arguing from the greater susceptibility of such fibres, when demyelinated, to the blocking effect of one such 'metabolic' insult, namely rising temperature.

Residual visual disturbance following the acute episode cannot be explained on the basis of conduction delay, since this consequence, based on persistence of delayed visual evoked responses, is almost invariable and independent of final visual acuity. Short-lived visual phenomena (Uhthoff 1890) following recovery, induced by temperature increase, would be likely to predominantly affect central vision, since the smaller fibres of the papillomacular bundle, when demyelinated, are more readily blocked by increasing temperature (Schauf and Davis 1974). Persistent vision loss is likely to be a manifestation of permanent conduction block, with or without the addition of axonal degeneration. The repeated emphasis on central vision loss in such cases would suggest that foveal fibres are particularly liable to undergo axonal degeneration following demyelination. Our own findings, however, and those of other recent studies suggest this view may represent an over-simplification. Frisen and Hoyt (1974) have described elongated scotomata between 10° and 25° from fixation in patients with retinal nerve fibre atrophy. Our own findings indicate that persistent paracentral and peripheral field defects predominate after recovery, suggesting that axonal degeneration, or at least conduction failure, is at least as common in arcuate fibres as for those in the papillomacular bundle.

Conclusions

Macular fibres are of smaller size but arranged at greater density than fibres in the remainder of the optic nerve. Retinal ganglion cells are divisible into three types on morphological and physiological criteria, and the optic nerve compound action potential is triphasic with peaks corresponding to fibres relaying from these cells. Conduction velocities are substantially slower for axons connected to foveal receptors than for those coming from the peripheral retina.

In optic neuritis all degrees of myelin loss are encountered, naked axons additionally showing a loss of oligodendrocytes. The nerve is infiltrated by fibrous astrocytes and phagocytes, and, in some of the latter, nuclear inclusion bodies have been described.

Demyelination of peripheral nerve can lead to conduction failure, conduction delay, or an inability to transmit a rapid train of impulses, and the optic nerve probably behaves similarly. Conduction delay cannot explain the clinical features of acute optic neuritis, and it seems likely that a reversible conduction block accounts for the behaviour of the visual disorder. Morphological factors alone do not account for the predominance of central visual impairment in the acute stages, suggesting that the smaller foveal fibres when demyelinated are more susceptible to a deranged metabolic environment. Their greater susceptibility to the blocking effect of temperature explains the frequency with which transient blurring of vision is noticed following recovery. Permanent visual impairment after optic neuritis is unusual and probably reflects conduction block with or without axonal degeneration. Though it has usually been considered to predominantly affect central vision, our own study suggests that conduction failure in arcuate fibres is at least as common, with a corresponding frequency of para-central field defects following clinical recovery.

REFERENCES

Arden, G. B. (1976). The retina-neurophysiology. In *The eye*, Vol. 2A, *Visual function in man* (2nd edn.), (ed. H. Davson), Chapter 7, pp. 229–356. Academic Press, New York.
Berliner, M. L. (1935). Acute optic neuritis in demyelinating diseases of the nervous system. *Archs Ophthal., N.Y.* **13**, 83–98.
Davis, F. A. and Schauf, C. L. (1975). Pathophysiology of multiple sclerosis. In *Multiple sclerosis research, Proceedings of a joint conference held by the Medical Research Council and the Multiple Sclerosis Society of Great Britain and Northern Ireland* (ed. A. N. Davison, J. H. Humphrey, A. L. Liversedge, W. I. McDonald, and J. S. Porterfield). HMSO, London.
de Preux, J. and Mair, W. G. P. (1974). Ultra-structure of the optic nerve in Schilder's disease, Devic's disease and disseminated sclerosis. *Acta neuropathol. (Berl.)* **30**, 225–42.
Duke-Elder, Sir Stewart and Wybar, K. C. (1961). The anatomy of the visual system. *System of ophthalmology* (ed. Sir Stewart Duke-Elder), Vol. 2. Henry Kimpton, London.
Ernest, J. T. (1976). Vasculature of the anterior optic nerve. *Am. J. Ophthal.* **82**, 509–10.
Frisén, L. and Hoyt, W. F. (1974). Insidious atrophy of retinal nerve fibers in multiple sclerosis. *Archs Ophthal., N.Y.* **92**, 91–7.
Gartner, S. (1953). Optic neuropathy in multiple sclerosis. Optic neuritis. *Archs Ophthal., N.Y.* **50**, 718–26.
Halliday, A. M. and McDonald, W. I. (1977). Pathophysiology of demyelinating disease. *Br. med. Bull.* **33**, 21–7.

Hayreh, S. S. (1969). Blood supply of the optic nerve head and its role in optic atrophy, glaucoma and oedema of the optic disc. *Br. J. Ophthal.* **53**, 721–48.

Holden, A. L. (1976). The central visual pathways. In *The eye*, Vol. 2A., *Visual function in man* (2nd edn.), (ed. H. Davson), Chapter 8, pp. 357–474. Academic Press, New York.

Hoyt, W. F. (1962). Anatomic considerations of arcuate scotomas associated with lesions of the optic nerve and chiasm. A nauta axon degeneration study in the monkey. *Bull. Johns Hopkins Hosp.* **111**, 57–71.

Lieberman, M. F., Maumenee, A. E., and Green, W. R. (1976). Histologic studies of the vasculature of the anterior optic nerve. *Am. J. Ophthal.* **82**, 405–23.

McAlpine, D. (1972). Clinical studies. In *Multiple sclerosis: a reappraisal* (2nd edn.), ed. D. MacAlpine, C. E. Lumsden, and E. D. Acheson), p. 157. Churchill Livingstone, Edinburgh.

Michael, C. R. (1968*a*). Receptive fields of single optic nerve fibers in a mammal with an all-cone retina. I: contrast—sensitive units. *J. Neurophysiol.* **31**, 249–56.

— (1968*b*). Receptive fields of single optic nerve fibers in a mammal with an all-cone retina. II: directionally selective units. *J. Neurophysiol.* **31**, 257–67.

Neary, D. and Eames, R. A. (1975). The pathology of ulnar nerve compression in man. *Neuropathol. and appl. Neurobiol.* **1**, 69–88.

Pearlman, A. L. and Hughes, C. P. (1973). Functional role of efferents to the retina. *Trans. Am. neurol. Ass.* **98**, 48–51.

Potts, A. M., Hodges, D., Shelman, C. B., Fritz, K. J., Levy, N. S., and Magnall, Y. (1972*a*). Morphology of the primate optic nerve. 1. Method and total fiber count. *Invest. Ophthal.* **11**, 980–8.

—————— (1972*b*). Morphology of the primate optic nerve. 2. Total fiber size distribution and fiber density distribution. *Invest. Ophthal.* **11**, 989–1003.

————— (1972*c*). Morphology of the primate optic nerve. 3. Fiber characteristic of the foveal outflow. *Invest. Ophthal.* **11**, 1004–16.

Schauf, C. L. and Davis, F. A. (1974). Impulse conduction in multiple sclerosis: A theoretical basis for modification by temperature and pharmacological agents. *J. Neurol. Neurosurg. Psychiat.* **37**, 152–61.

Uhthoff, W. (1890). Untersuchungen uber die bei der multiplen herdsklerose vorkommenden augenstorungen. *Arch. Psychiat. NervKrankh.* **21**, 55–116, 303–410.

Note. The abbreviations used in this book for titles of journals are those of the *World List of Scientific Periodicals, 1900–1960* (fourth edition 1963), Butterworths, London. For journals introduced since 1960, the notation of the *Cumulated Index Medicus*, published by the U.S. Department of Health, Education, and Welfare, has been followed.

1 Historical survey

They are characterized by failure of sight limited to one eye, often accompanied by neuralgic pain about the temple and orbit and by pain in moving the eye; many recover but permanent damage and even total blindness may ensue; there is at first little, sometimes no, ophthalmoscopic change, but the disc often becomes more or less atrophic in a few weeks, and occasionally there are slight retinal changes (Nettleship 1884).

The credit for the description of the syndrome of optic neuritis belongs to a number of authors besides Nettleship (Parinaud 1884; Uhthoff 1890; Buzzard 1893; Gunn 1897). Nettleship further delineated the syndrome by pointing out the tendency for the ocular pain to antedate the visual failure, and for the maximal visual field disturbance to be central.

Gunn (1897, 1904a, 1904b) published a number of articles, reviewing a series which eventually extended to 350 cases. The tendency for the visual failure to progress over one to three days and recover over a period of approximately six weeks was described, and the occasional failure to recover was also appreciated. Gunn confirmed the frequency of central field involvement and noted the common disturbance of colour vision; in addition, he described the paradoxical association of a normal visual acuity with a recent history of visual failure, although claiming that all such cases, if examined carefully, would have a colour scotoma at or near fixation.

Pain

Gunn reiterated the frequency of ocular pain (in one-third of his patients) and described an associated tenderness on pressure of the globe. Surprisingly, Benedict (1933) regarded pain as an uncommon symptom, but in a subsequent analysis (1942) he found it to be present in at least 50 per cent of cases. More recently, a frequency of 77 per cent has been recorded (Hutchinson 1976). Although the severity of the associated pain was initially regarded as an important factor in prognosis for visual recovery (Nettleship 1884; Swanzy 1897), this has not been subsequently confirmed.

The visual field defect

Traquair (1930) elaborated on the visual field changes, stressing the invariable involvement of the central field in the acute stages, and Adie (1932) also made a central scotoma a prerequisite for the diagnosis.

In a group of 12 patients with multiple sclerosis, but with a more insidious visual failure, Klingmann (1910) found multiple, predominantly temporal, paracentral scotomata, with relative preservation of central vision. Cases of acute optic neuritis with visual field changes suggesting chiasmal (Traquair 1925) or tract involvement (Rønne 1928) were subsequently described. In an analysis of 100 consecutive cases of optic neuritis, Chamlin (1953) placed less emphasis on central field changes; paracentral nerve fibre bundle defects were present in 24 per cent of his cases, although Traquair (1930) had previously regarded them as a rarity in this condition. The subtle quality of such visual field changes, emphasized in a recent paper by Frisén and Hoyt (1974), may well account for these differences. Although Bradley and Whitty (1967) initially excluded patients with atypical field defects from their review, subsequent analysis showed this group did not differ in terms of eventual visual recovery from those cases with central field involvement.

Fundal changes

Uhthoff (1904) recorded disc swelling in 5 per cent of his patients with optic neuritis. Subsequent authors (Paton 1914; Lillie 1934; Berliner 1935; Sugar 1939) tended to accord it a similar emphasis, although Adie (1932) described disc oedema, often of minor degree, in 30 per cent of 70 cases.

Retinal haemorrhages were less often described. They were, however, noted by both Lillie (1934) and Berliner (1935), but only accompanying more marked degrees of optic disc swelling.

Differing figures have been quoted for the development of optic atrophy after an attack of acute optic neuritis. Berliner (1935) regarded some degree of atrophy as almost invariable, whereas Hyllested and Moller (1961) found it in only 60 per cent of their 52 cases.

Uhthoff's syndrome

Uhthoff (1890) is generally credited with the first description of transient visual blurring in patients with multiple sclerosis, his four cases developing the symptoms with exercise. Gunn (1897, 1904b) observed the same phenomenon, in patients recovering from optic neuritis, in association with bright light, and, with remarkable prescience, attributed it to a 'physiological degeneration' in ill-nourished axis cylinders. Subsequently a number of factors, in particular heating, were recorded as being capable of causing a short-lived exacerbation of visual and other symptoms in patients with multiple sclerosis. Indeed, Davis (1966) regarded the phenomenon as being sufficiently specific to recommend the use of a hot-bath test as a diagnostic investigation. Nelson, Jeffreys and McDowell (1958) had, however, by then described visual blurring with heating in patients with diagnoses other than multiple sclerosis (Friedreich's ataxia, pituitary tumour, and posterior cerebral artery insufficiency) and recently Smith, Hoyt, and Susac (1973) reported a patient with Leber's optic atrophy who presented with exercise-induced visual blurring, confirming an earlier description, in two cases, by Norris (1884).

Cerebrospinal fluid changes

Although characteristic changes in the cerebrospinal fluid (CSF) were quickly appreciated as a valuable aid in the diagnosis of multiple sclerosis, the possible changes occurring in patients with isolated optic neuritis were seldom investigated. Watkins (1939) described the CSF findings in 40 patients with acute optic neuritis, but failed to distinguish those with established multiple sclerosis. Yahr, Goldensohn and Kabat (1954) found normal gamma globulin levels in the CSF in six patients with retrobulbar neuritis, despite recording elevated levels in 66·5 per cent of their cases of multiple sclerosis. Similarly, elevated gamma-globulin levels were found in only one of 11 patients with optic neuritis studied by Ivers, McKenzie, McGuckin, and Goldstein (1961). Sandberg and Bynke (1973) examined 25 cases of optic neuritis without other signs of central nervous system involvement. In a follow-up of unspecified duration, three developed evidence of multiple sclerosis. Four of the patients showed an elevated relative IgG concentration, and six showed an abnormal banding of the IgG on agarose electrophoresis (oligoclonal IgG), a feature present in approximately 95 per cent of patients with unequivocal multiple sclerosis (Link and Muller 1971). Only one of these patients with oligoclonal IgG subsequently developed evidence of multiple sclerosis during the follow up period. Whether this and other CSF characteristics could be used to predict the subsequent development of multiple sclerosis remains undetermined.

Aetiology

In early publications, the condition was often attributed, on inadequate evidence, to a variety of disorders, for example gout, although syphilis was recognized to be a frequent factor, being present, for example, in five of Nettleship's 28 cases. The role of focal sepsis was emphasized, and attention initially concentrated on the paranasal sinuses.

Sinusitis

The attempt to relate cases of optic neuritis to concomitant sinus disease was stimulated by description of the close anatomical relationship between the optic nerve and the paranasal sinuses (Onodi 1908; Loeb 1909). Examples of purulent sinusitis, from both operative and post-mortem examination, with perforation of adjacent bone and secondary optic nerve or chiasmatic involvement were used to support the concept of an association (Pickworth 1928; Doesschate 1928). Lesser degrees of sinus disease, often only apparent on biopsy examination, were held to be equally significant, neglecting the occurrence of such changes in individuals without visual symptoms.

Thus White (quoted by Gifford 1931) considered all his first 17 cases of optic neuritis were due to sinusitis and of 225 cases of retrobulbar neuritis from the Mayo Clinic analysed by Benedict (1933), over 60 per cent had had some form of intranasal sinus operation performed elsewhere. In his critical analysis, Gifford (1931) concluded that there was insufficient evidence to support the association, other than on rare occasions.

Focal sepsis

The increasing number of negative sinus explorations on patients with optic neuritis led to a search for focal sepsis elsewhere. By 1928 White favoured teeth and tonsils as the most likely sources but Traquair (1930) was unable to find a single personal case of retrobulbar neuritis attributable to tonsillar infection or dental abscess, and regarded rhinogenic retrobulbar neuritis as a rarity. Despite this, the acceptance of an association (Bossy and Jequier, 1961) and the confidence in the value of surgical intervention (Calvet, Calmettes, and Coll 1967) have persisted.

Toxic agents

An accumulating literature indicated the frequency with which a similar, if not identical, visual disturbance could be caused by disorders other than multiple sclerosis. The role of toxic agents and drugs was emphasized, and the recovery of vision following withdrawal of the offending agent—neglecting the natural history of the condition—used to support the association. The dangers inherent in such assumptions were revealed when cases of optic neuritis, attributed to drugs or toxic agents, subsequently progressed to multiple sclerosis. Lynn (1959) described such an experience where DDT had been held responsible for the initial visual disturbance.

Multiple sclerosis

The relationship of optic neuritis to multiple sclerosis was appreciated by Buzzard (1893) who found a history of an episode of visual failure in five of 18 cases of multiple sclerosis; he stressed the evanescent character of the visual symptoms in some instances and the problem of differentiating the condition from conversion hysteria. Buzzard found optic atrophy in 42·6 per cent of 68 hospital cases of multiple sclerosis, a figure similar to the 40 per cent of 100 cases obtained by Uhthoff (1890).

As soon as an association was recognized between optic neuritis and the subsequent development of multiple sclerosis, arguments arose as to the frequency with which one followed the other. Whilst Percival (1926) and Heckford (1934) had not encountered the progression, Adie (1930) believed that multiple sclerosis accounted for virtually every case of acute optic neuritis. More cautious observers opted for an intermediate position, and Adie himself wondered if an attack of optic neuritis 'could not be the only manifestation in a lifetime of the activity of the agent causing multiple sclerosis'. The length of follow-up was clearly critical in this assessment, as the average time elapsing between initial attack and subsequent extra-ocular manifestation was 8 years in Adie's series. By contrast, in a recent survey (Bradley and Whitty 1968) those patients with a previous history of optic neuritis in whom a subsequent, confident, diagnosis of multiple sclerosis could be made, had developed the necessary signs and symptoms to make such a diagnosis within 4 years of the original visual disturbance. Patients in whom the interval between visual and other episodes has been much longer (Adie (1930) had encountered an interval of 47 years in his search of the literature), and the findings at post-mortem examination of a much more extensive demyelinating process than had been apparent in life (Fog, Hyllested, and Anderson 1972), have suggested the possibility that in some patients with optic neuritis, plaques of demyelination in the rest of the nervous system, due to multiple sclerosis, may be asymptomatic.

The possibility of a similar occult demyelination of the optic nerves in multiple sclerosis has been raised by the discrepancy between the frequency of symptomatic involvement of the visual system in life, and the frequency of changes in the optic nerves at post-mortem examination.

Figures for the prevalence of clinically apparent optic nerve changes in cases of established multiple sclerosis vary according to the criteria used. Optic atrophy, for example, was found in 42·6 per cent of the cases examined by Buzzard (1893). On the other hand, Gartner (1953) found pathological evidence of optic nerve involvement in all 14 eyes examined from 10 patients in whom the diagnosis of multiple sclerosis had been confirmed histologically. Although Lynn (1959) was able, by the use of colour vision charts, to reveal evidence of optic nerve damage in a considerable number of patients without a history of visual symptoms in the same eye, the ability to record, in life, the true frequency of optic nerve demyelination in patients with multiple sclerosis, has awaited the introduction of electrophysiological techniques.

Treatment

The frequency with which normal visual acuity is regained after an attack of optic neuritis (75 per cent at six months in Bradley and Whitty's series (1967)) has led to difficulty in assessing the effects of treatment.

Optic nerve decompression

Compression of the inflamed optic nerve within the optic foramen, suggested by the post-mortem appearance of flattening of the nerve at this site (Samelsohn 1877, quoted by Percival 1926) was held responsible for the poor recovery of vision of some cases of optic neuritis (Nettleship 1884; Swanzy 1897), although Samelsohn's example was probably on a vascular basis.

White (1924, 1925) subsequently claimed that the prognosis of various optic neuropathies was related to the diameter of the optic foramen as assessed by radiological examination. This factor has not been considered by subsequent authors, although as recently as 1952, Miyazaki described surgical decompression of the nerve within the canal for the treatment of acute retrobulbar neuritis.

Corticosteroids

Amongst the large number of different treatments proposed for optic neuritis, attention has eventually concentrated on the use of corticosteroids. In a recent trial (Bowden, Bowden, Friedmann, Perkin, and Rose 1974), their use appeared to have no effect on the rate or degree of visual recovery.

REFERENCES

Adie, W. J. (1930). Acute retrobulbar neuritis in disseminated sclerosis. *Trans. ophthal. Soc. U.K.* **50**, 262–7.
— (1932). The aetiology and symptomatology of disseminated sclerosis. *Br. med. J.* **2**, 997–1000.
Benedict, W. L. (1933). Retrobulbar neuritis and disease of the nasal accessory sinuses. *Archs. Ophthal., N.Y.* **9**, 893–906.
— (1942). Multiple sclerosis as an etiologic factor in retrobulbar neuritis. *Archs. Ophthal., N.Y.* **28**, 988–95.
Berliner, M. L. (1935). Acute optic neuritis in demyelinating diseases of the nervous system. *Archs. Ophthal., N.Y.* **13**, 83–98.
Bossy, A. and Jequier, M. (1961). Sinusites, neurites optiques et sclerose en plaque. *Confinia neurol.* **21**, 217–22.
Bowden, A. N., Bowden, P. M. A., Friedman, A. I., Perkin, G. D., and Rose, F. C. (1974). A trial of corticotrophin gelatin injection in acute optic neuritis. *J. Neurol., Neurosurg. Psychiat.* **37**, 869–73.
Bradley, W. G. and Whitty, C. W. M. (1967). Acute optic neuritis: its clinical features and their relation to prognosis for recovery of vision. *J. Neurol. Neurosurg. Psychiat.* **30**, 531–8.
—., — (1968). Acute optic neuritis: prognosis for development of multiple sclerosis. *J. Neurol., Neurosurg. Psychiat.,* **31**, 10–18.

Buzzard, T. (1893). Atrophy of the optic nerve as a symptom of chronic disease of the central nervous system. *Br. med. J.* **2**, 779–84.

Calvet, J., Calmettes, L., and Coll, L. (1967). Le role des sinusites dans l'etiologie des nevrites optiques retro-bulbaires. *Revue Oto-Neuro-Ophtal.* **39**, 43–7.

Chamlin, M. (1953). Visual field changes in optic neuritis. *Archs. Ophthal., N.Y.* **50**, 699–713.

Davis, F.A. (1966). The hot bath test in the diagnosis of multiple sclerosis. *J. Mt Sinai Hosp.* **33**, 280–2.

*Doesschate, T. (1928). Pathologisch-Anatomische befunde bei rhinogenem sehnervenleiden. *Klin. Mbl. Augenheilk.* **80**, 831–2.

Fog, T., Hyllested, K., and Anderson, S. R. (1972). A case of benign multiple sclerosis, with autopsy. *Acta Neurol. Scand.* [Suppl.] **51** (Vol. 48) 369–70.

Frisén, L., and Hoyt, W. F. (1974). Insidious atrophy of retinal nerve fibres in multiple sclerosis. *Archs Ophthal., N.Y.* **92**, 91–7.

Gartner, S. (1953). Optic neuropathy in multiple sclerosis. *Archs Ophthal., N.Y.* **50**, 718–26.

Gifford, S. R. (1931). The relation of the paranasal sinuses to ocular disorders. *Archs Ophthal., N.Y.* **5**, 276–86.

Gunn, M. (1897). Discussion on retro-ocular neuritis. *Trans. ophthal.'Soc. U.K.* **17**, 107–217.

— (1904a). Discussion on retro-ocular neuritis. *Br. med. J.* **2**, 1285.

— (1904b). Retro-ocular neuritis. *Lancet* **2**, 412–13.

Heckford, F. (1934). In Discussion of some varieties of acute optic and retrobulbar neuritis (W. R. Brain). *Trans. ophthal. Soc. U.K.* **54**, 221–9.

Hutchinson, W. M. (1976). Acute optic neuritis and the prognosis for multiple sclerosis. *J. Neurol. Neurosurg. Psychiat.* **39**, 283–9.

Hyllested, K. and Moller, P. M. (1961). Follow up on patients with a history of optic neuritis. *Acta ophthal.* **39**, 655–62.

Ivers, R. R., McKenzie, B. F., McGuckin, W. F., and Goldstein, N. P. (1961). Spinal-fluid gamma globulin in multiple sclerosis and other neurologic diseases. Electrophoretic pattern in 606 patients. *J. Am. med. Ass.* **176**, 515–19.

Klingmann, T. (1910). Visual disturbances in multiple sclerosis. Their relation to changes in the visual field and ophthalmoscopic findings. Diagnostic significance. Report of twelve cases. *J. nerv. ment. Dis.* **37**, 734–48.

Lillie, W. I. (1934). The clinical significance of retrobulbar and optic neuritis. *Am. J. Ophthal.* **17**, 110–19.

Link, H. and Muller, R. (1971). Immunoglobulins in multiple sclerosis and infections of the nervous system. *Archs. Neurol., Chicago* **25**, 326–44.

Loeb, H. W. (1909). A study of the anatomic relations of the optic nerve to the accessory cavities of the nose. *Ann. Otol. Rhinol. Lar.* **18**, 243–73.

Lynn, B. H. (1959). Retrobulbar neuritis. A survey of the present conditions of cases occurring over the last fifty-six years. *Trans. ophthal. Soc. U.K.* **79**, 701–16.

Miyazaki, S. (1952). Opening of the optic nerve canal via the nasal route in the treatment of acute retrobulbar optic neuritis. *Acta Soc. ophthal. jap.* **56**, 190–3.

Nelson, D. A., Jeffreys, W. H., and McDowell, F. (1958). Effects of induced hyperthermia on some neurological diseases. *Archs Neurol. Psychiat., Chicago* **79**, 31–9.

Nettleship, E. (1884). On cases of retro-ocular neuritis. *Trans. ophthal. Soc. U.K.* **4**, 186–226.

Norris, W. F. (1884). Hereditary atrophy of the optic nerves. *Trans. Am. ophthal. Soc.* **3**, 662–78.

Onodi, A. (1908). The optic nerve and the accessory cavities of the nose. Contribution to the study of canalicular neuritis and atrophy of the optic nerves of nasal origin (Trans. H. Strauss). *Ann. Otol. Rhinol. Lar.* **17**, 1–52.

*Parinaud, H. (1884). Troubles oculaires de la sclerose en plaques. *J. Santé* **3**, 3–5.

Paton, L. (1914). Papilloedema in Disseminated Sclerosis. *Trans. ophthal. Soc. U.K.* **34**, 252–61.

Percival, A. S. (1926). Retrobulbar neuritis and associated conditions. *Trans. ophthal. Soc. U.K.* **46**, 392–8.

Pickworth, F. A. (1928). Perforation of the pituitary fossa by a septic lesion of the sphenoidal sinus associated with recent epilepsy and insanity. *J. Lar. Otol.* **43**, 186–90.

Rønne, H. (1928). On non-hypophyseal affections of the chiasma. *Acta ophthal.* **6**, 332–43.
Sandberg, H. and Bynke, H. (1973). Cerebrospinal fluid in 25 cases of optic neuritis. *Acta Neurol. Scand.* **49**, 443–52.
Smith, J. L., Hoyt, W. F., and Susac, J. O. (1973). Ocular fundus in acute Leber optic neuropathy. *Archs Ophthal. N.Y.* **90**, 349–54.
Sugar, S. (1939). Papillitis and papilloedema in multiple sclerosis. *Am. J. Ophthal.* **22**, 135–9.
Swanzy, H. R. (1897). In Discussion on retro-ocular neuritis. *Trans. ophthal. Soc. U.K.* **17**, 107–217.
Traquair, H. M. (1925). Acute retro-bulbar neuritis affecting the optic chiasma and tract. *Br. J. Ophthal.* **9**, 433–50.
— (1930). Toxic amblyopia, including retrobulbar neuritis. *Trans. ophthal. Soc. U.K.* **50**, 351–85.
Uhthoff, W. (1890). Untersuchungen uber die bei der multiplen herdsklerose vorkommenden augenstorungen. *Arch. Psychiat. NervKrankh.* **21**, 55–116, 303–410.
— (1904). Discussion on retro-ocular neuritis. *Br. med. J.* **2**, 1285–6.
Watkins, A. L. (1939). The cerebro-spinal fluid in cases of optic neuritis, toxic amblyopia, and tumours producing central scotoma. *Archs Neurol. Psychiat., Chicago* **41**, 418–22.
White, L. E. (1924). An anatomic and X-ray study of the optic canal in cases of optic nerve involvement. *Ann. Otol. Rhinol. Lar.* **33**, 121–50.
— (1925). The optic canal in optic atrophy. *Ann. Otol. Rhinol. Lar.* **34**, 1210–23.
— (1928). The location of the focus in optic nerve disturbances from infection. *Ann. Otol. Rhinol. Lar.* **37**, 128–64.
Yahr, M. D., Goldensohn, S. S., and Kabat, E. A. (1954). Further studies on the gamma globulin content of cerebrospinal fluid in multiple sclerosis and other neurological diseases. *Ann. N.Y. Acad. Sci.* **58**, 613–24.

*In this, and later chapters, an asterisk indicates references not personally consulted.

2 Methodology and epidemiology

At present the name retrobulbar neuritis is used indiscriminately when reference is being made to a number of manifestations—usually distinguishable clinically—of the effects of various unrelated pathological processes, the only common feature being that the signs indicate a lesion of the optic nerves (Adie 1932).

The diagnosis of optic neuritis remains a clinical one, so that comparison of published series of the condition is dependent on the diagnostic criteria used; where these vary the validity of any conclusions made will be lessened by the inclusion of a number of different pathological processes. When the optic neuritis is defined as an involvement of the optic nerve by any inflammatory, demyelinating, or degenerative process (Nikoskelainen and Riekkinen 1974), disorders of optic nerve function are included whose natural histories differ substantially. On the other hand, more rigid diagnostic criteria, for example the requirement of a central or para-central field defect (Bradley and Whitty 1967; Hutchinson 1976) may exclude cases with otherwise typical manifestations.

In an attempt to overcome this problem, we have analysed our material on the basis of defined clinical criteria, but at the same time, have considered whether atypical features, such as an abnormal field defect, alter the prognosis, either for recovery of visual function, or for the subsequent development of multiple sclerosis.

Case selection

The material on which our study has been based consists of patients referred to the Medical Ophthalmology Unit of the Royal Eye Hospital between 1963 and 1969.

Optic neuritis can be defined as a condition causing a relatively rapid onset of visual failure, in which no evidence for a toxic, vascular, or compressive aetiology can be discovered, and where local retinal lesions have been excluded. Bilateral cases are defined on the basis of the two eyes being involved simultaneously or within one month of each other. Attacks involving the second eye at an interval greater than one month, have been classified as recurrences, as have further episodes involving the originally affected eye.

The absence of pain, and the absence of a field defect (or the presence of a defect not involving central vision) have not barred inclusion, although such cases have also been considered separately, in order to determine whether such factors influenced visual recovery.

All cases meeting these criteria were admitted to the Medical Ophthalmology Unit, and subsequently followed in the out-patient department. A full neurological assessment was made at the original admission, and carried out subsequently when specific symptoms suggested it was appropriate. Of the 170 patients admitted during this period 148 were reassessed both neurologically and ophthalmologically during 1969.

During admission, cerebrospinal fluid examination was carried out on 164 patients, and radiological examination of the optic formina and paranasal sinuses in the majority.

Methodology

Visual acuity

This was assessed with Snellen charts, using refractive correction if necessary.

Visual fields

These were examined with the Friedmann analyser (Friedmann 1966). This instrument employs static perimetry and measures the threshold to flashes of white light shone through 46 holes set in a screen covering the central 25 degrees of vision. Dark adaptation was used. Threshold stimulation, measured in arbitrary log units, was varied according to the age of the patient, as shown in Table 2.1.

Table 2.1 Filter settings for the Friedmann analyser in relation to age

Filter setting (log units)	Age (years)
2.0	less than 40
1.8	41–50
1.6	51–60
1.4	over 60

Macular threshold

This was determined with the same instrument, using a white light source at fixation, and measured in the same log units, the minimal stimulus strength used being 2·8 units, and the maximal 0·0 units.

Colour vision

This was assessed with Hardy–Rand–Rittler pseudo-isochromatic plates (American Optical Corporation), under conditions of controlled illumination.

Pupil reactions

Pupil sizes were measured. Assessment of a reduction in the light reaction was generally made against the contralateral normal pupil. A Marcus Gunn pupil was defined on the basis of a paradoxical dilatation of the pupil during the swinging light test.

Fundus examination

This was always done through dilated pupils. Intraocular pressure was measured with the applanation tonometer. The descriptions of the optic disc appearance at the onset and at the time of the follow-up examination in 1969 were those agreed on by two independent observers. Ninety-two of the patients at follow-up had fundus photography performed.

Cerebrospinal fluid examination

This was performed on 164 patients. Cell counts were performed by standard procedures. The total protein concentration was measured by precipitation with salicylsulphonic acid (Denis and Ayer 1920), and a qualitative estimation of the globulin content made by the method of Pandy.

Neurological examination

The presence of abnormal neurological signs, at both the original admission and the follow-up examination in 1969, were determined by two independent assessors. Only those signs found by both observers were accepted as being present. The criteria used for the diagnosis of multiple sclerosis have been:

Definite

A history of optic neuritis and of remitting and relapsing symptoms with physical signs of at least two separate neurological lesions outside the visual system.

Probable

A history of optic neuritis and either:
a remitting and relapsing symptoms but physical signs of only one lesion;
b no history of remitting and relapsing symptoms but physical signs of two or more lesions.

Possible

A history of optic neuritis and either:
a remitting and relapsing symptoms without physical signs; or
b physical signs of one lesion without remitting and relapsing symptoms.

None

History of optic neuritis alone.

Age distribution

The age distribution at the time of the first symptom of the optic neuritis leading to admission is shown in Fig. 2.1. The mean age at the onset of visual symptoms was 33·5 years (range 10 to 60 years). In 143 of 170 patients (84·1 per cent) the onset was between the ages of 20 and 50. For males the mean age was 34·3 years (60 cases) and for females 33·1 years (110 cases). The difference is not significant.

Table 2.2 lists the age distribution in other reported series.

Although Marshall (1950) found a lower mean age for females with optic neuritis than for males, this was not our experience, nor did Bradley and Whitty (1967) find a difference in age distribution between the sexes. Other authors have generally not analysed their figures in this way, though a study

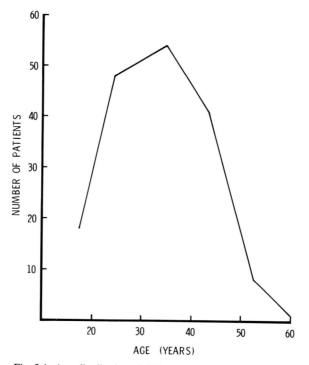

Fig. 2.1. Age distribution of 170 cases of optic neuritis.

Table 2.2 Mean age, or age distribution, of patients with optic neuritis reported elsewhere

Authors	No. of patients	Unilateral or bilateral cases	Mean age (years) or age distribution	Aetiology*
Lynn (1959)	200	Both	25	MS or unknown
Tatlow (1948)	46	Both	27.7	Mixed
Leibowitz et al. (1966)	38	Unilateral	28.8	Unknown
Alter et al. (1973)	15 (Orientals)	Both	29.4	Unknown
Marshall (1950)	152 (Females)	Both	30.5	Mixed
Traquair (1930)	160	Both	32	Mixed
Nikoskelainen (1975)	185	Both	32	Mixed
Alter et al. (1973)	13 (Caucasian)	Both	32.1	Unknown
Carroll (1940)	100	Both	32.7	Mixed
Leibowitz et al. (1966)	37	Unilateral	33.3	MS
Nettleship (1884)	28	Unilateral	35	Mixed
Taub and Rucker (1954)	28	Not stated	35	MS
Marshall (1950)	170 (Males)	Both	37	Mixed
Taub and Rucker (1954)	59	Not stated	38.2	Unknown
Bagley (1952)	133	Both	57.1 per cent between 25 and 55	Mixed
Earl and Martin (1967)	104	Not stated	Over 70 per cent between 20 and 50	MS or unknown
Hutchinson (1976)	144	Both	74 per cent between 20 and 50	MS or unknown
Nikoskelainen (1975)	185	Both	81 per cent between 20 and 49	Mixed
Bradley and Whitty (1967)	73	Both	82 per cent between 20 and 50	MS or unknown

* MS refers to multiple sclerosis. A mixed aetiology implies the inclusion of other forms of optic neuropathy—for example syphilis, Leber's optic atrophy.

of Nikoskelainen's results (1975) does not appear to support Marshall's finding.

Sex distribution

The majority of patients in this study were females (64·7 per cent) and, as Table 2.3 shows, this has generally been the finding with other published

Table 2.3 The sex distribution of patients with optic neuritis reported elsewhere

Authors	No. of patients	Unilateral or bilateral cases	Percentage of females	Aetiology*
Bagley (1952)	133	Both	40.9	Mixed
Leibowitz et al. (1966)	38	Unilateral	42.0	Unknown
Nettleship (1884)	28	Unilateral	44.0	Mixed
Griffith (1897)	27	Unilateral	44.4	Not stated
Marshall (1950)	322	Both	47.0	Mixed
Burke (1968)	31	Not stated	48.7	Not stated
Carroll (1940)	100	Both	54.0	Mixed
Tatlow (1948)	46	Both	54.3	Mixed
Alter et al. (1973)	39	Both	55.5	Unknown
Nikoskelainen (1975)	185	Both	57.0	Mixed
Giles and Isaacson (1961)	80	Not stated	61.3	Unknown
Hyllested and Moller (1961)	52	Both	61.5	Mixed
Traquair (1930)	160	Both	62.0	Mixed
Bradley and Whitty (1967)	73	Both	63.0	MS or unknown
Adie (1932)	?	Unilateral	63.7	MS
Adie (1932)	?	Unilateral	64.7	Unknown
Landy and Ohlrich (1970)	57	Both	64.9	MS or unknown
Percy et al. (1972)	30	Not stated	67.7	Unknown
Leibowitz et al. (1966)	37	Unilateral	68.0	MS
Swanzy (1897)	54	Unilateral	70.4	Not stated
Hutchinson (1976)	144	Both	73.0	MS or unknown
Earl and Martin (1967)	104	Not stated	77.9	MS or unknown

* See footnote to Table 2.2.

series. It is apparent that where a lower figure for the proportion of female patients has been found, optic neuropathies of a number of different aetiological types have been included. When such neuropathies have a male preponderance, for example, tobacco amblyopia and Leber's optic atrophy, the proportion of female patients in the final total will be lessened.

Leibowitz, Alter, and Halpern (1966) found a considerably lower percentage of female patients in a group of cases with optic neuritis alone, as compared with a group of patients with multiple sclerosis who had presented with optic neuritis. In a similar analysis, however, Adie (1932) found almost identical percentages in the two groups (64·7 and 63·7 respectively).

In our own series, there were 82 patients who had presented initially with optic neuritis and no other evidence of neurological disease, who were assessed at the follow-up examination. Of these, 44 subsequently showed some evidence of multiple sclerosis, whilst 38 did not. (The follow-up period for the two groups was comparable.) Of the former, 59·1 per cent were female, and of the latter 60·5 per cent. The difference is insignificant.

Nationality

Of the 170 patients, 156 (92 per cent) were born in Britain or Eire. Of 14 patients born elsewhere, only four were of non-Caucasian origin.

A.J., aged 40, female, Jamaican, resident in England for 5 years. Admitted February 1968 with an 18-day history of ocular pain and subsequent visual blurring. Vision was reduced to counting fingers in the right eye with evidence of optic disc swelling. Vision recovered to normal. There was no evidence of multiple sclerosis at the onset or one year later.

A.V., aged 40, male, Indian, resident in England for 10 years. Admitted April 1967 with a one-week history of pain and vision loss in the left eye. Visual acuity on admission was 6/18 and there was marked swelling of the optic disc with adjacent retinal haemorrhages. Vision returned to normal. There was no evidence of multiple sclerosis at the onset or two years later.

B.S., aged 38, male, Persian, temporary resident in England. Admitted May 1967 with a 5-week history of pain and visual blurring in the left eye. Visual acuity was 6/6 by the time of admission, though a relative central scotoma was apparent on field testing. The optic disc was normal. The patient complained of occasional paraesthesiae in the arms, but there were no abnormal neurological findings outside the visual system.

C.S., aged 41, female, Jamaican, resident in England for 6 years. Admitted April 1968 with an eleven-day history of blurring of vision in the left eye, associated with pain on eye movement. For 2 months the patient had noticed numbness of the right foot and aching in the right arm. There was a history of frequency of micturition. Vision was reduced to counting fingers and there was slight oedema of the optic disc. The neurological examination was otherwise normal. Her vision recovered. In June 1969 she developed a paraplegia with numbness of the left leg and urinary retention. Recovery occurred after 3 months. Assessment subsequently showed evidence of definite multiple sclerosis.

The numbers are insufficient to make any comparison between the clinical features of this group and the remainder, though all recovered normal vision. Alter, Good, and Okihiro (1973) compared the clinical features of optic neuritis in Orientals and Caucasians resident in Hawaii and found no significant differences, apart from a higher percentage of patients with good residual visual acuity in Orientals.

A confident diagnosis of definite multiple sclerosis was subsequently made in one, Jamaican, patient. The possibility of a Jamaican neuropathy was considered in this patient, but rejected for the following reasons:
a Remissions of the cord syndromes in this condition are seldom encountered (Montgomery, Cruickshank, Robertson, and McMenemey 1964).
b Optic nerve involvement tends to produce bilateral optic atrophy, with

insidious visual deterioration and persisting central or paracentral scotomata (Crews 1963; Montgomery *et al*, 1964; Mackenzie and Phillips 1968), though occasional cases with a more rapid onset of visual failure have been described in Nigerians (Osuntokun 1968).

Family history

Three patients had a family history of multiple sclerosis, in a father, sister, and maternal aunt respectively, giving a familial incidence of 1·76 per cent in patients with optic neuritis. This figure is somewhat lower than that generally quoted for the familial incidence of the disease in patients with multiple sclerosis.

Associated conditions

Migraine

Although, on direct questioning, 27 of 165 patients (16·4 per cent) gave a history of migraine, a critical evaluation of the symptoms complained of suggested a much lower figure. Using the criteria of Watkins and Espir (1969), nine patients (5·5 per cent) described periodic, predominantly unilateral headaches, often of a throbbing quality. Most of these patients had had, at some time, accompanying symptoms such as nausea, vomiting, visual disturbance, etc.

Watkins and Espir (1969) obtained a much higher figure in a group of 100 patients with multiple sclerosis; 27 per cent gave a history of migraine headaches compared with 12 per cent in age and sex-matched controls. Other sources give a lower figure for the incidence of migraine in the general population, a figure in fact analogous to the incidence in this group of patients with optic neuritis.

Atopy

Twenty-three of 166 patients (13·9 per cent) gave a history of hay fever, asthma, or eczema. Similar figures were found for patients at the follow-up examination having either definite multiple sclerosis (13·9 per cent) or no evidence of multiple sclerosis (15·6 per cent). McAlpine and Compston (1952) found a history of asthma, hay fever, urticaria, angio-neurotic oedema, food allergy, contact dermatitis, or eczema in 16 per cent of both 250 cases of multiple sclerosis, and a control group. Frövig, Presthus, and Sponheim (1967) however have concluded that a history of these conditions in a patient or his family is more common in multiple sclerosis than in the general population, though their finding for the incidence of hay fever, asthma, or eczema alone (16 per cent) is not dissimilar to our own. It seems unlikely that their conclusion can be applied to patients with a history of optic neuritis, whether or not they subsequently manifest evidence of multiple sclerosis.

Thyroid disorders

Four patients had a history of investigations or treatment for thyroid disease. In one the investigations had been normal and in another the results were unknown. The third patient had a history of thyrotoxicosis treated by partial thyroidectomy, and the fourth a history of thyrotoxicosis at the age of 14, which had resolved spontaneously. At the time of their admission, all four patients appeared euthyroid. Formal thyroid function tests were not performed.

Although the clinical status of the thyroid gland has not been studied in patients with multiple sclerosis a high incidence of adenomatosis and involutional change has been found at post-mortem examination (Lumsden 1970). The possible implications of this finding have not been established.

Precipitating factors

Trauma

McAlpine and Compston (1952) obtained a history of trauma (including dental extraction but not surgical operation) within 3 months of the onset of the first symptom in 14 per cent of 250 unselected cases of multiple sclerosis. In many of these, there was a correlation between the site of the injury and the initial lesion in the nervous system. In a control group interviewed in the medical and surgical wards, 5·2 per cent had received an injury within 3 months of the onset of their disease.

Nine of our patients had a history of trauma within 3 months of the onset of their optic neuritis (5·3 per cent), an almost identical percentage to that found in McAlpine's control group. Four had had dental extractions, one had been involved in a road traffic accident, whilst four had had injuries in or around the eye. Though, in three of these four cases, between 2 and 5 weeks had elapsed between the trauma and the onset of visual symptoms, in one patient, the interval was much shorter,

S.B. aged 19, Female. Six days before admission, whilst playing hockey, she received a blow to the left shoulder and face. Blurring of vision developed a few hours later followed by pain on eye movement. Two years before she had had an episode of right retrobulbar neuritis recovering over 6 months. On examination, the left disc was slightly swollen and the right was pale. Little recovery occurred in the left eye, however, and 3 years later her acuity was hand movements only. There was no evidence of multiple sclerosis at that time.

Similar cases have been described in the literature. McAlpine (1946) mentioned two cases of retrobulbar neuritis in whom minor trauma had occurred in the affected eye 24 and 72 hours before. Mackay (1953) described a patient in whom the diagnosis of multiple sclerosis was established at the age of 35, who had developed blindness of the left eye following a fall on her nose at the age of 4. Miller (1964) mentions similar cases. The reports were on patients with undoubted multiple sclerosis, though in Mackay's case, 31 years had elapsed before the diagnosis had been established. None of our four patients with optic neuritis and a history of injury in the region of the affected eye had evidence of multiple sclerosis at follow-up, though one had had an episode of retrobulbar neuritis previously in the other eye.

Other factors

Three patients were pregnant at the time of onset of their visual symptoms ($\frac{1}{2}$, 2, and 3 months respectively).

In one patient, an influenza vaccine had been given 3 weeks before the onset of visual symptoms.

Month of onset

Taub and Rucker (1954) were the first authors to consider the possibility of a seasonal variation in the incidence of optic neuritis. They were able to assess this in 74 cases of optic neuritis diagnosed 10 to 15 years before. They found a significantly lower proportion of cases occurring in the months from November to March; 47·3 per cent of their cases occurred between April and July inclusively.

Bradley and Whitty (1967) also considered this question in 73 cases of acute optic neuritis, some of which were bilateral. Forty-four per cent of their cases occurred between April and July, though this figure did not reach significance.

Hutchinson (1976) has recently noted a similar trend. Of 193 attacks of optic neuritis, some bilateral, in 144 patients, a significantly higher percentage of attacks occurred between April and July (48·2 per cent) compared with August to November (21·3 per cent).

We have analysed our own figures (Fig. 2.2) in a similar manner, but with differing results. Of our cases 27·6 per cent occurred between April and July, a percentage not differing significantly from the 32·9 per cent between August and November. Whereas 46·5 per cent of our cases occurred between November and March, the analogous figure for Taub and Rucker's (1954) series was 24·3 per cent.

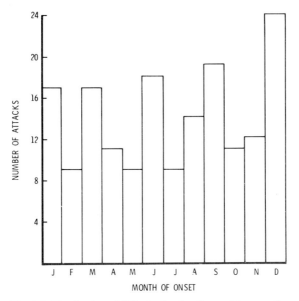

Fig. 2.2. Distribution of 170 attacks of optic neuritis according to month of onset. A significant excess ($P < 0.01$) of cases occurred in December, but not in the period from April to July ($27.6\% - 0.10 > P > 0.05$).

It is difficult to account for these discrepancies, as the cases in these four series appear similar in their clinical features.

All the patients in our series had been admitted to hospital, whereas, as far as one can tell, few of the patients in the other series were assessed on an in-patient basis. Many of our cases were already improving at the time of their admission; conceivably patients may be more willing to consider admission for an apparently benign condition during the winter than the summer months. If this is the case, our figures would be biased accordingly. Unfortunately we are unable to give figures for cases of optic neuritis not admitted during that period in order to test this hypothesis. Accordingly we are unable from our series of in-patient cases to confirm the seasonal incidence reported by others.

Conclusions

In general, the peak incidence of optic neuritis appears in the early thirties, and the vast majority of patients will be between the ages of 20 and 50. In this series, the mean age at presentation was similar for male and female patients.

Overall, female patients predominate, particularly if other forms of optic neuropathy are excluded. A suggestion that the female predominance disappears if cases of optic neuritis not progressing to multiple sclerosis are considered, was not confirmed in this study.

Only four patients of non-Caucasian origin were encountered, of whom one subsequently showed definite evidence of multiple sclerosis.

A history of migraine, when defined critically, was encountered no more frequently than is obtained in the general population.

The frequency of a history of atopy (as defined) did not differ greatly from that obtained by McAlpine and Compston (1952) in both a series of cases of multiple sclerosis and a control group. Previous episodes of possible disordered thyroid function were encountered infrequently.

The role of trauma in precipitating visual symptoms in this series was almost identical to that in a control group studied by McAlpine and Compston (1952). In one patient, however, the trauma and subsequent optic neuritis were closely related in time.

Despite the seasonal variation in the incidence of optic neuritis reported previously, this could not be confirmed. It is suggested that the contradiction may be explicable on the basis of differences in the proportion of patients admitted to hospital.

REFERENCES

Adie, W. J. (1932). The aetiology and symptomatology of disseminated sclerosis. *Br. med. J.* **2**, 997–1000.

Alter, M., Good, J., and Okihiro, M. (1973). Optic neuritis in Orientals and Caucasians. *Neurology, Minneap.* **23**, 631–9.

Bagley, C. H. (1952). An etiologic study of a series of optic neuropathies. *Am. J. Ophthal.* **35**, 761–72.

Bradley, W. G. and Whitty, C. W. M. (1967). Acute optic neuritis: its clinical features and their relation to prognosis for recovery of vision. *J. Neurol. Neurosurg. Psychiat.* **30**, 531–8.

Burke, W. J. (1968). Optic neuritis. *Proc. Aust. Assoc. Neurol.* **5**, 243–5.

Carrol, F. D. (1940). Retrobulbar neuritis. Observations on one hundred cases. *Archs. Ophthal. N.Y.* **24**, 44–54.

Crews, S. J. (1963). Bilateral amblyopia in West Indians. *Trans. ophthal. Soc. U.K.* **83**, 653–67.

Denis, W. and Ayer, J. B. (1920). A method for the quantitative determination of protein in cerebrospinal fluid. *Archs. intern. Med.* **26**, 436–42

Earl, C. J. and Martin, B. (1967). Prognosis in optic neuritis related to age. *Lancet* **1**, 74–6.

Friedmann, A. I. (1966). Serial analysis of changes in visual defects, employing a new instrument, to determine the activity of diseases involving the visual pathways. *Ophthalmologica, Basel* **152**, 1–12.

Frövig, A. G., Presthus, J. and Sponheim, N. (1967). The significance of allergy in the etiology and pathogenesis of multiple sclerosis. *Acta Neurol. Scand.* **43**, 215–27.

Giles, C. L. and Isaacson, J. D. (1961). The treatment of acute optic neuritis. *Archs Ophthal. N.Y.* **66**, 176–9.

Griffith, A. H. (1897). Discussion on retro-ocular neuritis. *Trans. ophthal. Soc. U.K.* **17**, 107–217.

Hutchinson, W. M. (1976). Acute optic neuritis and the prognosis for multiple sclerosis. *J. Neurol. Neurosurg. Psychiat.* **39**, 283–9.

Hyllested, K. and Moller, P. M. (1961). Follow-up on patients with a history of optic neuritis. *Acta ophthal.* **39**, 655–62.

Landy, P. J. and Ohlrich, G. D. (1970). Optic neuritis and its relationship to disseminated sclerosis. *Proc. Aust. Assoc. Neurol.* **7**, 67–70.

Leibowitz, U., Alter, M., and Halpern, L. (1966). Clinical studies of multiple sclerosis in Israel. IV. Optic neuropathy and multiple sclerosis. *Archs. Neurol., Chicago* **14**, 459–66.

Lumsden, C. E. (1970). The neuropathology of multiple sclerosis. In *Handbook of clinical neurology* (eds. P. J. Vinken and G. W. Bruyn), Vol. 9, pp. 217–309. North-Holland, Amsterdam.

Lynn, B. H. (1959). Retrobulbar neuritis. A survey of the present conditions of cases occurring over the last fifty-six years. *Trans. ophthal. Soc. U.K.* **79**, 701–16.

Mackay, R. P. (1953). Multiple sclerosis: its onset and duration. A clinical study of 309 private patients. *Med. Clins. N. Am.* **37**, 511–21.

Mackenzie, A. D. and Phillips, C. I. (1968). West Indian amblyopia. *Brain* **91**, 249–60.

McAlpine, D. (1946). The problem of disseminated sclerosis. *Brain* **69**, 233–50.

— and Compston, N. D. (1952). Some aspects of the natural history of disseminated sclerosis. *Q. Jl. Med.* **21**, 135–67.

Marshall, D. (1950). Ocular manifestations of multiple sclerosis and relationship to retrobulbar neuritis. *Trans. Am. ophthal. Soc.* **48**, 487–525.

Miller, H. (1964). Trauma and multiple sclerosis. *Lancet* **1**, 848–50.

Montgomery, R. D., Cruickshank, E. K., Robertson, W. B. and McMenemey, W. H. (1964). Clinical and pathological observations on Jamaican neuropathy. *Brain* **87**, 425–62.

Nettleship, E. (1884). On cases of retro-ocular neuritis. *Trans. ophthal. Soc. U.K.* **4**, 186–226.

Nikoskelainen, E. and Riekkinen, P. (1974). Optic neuritis—a sign of multiple sclerosis or other diseases of the central nervous system. *Acta Neurol. Scand.* **50**, 690–718.

— (1975). Symptoms, signs and early course of optic neuritis. *Acta ophthal.* **53**, 254–72.

Osuntokun, B. O. (1968). An ataxic neuropathy in Nigeria. A clinical, biochemical and electrophysiological study. *Brain* **91**, 215–48.

Percy, A. K., Nobrega, F. T., and Kurland, L. T. (1972). Optic neuritis and multiple sclerosis. *Archs Ophthal., N.Y.* **87**, 135–9.

Swanzy, H. R. (1897). Discussion on retro-ocular neuritis. *Trans. ophthal. Soc. U.K.* **17**, 107–217.

Tatlow, W. F. T. (1948). The prognosis of retrobulbar neuritis. *Br. J. Ophthal.* **32**, 488–97.

Taub, R. G. and Rucker, C. W. (1954). The relationship of retrobulbar neuritis to multiple sclerosis. *Am. J. Ophthal.* **37**, 494–7.

Traquair, H. M. (1930). Toxic amblyopia including retrobulbar neuritis. *Trans. ophthal. Soc. U.K.* **50**, 351–85.

Watkins, S. M. and Espir, M. (1969). Migraine and multiple sclerosis. *J. Neurol. Neurosurg. Psychiat.* **32**, 35–7.

3 Symptoms at presentation

Retrobulbar neuritis is one of the difficult subjects in ophthalmology. It tends to elude research, in the sense of laboratory work on pathological material, and to tempt towards speculation. It is, therefore, pre-eminently a subject for investigation by close and accurate clinical observation (Traquair 1930).

Despite the introduction of electro-physiological techniques, the diagnosis of optic neuritis depends on accurate clinical assessment.

Fig. 3.1 shows the duration of visual symptoms prior to admission, the information not being available in three patients. Two-thirds of the patients (113 out of 167) were admitted within 3 weeks of the onset of their visual symptoms. As expected, the longer the duration of symptoms before admission, the greater the proportion of patients who had improved (Fig. 3.2).

Surprisingly few authors have considered the factor of symptom-duration on initial examination and its relationship to the severity of visual disturb-

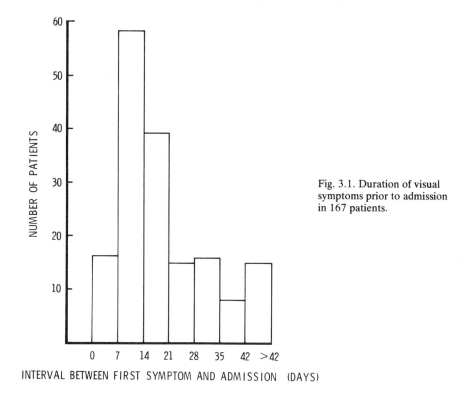

Fig. 3.1. Duration of visual symptoms prior to admission in 167 patients.

ance. Bradley and Whitty (1967) concluded that cases were usually improving by the end of the first week after the onset of visual symptoms, a finding previously recorded by Adie (1932). In a series of 185 cases (Nikoskelainen 1975), 16·2 per cent reported subjective improvement in visual blurring by the time of the first examination.

Pain

Nettleship (1884) was aware of ocular pain, tenderness of the globe, and pain on eye movement as accompaniments of the visual loss in this condition. More severe or longer lasting pain was thought to have an adverse affect on visual prognosis, an opinion shared by Swanzy (1897), whilst Gunn (1904*a*) attached the same significance to deep-seated pain. By 1932, Adie considered that 'some pain is almost always present at the onset, at rest, on voluntary movement, or on pressure of the eyeball'.

Frequency and site

In our series, pain was present in or around the eye in 87 per cent of cases (147/170). The pain was orbital in 131 and solely supra-orbital in 9; a combination of these sites occurred in 20 patients. Other sites affected were

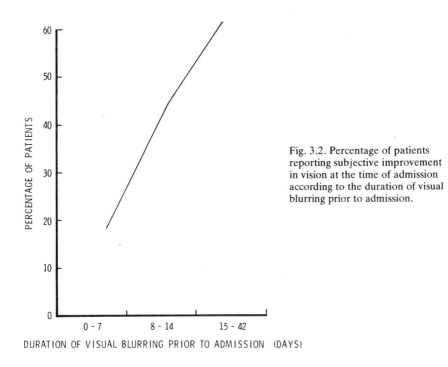

Fig. 3.2. Percentage of patients reporting subjective improvement in vision at the time of admission according to the duration of visual blurring prior to admission.

frontal (5 cases), temporal (2), maxillary (2), generalized (2), occipital (1), scalp (1), and lower jaw (1); patients with pain in these sites usually had orbital pain in addition. Pain was absent throughout in 16/170 (9 per cent).

The frequency with which pain has been recorded in optic neuritis has varied considerably, as can be seen from Table 3.1. The differences partly reflect varying clinical material, and partly the types of pain that have been included. Benedict (1942), with increasing awareness of the symptom,

Table 3.1 Frequency of pain in optic neuritis

Author	Percentage	Aetiology of optic neuritis
Carroll (1940)	20	Mixed
Marshall (1950)	22	Mixed
Carroll (1952)	23	Mixed
Lynn (1959)	25	MS or unknown
Gunn (1904*b*)	33	Mixed
Kurland *et al.* (1966)	36	MS or unknown
Benedict (1942)	50	MS
Nettleship (1884)	61	Mixed
Nikoskelainen (1975)	62	Mixed
Jessop (1907)	67	Unknown
Bradley and Whitty (1967)	68	MS or unknown
Sandberg and Bynke (1973)	72	Unknown
Hutchinson (1976)	77	MS or unknown
Adie (1932)	Almost always	MS

revised his own figures for its prevalence, and in four recent series, the symptom has been found with a frequency approaching our own (Bradley and Whitty 1967; Sandberg and Bynke 1973; Nikoskelainen 1975; Hutchinson 1976).

Tenderness of the globe and pain on eye movement

Pain on eye movement occurred in 145/170 (85 per cent) of our cases; only seven of these were not associated with pain in the eye at rest. In 107/145, a specific movement exacerbated the pain, elevation (33 per cent) and abduction (25 per cent) being the most common, followed by adduction (16 per cent) and a combination of elevation and abduction (16 per cent). Thirty-three (19 per cent) had tenderness in the eye which, in all cases, was associated with pain at rest or on eye movement.

Hock (1884), quoted by Nettleship (1884), stated that the type of field defect in optic neuritis could be predicted from the direction of eye movement that caused the most pain. Gunn (1897) and more recent authors have been unable to confirm this observation, nor did we find it in our own material.

Duration of pain and relationship to vision loss

In 99 patients (those receiving steroids were excluded) an accurate assessment of the duration of eye pain was possible (Fig. 3.3).

One patient, with right papillitis, and ocular pain persisting for 6 weeks, had evidence of mucopus in the right maxillary antrum, producing a fluid level on radiological examination. The use of Otrivine nasal spray (0·1 per cent Xylo metazoline) relieved the pain within 6 hours. Eighteen months later, neurological assessment showed evidence of probable multiple sclerosis.

In general, no correlation was found between the presence or duration of ocular pain and sinus abnormalities on radiological examination (see Chapter 6).

In 47 patients (29 per cent), pain coincided with the onset of visual blurring, in 65 (43 per cent) the pain preceded, and in 42 (27 per cent) followed visual blurring (Fig. 3.4).

Nettleship (1884) similarly found that pain tended to precede, or coincide with, the defect of vision, a view shared by Carroll (1952) and Lynn (1959),

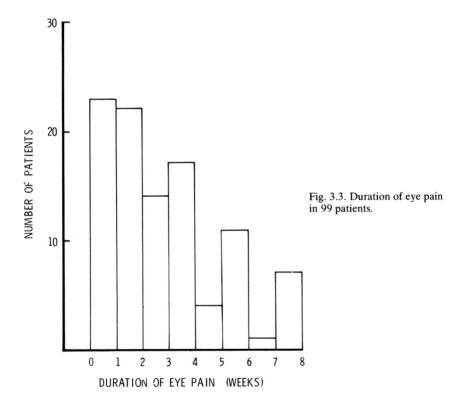

Fig. 3.3. Duration of eye pain in 99 patients.

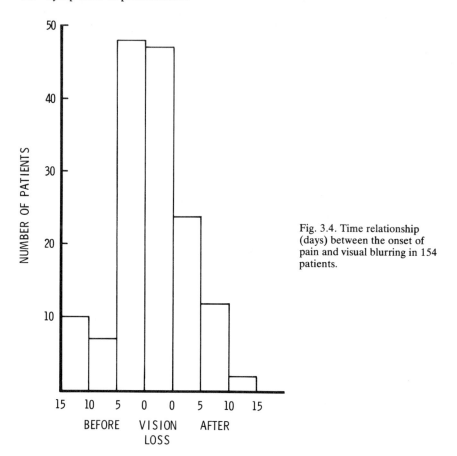

Fig. 3.4. Time relationship (days) between the onset of pain and visual blurring in 154 patients.

the former describing an interval of up to four weeks between the two symptoms. In Bradley and Whitty's experience (1967), on the other hand, they most commonly coincided, whilst Nikoskelainen (1975) described a decrease in visual acuity as the commonest initial symptom.

Contrary to early belief, there is no evidence that the character or duration of the pain has a significant effect upon visual outcome. On occasions, the pain may last several weeks and, in such circumstances, corticosteroid therapy appears capable of rapidly relieving it.

The origin of the pain remains uncertain, but a careful study of its characteristics, for example, site, radiation, aggravating factors, duration, and relationship to visual acuity may indicate the underlying pathology.

The optic nerve is pain insensitive, but its covering of meninges undoubtedly contains pain fibres. It has been suggested (Rose 1972) that the pain of optic neuritis is due to distension of these meninges by a swollen optic nerve, though if this is so, the speed of development of the swelling must be important, since the more gradual enlargement of the nerve by glioma is characteristically painless. Sudden enlargement of an optic nerve glioma, as indicated by rapidly deteriorating vision, can be painful (Spencer 1972), and pain is also a prominent feature of malignant optic gliomas occurring in adult life (Hoyt *et al.* 1973). Ultrasonography has revealed enlargement of the optic nerve in optic neuritis, as well as swelling of the adjacent extraocular muscles, probably oedematous in nature (Coleman and Carroll 1972). The origins of the superior and medial rectus particularly are closely associated with the optic nerve sheath (Duke-Elder 1961). Since abduction is more likely to cause pain than adduction it may be the oedematous swelling of extra-ocular muscles which is responsible for pain on eye movement in some cases. The fact that pain and blurring of vision are not necessarily closely related in time suggests that oedema of the optic nerve can occur without sufficient conduction block being present to produce visual blurring.

Visual symptoms

These were described usually as blurring or fogging of vision, although more positive visual phenomena were encountered in a small number of patients.

Mode of onset and progression

In 31 cases (18·2 per cent) the visual disturbance was present on waking and, in the remainder, developed during the day. Seventeen patients described the onset of visual blurring as sudden and, in 8 of these, further deterioration occurred. An accurate assessment of the period over which visual blurring progressed was obtained in 99 patients (Table 3.2).

Vail (1931) claimed that the acute visual disturbance secondary to sinus disease was always apparent on waking, but there is no evidence that this feature is of any value in differential diagnosis. In 185 cases of optic neuritis collected by Nikoskelainen (1975), a visual disturbance on waking was noticed by 15 per cent. Table 3.3 gives the findings of other authors regarding the progression of visual disturbance after onset.

In attempting to understand the pathogenesis of optic neuritis, the period during which vision continues to deteriorate could be of significance. The description of sudden vision loss must be treated with caution, since patients may only become aware of a unilateral visual disturbance by accident, when for some reason the remaining eye is covered. A comparison with figures obtained by McAlpine *et al.* (1972) in 219 patients with multiple sclerosis (Table 3.2), reveals that symptoms referrable to demyelination in other parts of the nervous system can similarly reach a maximum within a short period.

Table 3.2 A comparison of the time course of visual compared with other symptoms

Period of visual deterioration (99 patients)	Percentage
Sudden onset, or on waking without further deterioration	13.1
Less than 24 hours	3.0
1–2 days	16.2
3–7 days	43.4
1–2 weeks	17.2
Over 2 weeks	7.1

Time taken for symptoms (of multiple sclerosis) to reach maximum intensity (219 patients) McAlpine *et al.* 1972.

Less than 24 hours	39.2
1–7 days	29.2
1–8 weeks	14.2
3 months	5.9
3–12 months	2.7
Insidious and progressive	8.7

Table 3.3 Time for development of maximal deficit from onset of visual blurring

Author	Time for development of maximal visual deficit
Adie (1932)	Hours
Traquair (1930)	1–2 days
Griffith (1897)	2 days
Gunn (1904*a*)	1–3 days
Benedict (1942)	3–4 days
Marshall (1950)	4 days (40.4 per cent)
Hutchinson (1976)	Days (65 per cent)
Hyllested and Moller (1961)	1–14 days (65 per cent) Hours (29 per cent)
Nikoskelainen (1975)	1–2 days (20 per cent)
	3–7 days (23 per cent)

Subjective field defect

The vast majority of patients described generalized blurring of vision, although it was often predominantly central. And although 3·5 per cent complained of temporal or peripheral, 1·8 per cent of quadrantic, and 2·3 per cent of altitudinal defects, all tended to become generalized as the condition progressed. Marshall's findings (1950) were similar; 5·4 per cent of his cases had hemianopic or altitudinal defects, the remainder complaining of generalized or central impairment.

Positive visual phenomena

These were noted by eight patients (Table 3.4). None of these cases had a personal or family history of migraine and, of five followed for a minimum period of 1 year, two had possible, and three probable, multiple sclerosis on re-examination.

Table 3.4 Clinical details of eight patients with positive visual phenomena

Case	Type of visual symptom	Course of optic neuritis	Follow-up assessment
P.J. aged 38 Female	Flashing black squares 1 week before the onset of visual blurring	Recovery	Possible MS 4 years later
B.B. aged 43 Female	Flashes of light whilst looking at slides, 1 day before the onset of visual blurring	Recovery	Possible MS 4 years later
L.O. aged 21 Female	Flashing lights in affected eye when looking down in dark room, 3 weeks after onset of optic neuritis	Recovery	Probable MS 3 years later
A.F. aged 51 Male	Floaty red spots of light with the right eye closed, occurring at night, 1 week before the onset of optic neuritis	Recovery	Probable MS 1 year later
E.F. aged 48 Male	Flickering light in temporal field 24 hours before onset of visual blurring	Recovery	Probable MS 1 year later
M.M. aged 30 Female	Misty vision on waking associated with shimmering lights in central field	Recovery	Not followed up
A.M. aged 19 Female	With visual blurring, certain objects and colours appeared excessively bright	Visual acuity 6/12 after 6 months	Not followed up
P.E. aged 36 Female	Occasional flashes of light after onset of left optic neuritis	Recovery	Not followed up

Gunn (1897) commented that occasionally patients would complain of seeing objects as through a moving haze. According to Traquair (1930), the condition 'may be ushered in by a sensation of flashes or sparks of light or by a feeling of mistiness as if the patient was looking through dark smoke'. Such symptoms are, however, uncommon. Earl (1964) was only able to find a single example, the patient describing showers of sparks occurring in the upper field when certain eye movements were performed.

Davis, Bergen, Schauf, McDonald, and Deutsch (1976) have recently described the phenomenon in nine cases, the majority experiencing the symptoms only with horizontal eye movements. An analogy with Lhermitte's sign was suggested by the brief duration of the symptom and its tendency to fatiguability. Although the authors noted the ability of mechanical stimulation to temporarily depolarize myelinated nerve fibres, they were unable to explain the apparent susceptibility of demyelinated optic nerve fibres to mechanical stress.

The effect of bright light

Although several of our cases, following recovery, were aware of the deleterious effects of bright light, none had noted this phenomenon in the acute stages, as described by Gunn (1897). Lillie (1934) noted that vision was better at dawn, or dusk, or on cloudy days, and Carroll (1940) made similar observations.

Laterality

In our series, the right eye was first involved in 83 patients (49 per cent) and the left in 87 (51 per cent). Although individual authors have not always found such a symmetrical distribution (Table 3.5), a combination of several series produces figures comparable to our own.

Table 3.5 The distribution of unilateral attacks of optic neuritis

	Side involved	
	Left	Right
Nettleship (1884)	10	14
Bagley (1952)	10	8
Schlossman and Phillips (1954)	12	8
Hyllested and Moller (1961)	18	23
Kurland et al. (1966)	73	70
Bradley et al. (1967)	43	30
Rischbieth (1968)	51	48
Landy and Ohlrich (1970)	30	18
Total	247 (53%)	219 (47%)

Other symptoms

Five of the patients had had symptoms suggesting an upper respiratory tract infection within one week of the onset of visual symptoms. Four others had a purulent nasal discharge at the time of onset of other symptoms, but none of these had sinus abnormalities on radiological examination. (The relationship of sinus disease to optic neuritis is considered on pages 94–7.) In 12 patients, symptoms suggesting involvement of other parts of the central nervous system occurred within 1 month of the development of the optic neuritis.

Conclusions

Each eye is affected with equal regularity. The visual deficit develops rapidly in optic neuritis and, in the vast majority of cases, will have reached its maximum within 3–4 days. An equally early recovery is the rule, so that a considerable proportion of patients will have noted subjective improvement by the time of referral.

Visual blurring is usually central or generalized; a small number of patients complain of peripheral or altitudinal defects at onset, but these tend to become generalized later. Positive visual phenomena, such as a sensation of sparks and flashes of light induced by certain eye movements, are encountered infrequently. The visual defect is found on waking in 18 per cent and is noticed to begin abruptly on other occasions; the sudden, accidental, discovery of a defect probably inflates these figures.

Pain in the majority of cases antedates or coincides with visual blurring and is present in most patients if careful inquiry is made. Its duration is variable, but will exceed 4 weeks in only 25 per cent.

In the early stages, the disturbing effect of bright light on vision may be noted by the patient, but this becomes a more common complaint following recovery.

In this series there were no significant accompanying non-neurological symptoms.

REFERENCES

Adie, W. J. (1932). The aetiology and symptomatology of disseminated sclerosis. *Br. med. J.* **2**, 997–1000.
Bagley, C. H. (1952). An etiologic study of a series of optic neuropathies. *Am. J. Ophthal.* **35**, 761–72.
Benedict, W. L. (1942). Multiple sclerosis as an etiological factor in retrobulbar neuritis. *Archs Ophthal., N.Y.* **28**, 988–95.
Bradley, W. G., and Whitty, C. W. M. (1967). Acute optic neuritis: its clinical features and their relation to prognosis for recovery of vision. *J. Neurol. Neurosurg. Psychiat.* **30**, 531–8.
Carroll, F. D. (1940). Retrobulbar neuritis. Observations on one hundred cases. *Archs Ophthal., N.Y.* **24**, 44–54.
— (1952). Optic neuritis. A 15-year study. *Am. J. Ophthal.* **35**, 75–82.
Coleman, D. J., and Carroll, F. D. (1972). A new technique for evaluation of optic neuropathy. *Trans. Am. ophthal. Soc.* **70**, 154–60.
Davis, F. A., Bergen, D., Schauf, C., McDonald, W. I., and Deutsch, W. (1976). Movement phosphenes in optic neuritis: A new clinical sign. *Neurology, Minneap.* **26**, 1100–4.
Duke-Elder, S. (1961). *System of ophthalmology*, Volume 2, *The anatomy of the visual system* by S. Duke-Elder and K. C. Wybar, p. 420. Henry Kimpton, London.

Earl, C. J. (1964). Some aspects of optic atrophy. *Trans. ophthal. Soc. U.K.* **84**, 215–26.
Griffith, A. H. (1897). Discussion on retro-ocular neuritis. *Trans. ophthal. Soc. U.K.* **17**, 107–217.
Gunn, M. (1897). Discussion on retro-ocular neuritis. *Trans. ophthal. Soc. U.K.* **17**, 107–217.
— (1904*a*). Discussion on retro-ocular neuritis. *Br. med. J.* **2**, 1285.
— (1904*b*). Retro-ocular neuritis. *Lancet* **2**, 412–13.
Hoyt, W. F., Meshel, L. G., Lessell, S., Schatz, N. J., and Suckling, R. D. (1973). Malignant optic glioma of adulthood. *Brain* **96**, 121–32.
Hutchinson, W. M. (1976). Acute optic neuritis and the prognosis for multiple sclerosis. *J. Neurol. Neurosurg. Psychiat.* **39**, 283–9.
Hyllested, K. and Moller, P. M. (1961). Follow-up on patients with a history of optic neuritis. *Acta ophthal.* **39**, 655–62.
Jessop, W. H. H. (1907). Three cases of acute uni-ocular optic neuritis in boys with great loss of vision and subsequent complete recovery. *Trans. ophthal. Soc. U.K.* **27**, 170–7.
Kurland, L. T., Beebe, G. W., Kurtzke, J. F., Nagler, B., Auth, T. L., Lessell, S., and Nefzger, M. D. (1966). Studies on the natural history of multiple sclerosis. 2. The progression of optic neuritis to multiple sclerosis. *Acta Neurol. Scand.* [Suppl] **19** (Vol. 42), 157–76.
Landy, P. J. and Ohlrich, G. D. (1970). Optic neuritis and its relationship to disseminated sclerosis. *Proc. Aust. Assoc. Neurol.* **7**, 67–70.
Lillie, W. I. (1934). The clinical significance of retrobulbar and optic neuritis. *Am. J. Ophthal.* **17**, 110–19.
Lynn, B. H. (1959). Retrobulbar neuritis. A survey of the present condition of cases occurring over the last fifty-six years. *Trans. ophthal. Soc. U.K.* **79**, 701–16.
McAlpine, D., Lumsden, C. E. and Acheson, E. C. (1972). *Multiple sclerosis: a reappraisal* (2nd edn). Churchill Livingstone, Edinburgh.
Marshall, D. (1950). Ocular manifestations of multiple sclerosis and relationship to retrobulbar neuritis. *Trans. Am. ophthal. Soc.* **48**, 487–525.
Nettleship, E. (1884). On cases of retro-ocular neuritis. *Trans. ophthal. Soc. U.K.* **4**, 186–226.
Nikoskelainen, E. (1975). Symptoms, signs and early course of optic neuritis. *Acta ophthal.* **53**, 254–72.
Rischbieth, R. H. C. (1968). Retrobulbar neuritis in the state of South Australia. *Proc. Aust. Assoc. Neurol.* **5**, 573–5.
Rose, F. C. (1972). The optic nerve (ed. J. S. Cant). Henry Kimpton, London.
Sandberg, M. and Bynke, H. (1973). Cerebrospinal fluid in 25 cases of optic neuritis. *Acta Neurol. Scand.* **49**, 443–52.
Schlossman, A. and Phillips, C. C. (1954). Optic neuritis in relation to demyelinating diseases. A clinical study. *Am. J. Ophthal.* **37**, 487–94.
Spencer, W. H. (1972). Primary neoplasms of the optic nerve and its sheaths: Clinical features and current concepts of pathogenetic mechanisms. *Trans. Am. ophthal. Soc.* **70**, 490–528.
Swanzy, H. R. (1897). Discussion on retro-ocular neuritis. *Trans. ophthal. Soc. U.K.* **17**, 107–217.
Traquair, H. M. (1930). Toxic amblyopia, including retrobulbar neuritis. *Trans. ophthal. Soc. U.K.* **17**, 107–217.
Vail, H. H. (1931). Retrobulbar optic neuritis originating in nasal sinuses: New method of demonstrating relation between sphenoid sinus and optic nerve. *Archs. Otolar.* **13**, 846.

4 Visual signs at presentation

It is the general opinion that visible reaction in the nerve is rare in multiple sclerosis, but I believe that with more careful neurologic examination and with more exact studies of the fundus this idea will change (Berliner 1935).

Visual acuity at presentation

The distribution of visual acuity amongst 165 cases at presentation is shown in Fig. 4.1. Those patients with previous attacks in the same eye have been excluded. The groups with less impaired vision had a longer duration of visual symptoms (Fig. 4.2) suggesting that, in many, improvement had

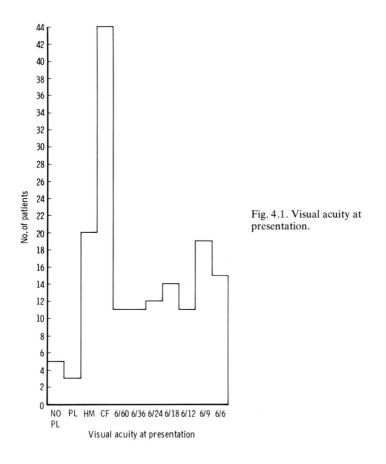

Fig. 4.1. Visual acuity at presentation.

already begun by the time of admission. Thus, for 14 patients with an acuity of 6/6, the mean duration of visual symptoms was 31 days, compared with 9·4 days for five patients with no perception of light. Table 4.1 compares the distribution of visual acuity at presentation in our own series with those of Marshall (1950) and Nikoskelainen (1975).

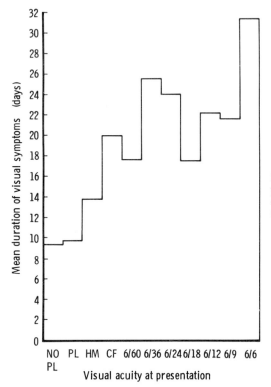

Fig. 4.2. Visual acuity at presentation according to duration of visual symptoms (*P* < 0·01).

Nettleship's (1884) series of 28 cases was clearly not typical, since six (21·4 per cent) suffered permanent complete vision loss. In Gunn's experience (1904), 'all degrees of failure of vision were met with up to absolute blindness'. Carroll (1940) concluded that in most cases there was a marked reduction in visual acuity, whilst Benedict (1942) considered that in the majority vision decreased to complete blindness for a period of 24 to 48 hours. Bradley and Whitty's (1967) findings support our own, indicating that the proportion of patients with poor vision falls rapidly as time elapses from the onset of symptoms. For example, 60 per cent of those seen within 24 hours had poor vision (6/60 or worse) whereas after 7 days from onset, 40 per cent had poor and 40 per cent fair vision (6/12–6/36).

It has long been recognized that a history suggestive of optic neuritis might

Table 4.1 Distribution of visual acuity at presentation in patients with optic neuritis (per cent)

Visual angle (degrees)	Percentage of patients			
	Nikoskelainen (1975)†	Marshall (1950)‡		Present series§
		Left*	Right	
1.0–1.3	17	24.2	21.3	9.1
1.4–2.5	19	16.3	18.5	18.2
3.3 or more	64	59.3	60.2	72.7

† Results were expressed as visual acuities of 0.8 or above; 0.4–0.7; or 0.3 or less.
‡ Results were expressed as visual acuities of 20/25 or above; 20/50–20/30; or 20/70 or less.
§ Equivalent grouping by visual acuity would be 6/6 or 5/6; 5/12–6/9; and 6/18 or less.
*The figures for the L eye did not add up to 100 per cent in the original publication.

be associated with normal or near normal visual acuity, even with early examination. Gunn (1897) believed that a colour scotoma at or near fixation could be found with an acuity of 6/6, and Carroll (1940) encountered some patients with visual blurring and scotoma despite vision of 20/20. The frequency with which near normal vision is found is largely dependent on how often a scotoma fails to involve central vision. The extreme views are exemplified by Gunn (1904), who stated the central portion of the visual field was always involved, and Chamlin (1953), who concluded that as many as 21 per cent of cases might be expected to show sparing of fixation with normal or near normal visual acuity. Daroff and Lawton Smith (1965) have recorded three such cases, combining papillitis with nerve fibre bundle defects.

Pupil asymmetry

In this series, excluding patients with previous attacks of optic neuritis, anisocoria occurred in 28·7 per cent, its extent being recorded in 17 cases (Table 4.2). In each the dilated pupil coincided with the eye affected by optic neuritis and was accompanied by an abnormality of the direct light response. Patients with anisocoria tended to have worse vision than average (Table 4.3).

Table 4.2 Degree of anisocoria in 17 patients

No. of patients	Degree of anisocoria (mm)
3	0.5
10	1.0
3	2
1	3

Table 4.3 Distribution of visual acuities on admission in patients with and without anisocoria

Visual acuity	Number of patients (per cent)	
	Without anisocoria	With anisocoria
No PL or CF	41 (35.1%)	31 (64.6%)
6/60–6/18	37 (31.6%)	11 (22.9%)
6/12–6/6	39 (33.3%)	6 (12.5%)

The differences are significant at $P<0.01$, $\chi^2=13.12$; $\nu=2$
PL=perception of light   CF=counting fingers

Marshall (1950) found anisocoria in only 3·2 per cent of cases, though it was present in six of 28 patients described by Nettleship (1884). In that series, however, many differing aetiologies were included, and indeed a constricted pupil on the affected side was as common as a dilated one. Nikoskelainen (1975) encountered anisocoria in 18 of 131 affected eyes (14 per cent), in all but one the dilated pupil belonging to the involved eye. Kurland, Beebe, Kurtzke, Nagler, Auth, Lessell, and Nefzger (1966) reported anisocoria in 10·8 per cent of 223 affected eyes. According to McAlpine, Lumsden, and Acheson (1972) the pupil is usually dilated to some degree on the affected side, though no references were quoted to support this statement.

The concept of amaurotic mydriasis is controversial, being considered a well-known phenomenon by one authority (Duke-Elder and Scott 1971) but its existence being denied by another (Walsh and Hoyt 1969). As we have indicated, though the phenomenon is more frequent in those with poor acuity it can occur despite nearly normal vision. In all cases, however, it coincided with an abnormality of the pupillary light response.

The pupillary reaction

Some form of impairment of the direct pupillary response was found in 75·8 per cent of 165 patients (including a depressed or ill-sustained reaction or a Marcus Gunn response found with the swinging light test). There was no absolute relationship to the severity of the visual defect as measured by acuity, for example six patients with an acuity of 6/6 had an abnormal pupillary response. However, for 71 patients with an acuity of counting fingers or less, an abnormal reaction was present in 90 per cent, compared with 61 per cent for 46 patients with an acuity of 6/12 or better (Fig. 4.3).

Opinions have varied as to the frequency of this finding. Gunn (1904) believed the light reaction to be invariably impaired when there was a decided amblyopia, though paradoxically he did not describe the phenom-

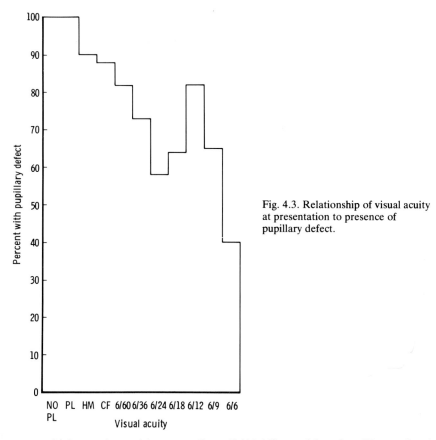

Fig. 4.3. Relationship of visual acuity at presentation to presence of pupillary defect.

enon which now bears his name. Carroll (1940) considered an ill-sustained light reaction to be an unreliable sign, whilst Marshall (1950) reported a normal pupil in 81·4 per cent of cases. Nikoskelainen (1975) discovered a depressed or absent light response in 26 per cent of patients, though of 72 eyes examined for a Marcus Gunn sign, 44 per cent were positive.

Macular threshold

This was measured in 71 patients (Fig. 4.4) and correlated well with visual acuity (Fig. 4.5).

Fundus appearance

The optic disc appearance (excluding patients with optic atrophy) was classified as normal, slightly blurred (often confined to the nasal regions),

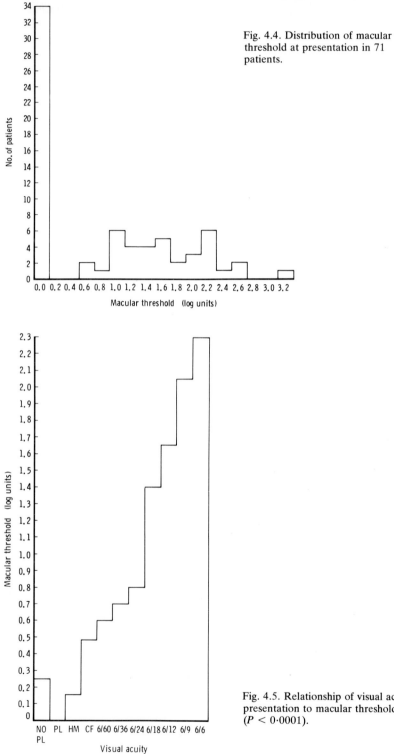

Fig. 4.4. Distribution of macular threshold at presentation in 71 patients.

Fig. 4.5. Relationship of visual acuity at presentation to macular threshold ($P < 0.0001$).

and markedly blurred, sometimes with peripapillary haemorrhages (neuroretinitis). The results and a comparison with other series are given in Table 4.4.

Table 4.4 Fundus changes in this and other series of optic neuritis (per cent)

	No of eyes examined	Normal	Slight disc blurring	Marked disc blurring	Disc blurring with haemorrhages
Present series	151	42.4	35.1	8.6	13.9
Uhthoff (1904)	100		———	5	———
Benedict (1942)	90		———	8.9	———
Paton (1914)			———	13	———
Hyllested and Moller (1961)	52		———	15.6	———
Marshall (1950)*		64.4	———	19.2 ———	3.2
Adie (1932)	70		———	30	———
Hutchinson (1976)*	175	60	18	17	
Bradley and Whitty (1967)*	78	55.1	———	24.4 ———	16.7
Nikoskelainen (1975)*	240	46	18	23	2

* Percentages made up to 100 by cases with evidence of optic atrophy.

Although Uhthoff (1904) described papillitis in only 5 per cent of multiple sclerosis patients, he thought it likely that a transitory inflammation of the papilla and nerve trunk was much more frequent, an observation borne out by subsequent findings and supported by Gunn (1904). Jessop (1907) reported three, and Buchanan (1923) four, cases of papillitis with good recovery of vision. Paton (1914) considered that 13 per cent of patients with optic nerve disease had disc swelling, and discussed the problems in differential diagnosis in the small number of cases where the papillitis was of sufficient severity to simulate papilloedema. A search of the literature by Sugar (1939) revealed 36 cases of multiple sclerosis with disc swelling, the author adding several personal cases.

The evolution of the optic disc changes has been examined in detail (Berliner 1935). Venous engorgement is the earliest reaction, followed by oedema appearing first in the upper nasal quadrant, but seldom exceeding one or two dioptres. Fluorescein photography (Rosen and Ashworth 1968) similarly demonstrates leakage of dye, sometimes remaining confined to a small segment, and first occurring at the nasal margin. Carroll (1940) concluded that marked degrees of disc swelling with or without haemorrhages were uncommon, a view supported by the frequency of the finding recorded by Benedict (1942) and Lynn (1959). More recent studies, however, have given it greater prominence (Table 4.4), and Bradley and Whitty (1967) reported haemorrhages as frequently as ourselves. The timing of the examination is relevant here, since initially dubious disc swelling may later progress to florid papillitis. Tables 4.5 and 4.6 illustrate the distribution of visual acuities and macular thresholds respectively, according to the appearances of the optic disc.

Table 4.5 Relationship of optic disc appearance to presenting visual acuity (per cent)

	Visual acuity at presentation		
	6/6–6/18	6/24–6/60	CF–no PL
Neuro-retinitis and severe papillitis	7 (20.6%)	4 (11.8%)	23 (67.6%)
Slight papillitis	14 (27%)	8 (15%)	31 (58%)
Normal disc	30 (46%)	17 (27%)	17 (27%)

$P<0.001$; $\chi^2=19.37$; $v=4$

Table 4.6 Relationship of optic disc appearance to presenting macular threshold

Macular threshold at presentation (log units)	Number of patients (per cent)		
	Neuro-retinitis and severe papillitis	Slight papillitis	Normal disc
2.8–2.0	2 (9.5%)	1 (6.7%)	8 (33.3%)
1.8–1.0	5 (23.8%)	4 (26.7%)	8 (33.3%)
0.8–1.0	14 (66.7%)	10 (66.6%)	8 (33.3%)

NS: $\chi^2=8.32$; $v=4$ but comparing patients with normal against abnormal discs, for macular thresholds above or below 1.0; $P<0.05$; $\chi^2=5.16$; $v=1$

Although severe disc swelling with or without haemorrhages is generally associated with markedly reduced vision and macular threshold, patients with severe papillitis and acuities of 6/6, or neuro-retinitis with acuities of 6/9 or 6/12 were seen, an association previously reported by Daroff and Lawton-Smith (1965).

Visual fields

Table 4.7 summarizes the types of field defect at presentation in 165 patients. Differentiation of central from centro-caecal scotomata has not been attempted.

Central scotoma to 5° (Fig. 4.6)

G.B., aged 49. Five-week history of pain on ocular movement in the left eye, followed after 1 week by visual blurring. There was a past history of transient peripheral paraesthesiae. Visual acuity was 6/18 with normal pupillary responses and fundus appearance. Visual fields showed a scotoma confined to the central 5°. Evidence of definite multiple sclerosis was found at follow-up 2 years later.

Table 4.7 Visual field analysis at presentation in 165 patients

		Number	%
Central field defects alone	5°	4	
	10°	13	30.9
	15°	22	
	Unspecified	12	
Central field defects with peripheral extension to 25°	Generalized	29	
	Altitudinal	7	24.2
	Sectorial	3	
	Hemianopic	1	
Generalized (25°) depression of visual field		15	9.3
Junctional defect		1	0.6
Arcuate		5	3.0
Peripheral defects with central sparing	Peripheral (diffuse)	3	
	Altitudinal	3	4.2
	Sectorial	1	
Field not possible due to severity of vision loss		8	4.8
Unsatisfactory or unreliable examination		32	19.4
Normal field		6	3.6

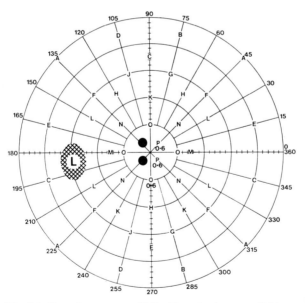

Fig. 4.6. Central scotoma to 5°. In this and subsequent fields, a black dot refers to an absent response. An unnumbered letter indicates a normal threshold at that site. Low figures indicate a severely depressed threshold, and vice versa for higher figures.

Central scotoma to 10° (Fig. 4.7)

A.A., aged 60. Three weeks prior to admission, developed blurring of vision of the left eye on waking, without ocular pain. Fourteen years before, the patient had developed diplopia with left facial numbness and limb ataxia with subsequent left sided trigeminal neuralgia. Visual acuity was 6/24 with a depressed pupillary light response and slight swelling of the optic disc. Visual fields showed a central scotoma to 10°. Neurological examination was normal.

Central scotoma to 15° (Fig. 4.8)

M.G., aged 42. Admitted with 10-day history of vision loss and aching in the left eye. Visual acuity was 6/9 with a Marcus Gunn response. Fundus examination was normal. Visual fields showed a central defect, predominantly to 5° but extending to 15°. Neurological examination 1 year later revealed evidence of definite multiple sclerosis.

Central scotoma with peripheral extension (Fig. 4.9)

P.H., aged 24. Three weeks before admission developed pain around the right eye followed one day later by visual blurring. Visual acuity was counting fingers with a depressed pupillary response and swelling of the nasal margin of the optic disc. Visual fields showed a dense central, 10°, scotoma extending to a lesser degree of severity to the periphery. Neurological examination was normal.

Central and altitudinal defect

E.G., aged 38 (Fig. 4.10). Sudden blurring of vision in the right eye 1 month before admission had been followed by retro-orbital pain exacerbated by movement. There was a history of transient vertigo 12 years previously. Visual acuity was 6/36 with slight swelling of the disc margins. Visual fields showed a central scotoma extending predominantly into the upper quadrants. The neurological examination was normal.

M.H., aged 50 (Fig. 4.11). Twelve days before admission developed blurring of the vision with pain in the left eye. There was a history of a previous episode of vertigo with ataxia. Visual acuity was 6/12 with a depressed pupillary reaction and slight blurring of the nasal margin of the optic disc. Visual fields showed a central defect extending altitudinally. The deep tendon reflexes were exaggerated.

Central and hemianopic defect (Fig. 4.12)

C.G., aged 42. Loss of vision on waking had occurred, without pain, 10 days prior to admission. Visual acuity in the right eye was counting fingers with a depressed pupillary response and pallor of the optic disc. Visual fields showed a predominantly nasal hemianopic defect with central involvement. Neurological examination was normal.

Junctional scotoma (Fig. 4.13)

W.H. aged 46. Sudden pain behind the left eye 3 weeks prior to admission had been associated with visual blurring confined to that eye. Visual acuity on the left was 6/18

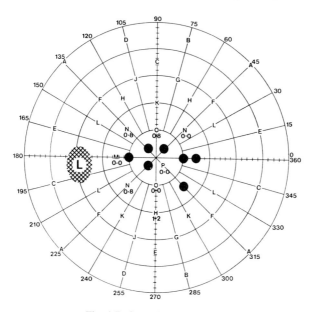

Fig. 4.7. Central scotoma to 10°.

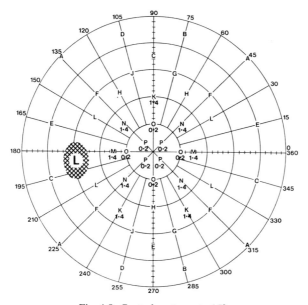

Fig. 4.8. Central scotoma to 15°.

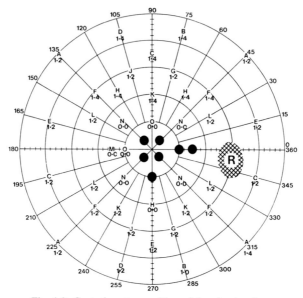

Fig. 4.9. Central scotoma with peripheral extension.

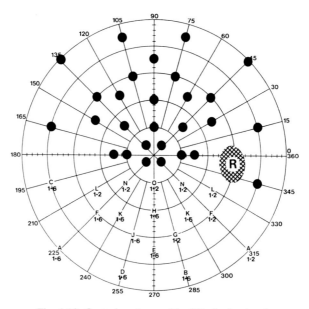

Fig. 4.10. Central scotoma with altitudinal extension.

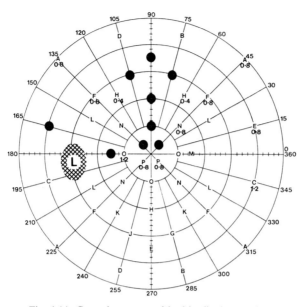

Fig. 4.11. Central scotoma with altitudinal extension.

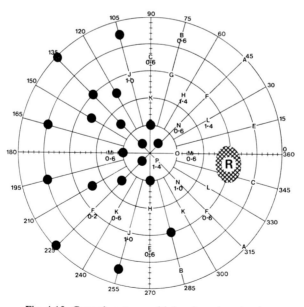

Fig. 4.12. Central scotoma with hemianopic extension.

and on the right 6/12. The left pupil showed a Marcus Gunn response. The right fundus appearances were normal, whilst the left disc was swollen with peripapillary haemorrhages. Visual fields showed a dense defect on the left extending to 25°, with, in the right eye, a small, temporal, paracentral scotoma. Both defects subsequently resolved. The neurological examination was normal.

Arcuate defects

M.R., aged 25 (Fig. 4.14). Pain behind the right eye, 6 days before admission, had been followed by patchy blurring of vision. There had been previous episodes of transient diplopia and clumsiness of the left hand. Visual acuity was 6/9 with a normal pupillary response, but mild swelling of the optic disc. Visual fields showed inferior and superior arcuate defects, subsequently resolving. Neurological examination showed evidence of definite multiple sclerosis.

J.S., aged 39 (Fig. 4.15). Nineteen days before admission, developed pain above the left eye followed within 24 hours by visual failure. The eye had been affected by a similar episode 13 years before, with subsequent bouts of limb paraesthesiae. Visual acuity was 6/9 with a depressed light reaction and swelling of the optic disc. Visual fields showed superior and inferior arcuate defects with relative central sparing. Neurological examination was normal.

R.C., aged 19 (Fig. 4.16). Blurred vision on waking 10 days before had been associated with mild frontal headache. Visual acuity was 6/24 with depression of the pupillary response and normal fundus examination. Visual fields showed a superior arcuate defect in the right eye. One year later, the patient suffered a transient sixth nerve palsy.

Peripheral defects (Fig. 4.17)

D.G., aged 19. Blurring of vision in the right eye had persisted for 8 weeks before admission, without associated pain. Visual acuity was 6/12 with normal pupillary reactions and fundus appearance. A further episode of visual blurring with pain occurred 3 months later and examination 6 years later showed evidence of definite multiple sclerosis.

Altitudinal defect (Fig. 4.18)

A.P., aged 37. Admitted with a 5-week history of hazy vision in the right eye without ocular pain. Visual acuity was 6/6, there was no pupillary defect and fundus examination was normal. Visual fields showed an altitudinal defect. There was a previous history of diplopia and episodic clumsiness with paraesthesiae in the right hand, and neurological examination showed evidence of definite multiple sclerosis.

Sectorial defect (Fig. 4.19)

A.V., aged 40. One week before admission rapid visual failure in the left eye had been accompanied by eye pain. Visual acuity was 6/18 with a depressed light response. The optic disc was markedly swollen with peripapillary haemorrhages. Visual fields showed a predominantly nasal sectorial defect. Neurological examination was normal.

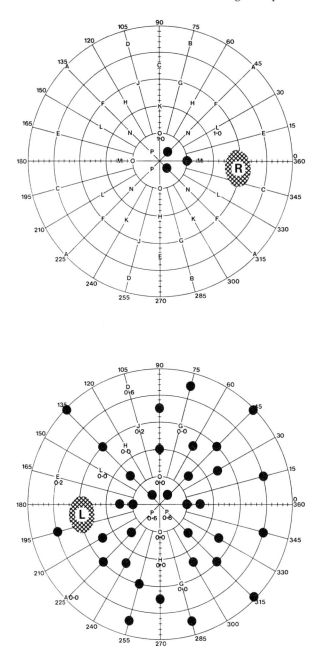

Fig. 4.13. L eye—generalized impairment; R eye—junctional defect.

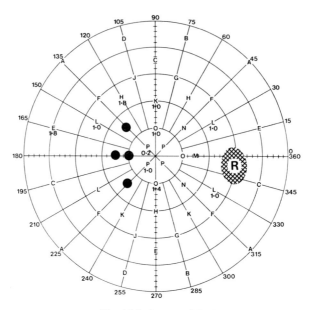

Fig. 4.14. Arcuate defect.

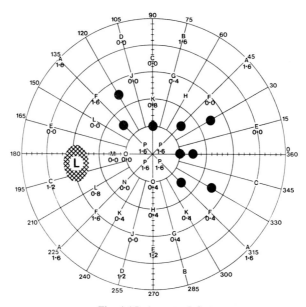

Fig. 4.15. Arcuate defect.

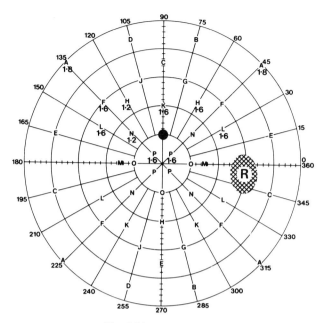

Fig. 4.16. Arcuate defect.

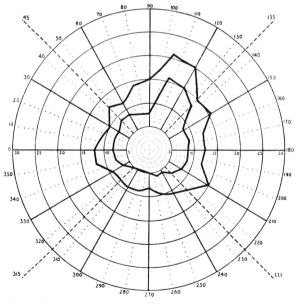

Fig. 4.17. Peripheral constriction; visual acuity 6/12; white 3/2000; red 8/2000.

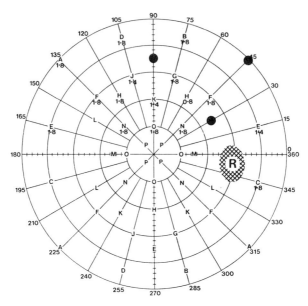

Fig. 4.18. Altitudinal defect.

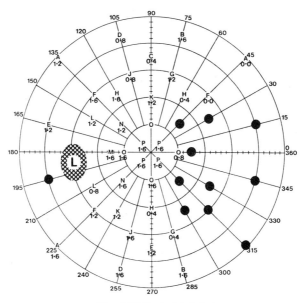

Fig. 4.19. Sectorial defect.

Fluctuating fields according to time of examination

The type of field defect demonstrated may vary according to the time of examination.

I.R. aged 40. Two weeks before admission developed blurring of vision in the left eye followed 1 week later by pain on lateral gaze. Five years before there had been an episode of mild bilateral visual blurring with recovery over 2 months. Visual acuity on the left was 6/36 with a Marcus Gunn pupil. Both optic discs showed mild pallor. The first visual field (Fig. 4.20) showed a diffuse defect to 25° with slight central sparing, evolving over the next 6 days (Figs. 4.21 and 4.22) to a predominantly altitudinal defect.

Table 4.7 indicates the types of field defect found in 165 patients at presentation. Patients with previous episodes of optic neuritis in the same eye have been excluded.

Early descriptions focused on central field defects in optic neuritis. Nettleship (1884) reported central scotomata in the majority and both Griffith (1897) and Gunn (1904) considered the central field to be always affected. Berliner (1935) and Carroll (1940) recorded typical central or paracentral defects, though the latter found some cases with an associated peripheral constriction or with extensions of central defects to the periphery. Central or paracentral scotomata, with or without peripheral extension, accounted for 90·8 per cent of Marshall's (1950) series, with a further 5 per

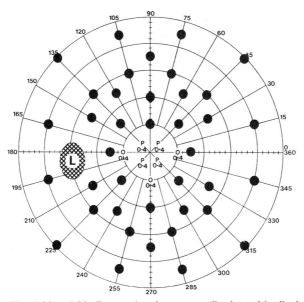

Fig. 4.20 – 4.22. Progression from generalized to altitudinal defect.

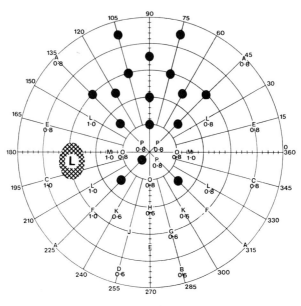

Fig. 4.21.

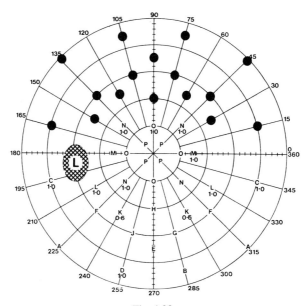

Fig. 4.22.

Visual signs at presentation 63

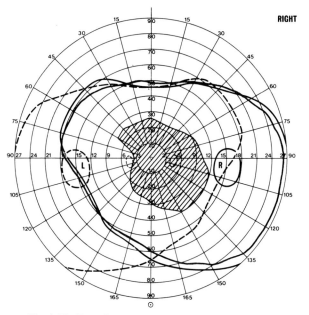

Fig. 4.23. Central scotoma in optic neuritis (white 2/330).

A woman, age 29, complained of pain in the left eye, especially on movement. After 1 week she noticed a 'scum' over the eye. Fields of vision showed a large central scotoma. Right V.A. 6/6 left 6/24. Neurological and general examination negative. In November 1953, a similar attack occurred in the right eye, with weakness of the right arm. V.A. was reduced to counting of fingers, on the left 6/5. (From Lynn 1959.)

cent reported to have hemianopic defects. Similarly, Hyllested and Moller (1961) found such defects in 98·5 per cent of their cases. Bradley and Whitty (1967) encountered six patients without central field changes, who in other respects had typical optic neuritis, but in a recent series (Hutchinson 1976) all such patients were excluded.

As early as 1904, Uhthoff concluded that some 8 per cent of patients might have peripheral constriction alone, though he included patients with syphilis, and hereditary and other disorders. Benedict (1942) found central scotomata in only 50 per cent, with centrocaecal defects in a further 25 per cent, the remainder being made up by a number of differing types, including hemianopic defects. Schlossman and Phillips (1954) commented on patients who had no loss of visual acuity but who nevertheless showed signs of optic neuritis. Field defects found in such patients included enlarged blind spots and paracentral or nerve-fibre-bundle defects sparing fixation. Although, Lynn (1959) stressed central field changes amongst 200 patients (Fig. 4.23), three patients with arcuate defects (Fig. 4.24), two with peripheral constriction plus central loss, two with peripheral constriction alone (Fig. 4.25), and one with an altitudinal loss (Fig. 4.26) were recorded. Chamlin (1953) had questioned reports of the relative rarity of other than central defects, based on an analysis of 100 personal cases. The delay from onset to examination was not indicated, though the author accepted that some central defects might have cleared during that period. Centrocaecal defects were found in 52 cases (Fig. 4.27) of whom only 31 were seen personally or had been examined in the acute stages. Twenty-four patients had paracentral nerve-fibre-bundle defects (Fig. 4.28) sparing fixation, with, in a further nine, similar defects extending to the periphery. Again only 18 of these 33 cases

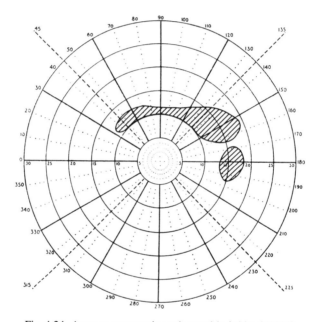

Fig. 4.24. Arcuate scotoma in optic neuritis (white 2/1000).
June 1954. A man of 37 years of age woke up one morning to find that vision in the right eye was blurred. There was a slight ache at the back of this eye, and when he closed his left eye, vision was restricted to the upper part of the field. The vision continued to deteriorate, so that in two more days it was completely lost. Visual acuity on the left was 6/5, J1. Neurological and general examination were negative, as were X-rays of skull, optic foramina and nasal accessory sinuses. In October 1957, a large arcuate scotoma still persists, together with a partial red/green blindness and pallor of the temporal side of the disc. Visual acuity right 6/6, J1; left 6/5, J1. (From Lynn 1959.)

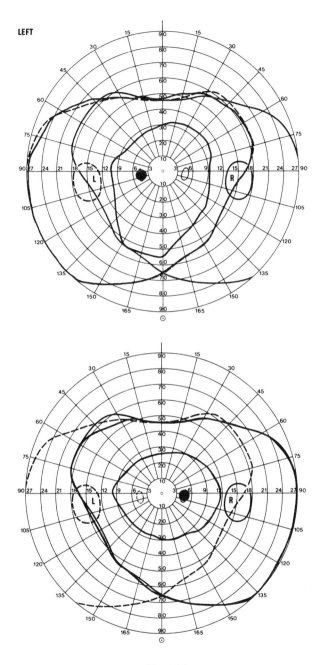

Fig. 4.25.

Pain and sudden loss of vision (P.L.) in the right eye in a young
woman of 23 years followed by a similar attack in the left (6/60) 3
weeks later with recovery to 6/9, 6/12; 2/330. (From Lynn 1959.)

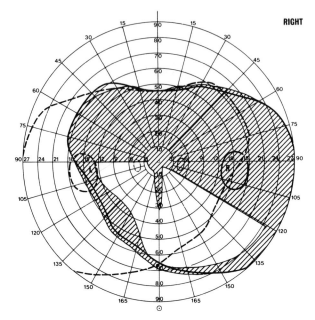

Fig. 4.26.

February 1958. Visual acuity (right) was fingers at 1 foot. The whole upper field was lost for 23/330 white in right eye. The left field showed no abnormality for 2/330 white. (From Lynn 1959.)

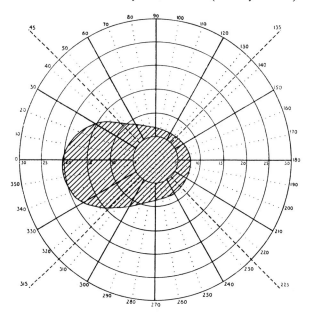

Fig. 4.27. Schematic sketch of typical cecocentral scotoma involving fixation (52 cases) (from Chamlin 1953).

were seen at the onset, with no fewer than 12 already having optic atrophy at the first examination. A further 11 cases had nerve-fibre-bundle defects involving fixation and the periphery, and four had peripheral defects alone, though none of these had evidence of multiple sclerosis, and indeed one had an elevated cerebrospinal fluid pressure.

Nikoskelainen (1975) analysed the field defects at presentation in 240 eyes of 185 patients, with findings comparable to our own (Table 4.8), suggesting that the higher incidence of arcuate and other defects found by Benedict (1942) and Chamlin (1953) might reflect a delay in examining the patient. Support for this concept comes from a comparison of the prevalence of optic atrophy in these series. Whereas it occurred in 11 per cent of Nikoskelainen's (1975) cases, and in 9·7 per cent of our own, it was recorded by Chamlin (1953) in 39 per cent (33 of 85 cases where details given).

Field defects in the clinically unaffected eye

In 161 patients, there was no history of a previous visual disturbance in the clinically unaffected eye. Of these, 100 had visual fields available for review and confirmed to be normal, 46 were reported to have had normal fields, though these were not available, and 15 (9·3 per cent) had some form of visual defect. Interpretation of isolated abnormalities on the Friedmann analyser may be difficult. Accordingly a field has only been considered abnormal if thresholds depressed by at least 0·2 log units were found at at least three separate sites. In some cases, the defects were more striking. A junction scotoma (Fig. 4.13) has already been referred to, whilst in another patient a considerable inferior defect was found.

W.P., aged 49. Admitted with a 6-month history of blurred vision in the right eye, unaccompanied by pain. There were no visual symptoms in the left eye. Visual acuity was counting fingers (right) and 6/18 (left), with bilateral optic atrophy. No field could be measured on the right because of the severity of vision loss. That on the left (Fig. 4.29) showed an infero-nasal defect with relative central sparing. At follow-up examination, 5 years later, there was evidence of definite multiple sclerosis. Vision had improved to 6/18 on the right but remained unaltered on the left, though the field defects had improved considerably on both sides.

In most of these 15 patients, the abnormalities consisted of scattered points of reduced threshold, not clearly corresponding to a particular type of field defect. Comparison with the abnormalities found in the unaffected eye by various electrophysiological techniques of patients with unilateral optic neuritis is probably an over-simplification. However, of 19 such patients studied by Halliday, McDonald, and Mushin (1973), two (10·5 per cent) had delayed responses, whereas three of 14 cases (21·4 per cent) reported by Galvin, Regan, and Heron (1976) had delayed temporal resolution of vision.

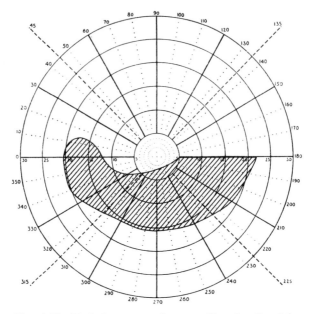

Fig. 4.28. Typical paracentral nerve fiber bundle defect (schematic) sparing fixation (24 cases) (from Chamlin 1953).

Table 4.8 A comparison of the distribution of visual field defects in our series and that of Nikoskelainen (1975) (Figures in per cent)

	Present study	Nikoskelainen (1975)
No. of eyes examined	165	240
Central defects with or without peripheral extension	64.4	68
Arcuate defects	3.0	3.0
Peripheral defects (all types)	4.2	5.0*
Too severe vision loss to enable field examination	4.8	5.0
Normal fields	3.6	5.0
Junctional defect in one eye with central loss in clinically affected eye	0.6	0
Unsatisfactory or unreliable examination	19.4	14

* Includes paracentral defects.

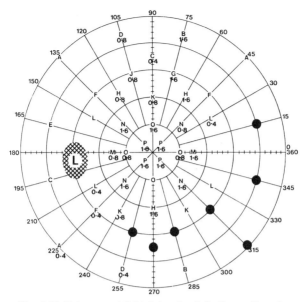

Fig. 4.29. Infero-nasal field defect in clinically unaffected eye.

Other types of field defect

Junction scotomata

We have already referred to a patient with unilateral visual failure and a junction scotoma in the clinically unaffected eye (Fig. 4.13). Traquair (1923) considered such scotomata to be due to a lesion of the crossing macular fibres at the junction of nerve and chiasm, giving an example (Fig. 4.30) in a patient with multiple sclerosis.

Chiasmatic lesions

Plaques of demyelination in the chiasm or retro-chiasmal part of the optic nerve have been described at post-mortem examination (Gartner 1953; Schlossman and Phillips 1954), though no clinical examples were encountered in this series. Rønne (1928) considered chiasmatic lesions to be not uncommon in multiple sclerosis, usually manifesting as a hemianopic central scotoma. Traquair (1925) described 3 cases, all with recovery, though none had progressed to multiple sclerosis. Ashworth (1967) has recorded one patient with a chronic chiasmal neuropathy, with evidence of multiple sclerosis appearing 18 years after the onset of visual symptoms.

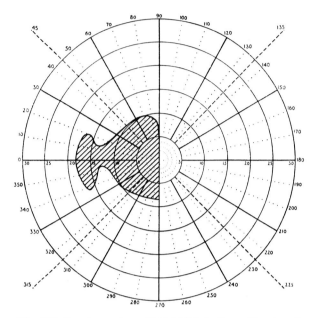

Fig. 4.30. Junction scotoma (2,20/1000); Left eye. Visual acuity
6/24; Miss R. Multiple sclerosis (from Traquair 1923).

Retrochiasmal lesions

Traquair (1925) described a patient with an inferior homonymous
hemianopia and subsequent recovery, who was well at follow-up three years
later. Marshall (1950) found hemianopic defects in 5 per cent of his cases. In
a vast survey of the literature, Savitsky and Rangell (1950) commented on
the paucity of cases of multiple sclerosis with homonymous hemianopia,
despite the pathological evidence of tract involvement. In 415 personally
observed cases of multiple sclerosis, they were unable to find a single
example. Chamlin and Davidoff (1954), however, collected four cases, all
with evidence of a more generalized neurological disturbance suggestive of
multiple sclerosis. In two cases, recovery led to paracentral homonymous
defects of a type suggesting lesions close to the occipital cortex. Vedel-
Jensen (1959) recorded two examples of optic tract neuritis in multiple
sclerosis, though in neither case had that diagnosis been definitely established. He was able to collect 16 cases from the literature. Boldt, Haerer,
Tourtellotte, Henderson, and De Jong (1963) analysed 365 consecutive
cases of multiple sclerosis and found homonymous field defects in five. They
felt unable, on the basis of the abnormalities, to locate the site of the lesions
more accurately.

Table 4.9 Patients with evidence of ocular inflammatory disease

Patient	Age	Evidence of MS		Optic neuritis	Type of ocular disease
		onset	follow-up		
S.H.	42	1	2	Pain Vision CF recovery to 6/6 Central scotoma Disc pallor	Healed choroiditis
W.W.	38	0	0	Pain Vision CF recovery to 6/6 Field not possible Disc swelling	Vitreous opacities and cells, later cells and flare in anterior chamber? 'cat-scratch disease (p. 110)
A.W.	25	0	1	Pain Vision HM recovery to 6/6 Central scotoma Disc normal	Venous sheathing—no further details
W.G.	20	1	1	Pain Vision HM recovery to 6/6 Fields not recorded Disc swelling	Choroiditis—no further details
E.G.	38	1	1	Pain Vision 6/36 recovery to 6/6 Central scotoma Disc swelling	Old keratitis
N.M.	23	1	1	Pain Vision 6/36 ? recovery Paracentral scotoma Slight temporal pallor	Vitreous opacity with adjacent retinal scar
P.G.	36	1	1	Pain Vision 6/18 recovery to 6/6 Paracentral scotoma Disc swelling	Vitreous changes and retinal vasculitis—not specified
M.K.	21	0	?	Pain Vision no PL recovery to 6/24 Field not possible Disc swelling	Venous sheathing, cells in posterior vitreous

For evidence of MS: 1=possible   2=probable   3=definite

Uveitis and retinal venous sheathing

In nine patients, there was some evidence of ocular inflammatory disease, details of which are given in Table 4.9. Information in some was sparse, though all of them, including the possible case of cat-scratch disease, had a typical history of optic neuritis. The relationship of optic neuritis to these disorders will be considered in Chapter 12.

Other ophthalmological findings

Eight patients were noted to have nystagmus on admission, in one probably congenital in origin. One patient had a sixth nerve palsy.

Conclusions

Visual acuity is usually markedly depressed in optic neuritis, particularly if the patients are seen soon after onset, but a significant minority of cases will have near normal vision despite a typical history. Pupil asymmetry has been encountered frequently in this series, though its existence in cases of unilateral optic nerve disease has been questioned. It is invariably associated with an abnormality of the pupillary light response and is more likely in those with severely reduced vision, as indeed is a depressed light reaction.

With experience, various degrees of disc swelling in the acute stages has been recognized increasingly frequently. Both neuro-retinitis and severe papillitis tend to be associated with a more abnormal visual acuity and macular threshold.

Central field defects predominated in this series and the overall frequency of field changes was similar to that found in another large, recently published collection. The higher incidence of arcuate and para-central defects reported by some authors may reflect a delay in assessment after onset of visual symptoms. Although chiasmal and retro-chiasmal field defects have been reported in multiple sclerosis, they were not seen in our patients apart from a junction scotoma in a clinically unaffected eye. Other field abnormalities were encountered in the 'normal' eye in 9·3 per cent of this series, though without adhering to a specific pattern.

Evidence of ocular inflammatory disease, a subject to be discussed in Chapter 12, was seen infrequently.

REFERENCES

Adie, W. J. (1932). The aetiology and symptomatology of disseminated sclerosis. *Br. med. J.* **2**, 997–1000.
Ashworth, B. (1967). Chronic retrobulbar and chiasmal neuritis. *Br. J. Ophthal.* **51**, 698–702.
Benedict, W. L. (1942). Multiple sclerosis as an etiologic factor in retrobulbar neuritis. *Archs Ophthal. N.Y.* **28**, 988–95.
Berliner, M. L. (1935). Acute optic neuritis in demyelinating diseases of the nervous system. *Archs Ophthal. N.Y.* **13**, 83–98.
Boldt, H. A., Haerer, A. F., Tourtellotte, W. W., Henderson, J. W., and De Jong, R. N. (1963). Retrochiasmal visual field defects from multiple sclerosis. *Archs Neurol., Chicago* **8**, 565–75.
Bradley, W. G. and Whitty, C. W. M. (1967). Acute optic neuritis: its clinical features and their relation to prognosis for recovery of vision. *J. Neurol. Neurosurg. Psychiat.* **30**, 531–8.
Buchanan, L. (1923). Monocular optic neuritis. *Br. J. Ophthal.* **7**, 170–4.
Carroll, F. D. (1940). Retrobulbar neuritis. Observations on one hundred cases. *Archs Ophthal. N.Y.* **24**, 44–54.

Chamlin, M. (1953). Visual field changes in optic neuritis. *Archs Ophthal., N.Y.* **50**, 699–713.
— and Davidoff, L. M. (1954). Homonymous hemianopia in multiple sclerosis. *Neurology, Minneap.* **4**, 429–37.
Daroff, R. B. and Lawton-Smith, J. (1965). Intraocular optic neuritis with normal visual acuity. *Neurology, Minneap.* **15**, 409–12.
Duke-Elder, Sir Stewart and Scott, G. I. (1971). *System of ophthalmology* Volume XII, *Neuro-Ophthalmology,* p. 618. Henry Kimpton, London.
Galvin, R. J., Regan, D., and Heron, J. R. (1976). Impaired temporal resolution of vision after acute retrobulbar neuritis. *Brain* **99**, 255–68.
Gartner, S. (1953). Optic neuropathy in multiple sclerosis. *Archs Ophthal., N.Y.* **50**, 718–26.
Griffith, A. H. (1897). In Discussion on retro-ocular neuritis. *Trans. ophthal. Soc. U.K.* **17**, 107–217.
Gunn, R. M. (1897). Discussion on retro-ocular neuritis. *Trans. ophthal. Soc. U.K.* **17**, 107–217.
— (1904). Discussion on retro-ocular neuritis. *Br. med. J.* **2**, 1285.
Halliday, A. M., McDonald, W. I., and Mushin, J. (1973). Delayed pattern-evoked responses in optic neuritis in relation to visual acuity. *Trans. ophthal. Soc. U.K.* **93**, 315–24.
Hutchinson, W. M. (1976). Acute optic neuritis and the prognosis for multiple sclerosis. *J. Neurol. Neurosurg. Psychiat.* **39**, 283–9.
Hyllested, K. and Moller, P. M. (1961). Follow-up on patients with a history of optic neuritis. *Acta ophthal.* **39**, 655–62.
Jessop. W. H. H. (1907). Three cases of acute uni-ocular optic neuritis in boys with great loss of vision and subsequent complete recovery. *Trans. ophthal. Soc. U.K.* **27**, 170–7.
Kurland, L. T., Beebe, G. W., Kurtzke, J. F., Nagler, B., Auth, T. L., Lessell, S., and Nefzger, M. D. (1966). Studies on the natural history of multiple sclerosis. 2. The progression of optic neuritis to multiple sclerosis. *Acta Neurol. Scand.* [Suppl] **19** (Vol. 42), 157–76.
Lynn, B. H. (1959). Retrobulbar neuritis. A survey of the present condition of cases occurring over the last fifty-six years. *Trans. ophthal. Soc. U.K.* **79**, 701–16.
McAlpine, D., Lumsden, C. E., and Acheson, E. D. (1972). *Multiple sclerosis. A reappraisal* (2nd ed.), p. 155. Churchill Livingstone, Edinburgh.
Marshall, D. (1950). Ocular manifestations of multiple sclerosis and relationship to retrobulbar neuritis. *Trans. Am. ophthal. Soc.* **48**, 487–525.
Nettleship, E. (1884). On cases of retro-ocular neuritis. *Trans. ophthal. Soc. U.K.* **4**, 186–226.
Nikoskelainen, E. (1975). Symptoms, signs and early course of optic neuritis. *Acta ophthal.* **53**, 254–72.
Paton. L. (1914). Papilloedema in disseminated sclerosis. *Trans. ophthal. Soc. U.K.* **34**, 252–61.
Rønne, H. (1928). On non-hypophyseal affections of the chiasma. *Acta ophthal.* **6**, 332–43.
Rosen, E. S. and Ashworth, B. (1968). Serial fluorescein photography in acute retrobulbar neuritis. *J. Neurol. Neurosurg. Psychiat.* **31**, 253–8.
Savitsky, N. and Rangell, L. (1950). On homonymous hemianopia in multiple sclerosis. *J. nerv. ment. Dis.* **111**, 225–31.
Schlossman, A. and Philips, C. C. (1954). Optic neuritis in relation to demyelinating diseases. *Am. J. Ophthal.* **37**, 487–94.
Sugar, S. (1939). Papillitis and papilloedema in multiple sclerosis. *Am. J. Ophthal.* **22**, 135–9.
Traquair, H. M. (1923). The Doyne Memorial Lecture: The differential characters of scotomata and their interpretation. *Trans. ophthal. Soc. U.K.* **43**, 480–533.
— (1925). Acute retrobulbar neuritis affecting the optic chiasma and tract. *Br. J. Ophthal.* **9**, 433–50.
Uhthoff, W. (1904). Discussion on retro-ocular neuritis. *Br. med. J.* **2**, 1285–6.
Vedel-Jensen, N. (1959). Optic tract neuritis in multiple sclerosis. *Acta ophthal.* **37**, 537–45.
Walsh, F. B. and Hoyt, W. F. (1969). *Clinical neuro-ophthalmology* (3 vol. edn.), Vol 1, p. 501. The Williams and Wilkins Company, Baltimore.

5 Differential diagnosis: Optic nerve compression

Intracranial tumours have too frequently been missed by over zealous enthusiasts searching for optic neuritis (Dandy 1922).

The clinical differentiation of optic neuritis from a prechiasmal tumour was considered by Dandy (1922) to depend on the rapidity of the visual loss and on the type of field defect. Both Traquair (1930) and Lillie (1934) stressed the importance of the time taken for the evolution of the field loss in compressive lesions, although the latter recognized that this factor alone could not invariably distinguish such cases from the visual failure due to optic neuritis. Amongst examples of central scotomata produced by meningioma, pituitary tumour, craniopharyngioma, and posterior communicating aneurysm (Walsh and Ford 1940), some had been of sudden onset, with considerable fluctuation in the degree of visual defect. Although a history of sudden vision loss with a central field defect usually indicates an optic neuritis, both can occur with a tumour, as can spontaneous improvement in visual function (Walsh 1956). The absence of optic atrophy despite an impairment of vision lasting several months strongly suggests an extrinsic tumour involving the optic nerves or chiasm, particularly craniopharyngioma (Walsh 1956). Meadows (1949) reported optic nerve compression with a sudden onset of visual failure; although many of his cases had a central scotoma, in the majority the defect had broken through to the periphery by the time of examination. One of his cases (due to aneurysm) described visual hallucinations, with sudden blue stars surrounded by a red rim. Although the absence of ocular pain has been considered an important feature of the visual failure produced by meningioma, Burke (1968) encountered the combination of periocular pain and loss of central vision in a case of sphenoidal wing meningioma, and with pituitary adenoma and internal carotid aneurysm.

Knight, Hoyt, and Wilson (1972) considered in detail the characteristic features of prechiasmal optic nerve compression, exemplified by three cases of meningioma, two of chromophobe adenoma and one of aneurysm. In all, the onset of unilateral visual blurring was insidious, although one patient first noted the symptom while driving in hot weather; the authors considered this an example of Uhthoff's syndrome, but the visual disturbance subsequently remained, and tests of temperature sensitivity were not performed. In two patients short-term fluctuations in the degree of visual blurring took place. Visual acuity was either normal or only marginally depressed, but tests of colour vision, using Hardy–Rand–Rittler charts, revealed marked impairment in all cases. Disc pallor generally followed the visual loss after several months, particularly in the cases of meningioma, but an afferent pupillary defect was invariably found. The presence of a central scotoma can lead to a diagnosis of retrobulbar neuritis in these cases, but in time, the scotoma enlarges and tends to break into the periphery. A combination of such clinical features should alert the clinician to the possibility of optic nerve compression and stimulate further investigation. Although routine X-rays of the skull and optic foramina are often normal, polytomography of the optic canals and sella reveals the presence of bone erosion in most cases, and with early diagnosis and surgical intervention, the prognosis for recovery of vision is excellent.

Optic nerve glioma

These tumours are associated with evidence of generalized neuro-fibromatosis in approximately 16 per cent of cases (Walsh 1956). The majority occur in the first two decades, but occasional cases are described in a much older age group (Condon and Rose 1967).

The character of the visual symptoms

The usual clinical picture is of a slowly progressive visual failure with subsequent proptosis. The resistance of axonal function to compression by astrocytic proliferation (Glaser, Hoyt, and Corbett 1971) probably accounts for the tendency of established visual defects to remain static for long periods of time.

Pain is generally absent in the optic gliomas of childhood but a sudden increase in size of the tumour, indicated by rapid visual deterioration, may be accompanied by pain (Spencer 1972). Pain is a more prominent feature of the malignant astrocytomas of the optic nerve and chiasm of adult life (Meadows 1949; Pfaffenbach, Kearns, and Hollenhorst, 1972; Hoyt, Meshel, Lessell, Schatz, and Suckling 1973; Hamilton, Garner, Tripathi, and Sanders 1973). It is usually supra- or retro-orbital in location (Hoyt *et al.* 1973) and may be accompanied by tenderness of the globe (Hamilton *et al.* 1973), or pain on ocular movement (Pfaffenbach *et al.* 1972). Visual hallucinations, consisting of coloured lights, have been described (Hudson 1912).

The type of field defect

An extensive unilateral field defect is usual, sometimes accompanied by a temporal hemianopia contralaterally when chiasmatic involvement has taken place.

Pupils and fundus appearance

A depression of the pupillary response usually correlates with the severity of the visual defect. Optic atrophy is commonly present in the tumours arising in childhood, whereas disc oedema often progressing to a picture of central retinal venous occlusion, is the usual finding in the more malignant astrocytomas of adults.

Natural history and response to steroids

The visual defect may fluctuate considerably and both the pain and visual disturbance of the tumours of adult life can show a marked steroid responsiveness (Pfaffenbach *et al.* 1972; Hoyt *et al.* 1973).

Other clinical features

Although proptosis is a characteristic feature, it may appear late, and was

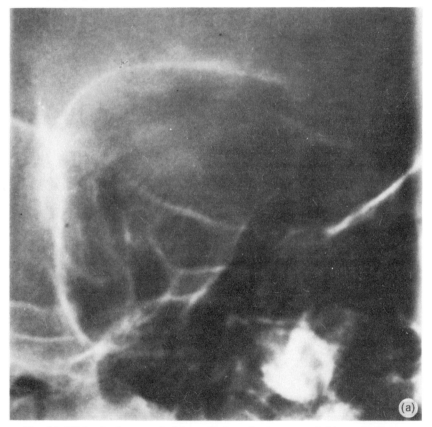

Fig. 5.1. Bilateral enlargement of the optic foramina in a case of chiasmatic glioma.

only present in a third of the cases in one series (Hoyt *et al*. 1973). Enlargement of the optic foramen (Fig. 5.1) generally indicates spread of tumour
into the cranial cavity, but rarely indicates meningeal proliferation alone
(Spencer 1972).

Meningioma

Meningiomas at various sites may involve the visual pathway, the resulting
visual disturbance being sometimes the sole neurological abnormality.
Although the lack of pain is of considerable help in differential diagnosis, the
combination of a visual deterioration, which may be rapid, a central
scotoma, and negative neuro-radiological investigations (Meadows 1949)
explain the frequent mis-diagnosis of these tumours in the initial stages
(Bardram and Møller 1952; Garfield and Neil-Dwyer 1975).

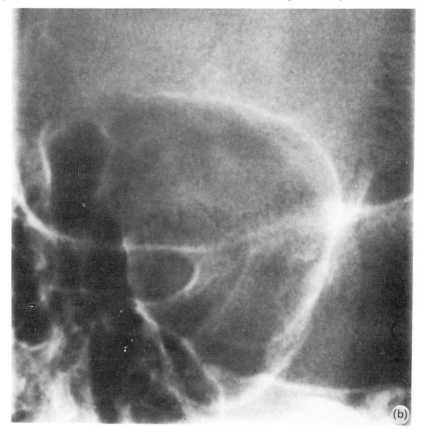

The character of the visual symptoms

Slowly progressive visual failure characterizes these tumours, but a sudden onset is well recognized, sometimes being discovered on waking (Schlezinger, Alpers, and Weiss 1946) or during pregnancy (Hagedoorn 1937). An exacerbation of the visual defect by bright light has been described in a case of suprasellar meningioma (Hagedoorn 1937) and in another patient with a tumour at this site, short-lived episodes of dimness of vision lasting approximately 30 minutes antedated the development of a more permanent vision loss (Ehlers and Malmros 1973).

Although Meadows (1949) did not record pain amongst the symptoms of his patients, it may occur with orbital optic nerve meningiomas (Spencer 1972) and as an occasional feature of suprasellar tumours, sometimes being accentuated by eye movement (Ehlers and Malmros 1973).

The type of field defect

All 3 cases of prechiasmatic compression by meningioma described by Knight *et al.* (1972) had paracentral or peripheral field defects at the initial examination (Fig. 5.2 a, b, and c). A central scotoma may occur with a subfrontal (Lillie 1934) or suprasellar meningioma (Hagedoorn 1937;

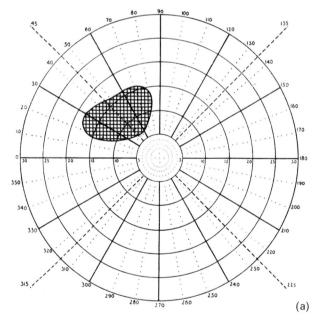

(a)

Fig. 5.2. (a) (b) (c) Progression of left monocular visual field defect during incipient optic nerve compression by prechiasmal meningioma (from Knight *et al.* 1972). 1/1000 white.

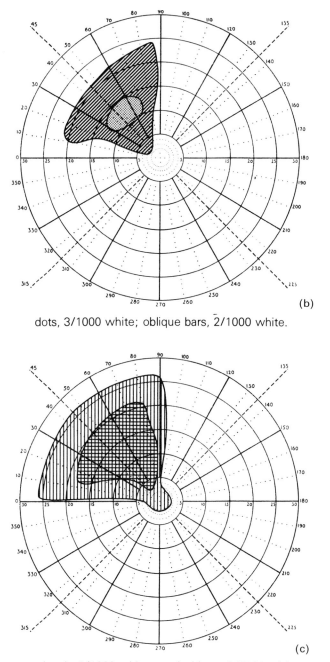

(b)

dots, 3/1000 white; oblique bars, 2/1000 white.

(c)

cross-hatch, 5/1000 white; vertical bars, 2/1000 white.

Schlezinger *et al*. 1946; Larsson and Nord 1947; Meadows 1949) although the experience of Ehlers and Malmros (1973) was that suprasellar meningiomas were more likely to cause a generalized depression of the visual field.

Pupils and fundus appearance

An afferent pupillary defect is common, although in the early stages it may be barely perceptible (Knight *et al*. 1972). Optic atrophy can be a late sign with intracranial tumours, but a combination of disc pallor and swelling with evidence of a retino-choroidal shunt has been suggested as a characteristic feature of those meningiomas arising from the orbital optic nerve (Spencer 1972).

Natural history and response to steroids

Tumours arising within the orbit are uncommon and tend to predominate in women (Hudson 1912; Spencer 1972). A progressive axial proptosis is usual with anterior lesions but may be late or absent throughout in tumours arising in the posterior orbit. The progressive, unilateral visual failure due to an intracanalicular meningioma is seldom mistaken for optic neuritis, but great diagnostic problems are posed with bilateral optic nerve lesions. Such a picture is not uncommon in multiple sclerosis but, in an early search of the literature, Hudson (1912) found one example of bilateral optic nerve sheath meningiomas, and Dandy (1922) gave a detailed account of a case diagnosed at craniotomy, the tumours arising immediately behind the optic foramina and extending forwards into the optic canals (Fig. 5.3). Meadows (1954) reported a similar case, visual failure affecting one eye and then the other, with an interval of three years.

The visual defect caused by meningioma may frequently remit, either spontaneously (Schlezinger *et al*. 1946; Larsson and Nord 1947; Ehlers and Malmros 1973) or following pregnancy (Hagedoorn 1937; Walsh and Ford 1940; Walsh 1956). Separate episodes of visual loss, with recovery, in each eye, led to a diagnosis of bilateral retrobulbar neuritis in a case of planum sphenoidale meningioma described by Lynn (1959). A response of the visual defect to corticosteroid therapy has not been recorded.

Other clinical features

Plain X-ray changes are unlikely with meningiomas arising from the anterior part of the intra-orbital optic nerve (Lloyd 1971), but orbital pneumography and particularly computerized axial tomography are likely to demonstrate them. Foraminal meningiomas have often been reported without radiological abnormalities, although all the examples collected by Lloyd (1971) were diagnosed without recourse to contrast radiology (Fig. 5.4, 5.5 a and b). In cases of prechiasmatic meningioma where routine foraminal views have

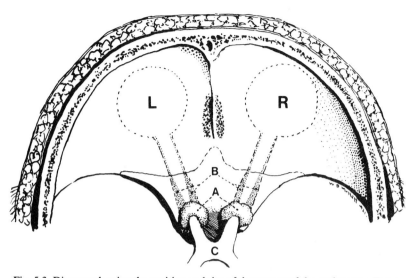

Fig. 5.3. Diagram showing the position and size of the tumors of the optic nerve. Tumors are symmetric collar like growths surrounding each optic nerve at the optic foramen and passing forward into the orbit.
A = exposed tumor, B = tumor on dural sheath of nerve in orbit, C = optic chiasma.
(From Dandy 1922.)

been normal, hypocycloidal polytomography can demonstrate either expansion or hyperostosis of the optic foramen (Knight *et al*. 1972). Small intracranial tumours may pose similar radiological problems, since suprasellar meningiomas with a diameter of less than 3 cm show plain X-ray changes in only a minority of cases (Jane and McKissock 1962).

Pituitary tumours

The character of the visual symptoms

The progression of visual disturbance is usually gradual, except in pituitary apoplexy, or on occasions during pregnancy (Enoksson, Lundberg, Sjöstedt, and Skanse 1961). The combination of ocular pain with unilateral visual loss, simulating retrobulbar neuritis, has been observed in cases of pituitary adenoma (Kelly 1962; Burke 1968).

The type of field defect

Nettleship (1897) drew attention to the association of central field defects with chiasmal tumours, but his case descriptions were inadequate, and pathological confirmation of the diagnosis was confined to a single case, probably a craniopharyngioma. In a review of the field defects associated

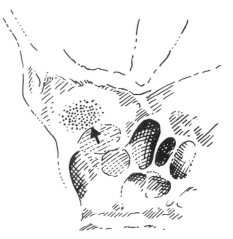

Fig. 5.4. Foraminal sheath meningioma. Area of calcification in the apex of the left orbit shown by hypocycloidal tomography (from Lloyd 1971).

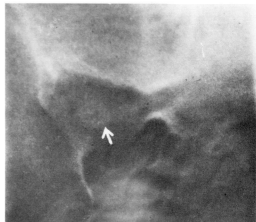

with hypophyseal disease, De Schweinitz and Holloway (1912) did not describe any classical central scotomata, although in a later communication (De Schweinitz 1923) such examples were given. By then Cushing and Walker (1915) had described cases of pituitary tumour with central field involvement and normal or near normal peripheral fields. Of a group of 15 patients with pituitary tumour and optic nerve involvement (Woods and Rowland 1931) two had relative central and paracentral scotomata with normal peripheral fields. Henderson (1939) surveyed Harvey Cushing's 338 cases of pituitary adenoma and found six patients with bilateral and three with unilateral central scotomata. Wilson and Falconer (1968) found bitemporal hemicentral scotomatous hemianopias in nearly half their cases, and described two patients with a unilateral central scotoma.

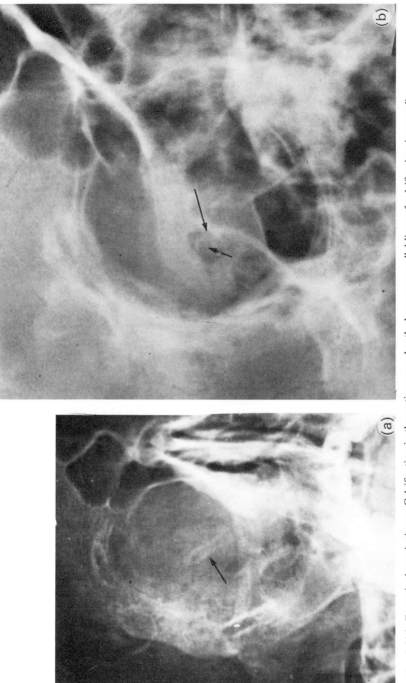

Fig. 5.5(a). Foraminal meningioma. Calcification in the optic nerve sheath shown as parallel lines of calcification (arrowed).
Fig. 5.5(b). In optic canal projection, the calcification is seen as a circular opacity within the outline of the optic foramen (from Lloyd 1971).

Natural history and response to steroids

Transient impairment of vision may occur with pituitary tumour (De Schweinitz 1923) as may spontaneous improvement (Williamson-Noble 1939; Walsh and Ford 1940). Spontaneous improvement of a unilateral central field defect, but with subsequent progression to a typical bitemporal hemianopia has also been noted (Rychener 1949). On occasions visual failure due to pituitary adenoma may respond to corticosteroids even to the extent of returning to normal (Senelick and Van Dyke 1974).

Craniopharyngioma

These tumours may also simulate an optic neuritis by the production of a central field defect, although the example quoted by Walsh and Ford (1940) was not supported by the fields used in the text. Isolated examples of unilateral or bilateral central scotomata have been reported (Larsson and Nord 1947) and represented nearly 50 per cent of the field changes in one series (Wagener and Love 1943). Spontaneous recovery of the field defect in these tumours may suggest a diagnosis of optic neuritis (Walsh 1956; Bardram and Møller 1952). In the patient of Franceschetti and Blum (1951) a unilateral central scotoma recovered spontaneously but later recurred in association with a bitemporal field defect and a Foster-Kennedy syndrome. Pregnancy may also influence the visual defect from these tumours (Hagedoorn 1937; Bradley 1968).

Metastatic tumour involving the optic nerve

Metastatic involvement of the optic nerve may lead to infiltration of the nerve or be confined to the optic nerve sheath. The latter may be asymptomatic, being demonstrated incidentally at post-mortem examination (Goldstein and Wexler 1931). Isolated metastasis within the substance of the optic nerve is rare, carcinoma of the breast being the commonest primary site in women, and carcinoma of the bronchus in men (Walsh 1956). With involvement of the optic nerve-head, fundoscopic evidence of the tumour is likely (Cherrington 1961) spread possibly occurring from tumour embolus of the central retinal vessels of the circle of Zinn (Gallie, Graham, and Hunter 1975). Infiltration of the optic nerve sheath by tumour is frequently associated with visual loss, particularly when the intracranial portion of the nerve is affected (Goldstein and Wexler 1931). Carcinomatous meningitis is associated with visual failure, often to a profound extent, in up to one-third of cases (Fischer-Williams, Bosanquet, and Daniel 1955). Unilateral cases are rare (Walshe 1923), the visual disturbance being usually bilateral, although as long as a month may elapse before the second eye shows involvement (Susac, Smith, and Powell 1973). Severe degrees of optic nerve demyelination and axonal degeneration can occur with arachnoid infiltration alone (Fischer-Williams *et al*. 1955) and, with tumour infiltration of the nerve, predominate in the adjacent areas (Katz, Valsamis, and Jampel 1961; Altrocchi and Eckman 1973). Rarely, optic nerve cuffing by tumour has been confined to the intraorbital nerve, with sparing of the intracranial segment (Altrocchi and Eckman 1973).

The character of the visual symptoms

Visual failure is often rapid and almost always bilateral. Pain is usually absent unless secondary glaucoma has developed (Gallie *et al*. 1975). Visual hallucinations in the form of golden lights have been described (Altrocchi and Eckman 1973).

The type of field defect

Formal fields have often not been reported or not attempted because of the severity of the visual loss, but both central (Fischer-Williams *et al*. 1955; Susac *et al*. 1973) and paracentral scotomata (Altrocchi and Eckman 1973) are described (Fig. 5.6, a and b).

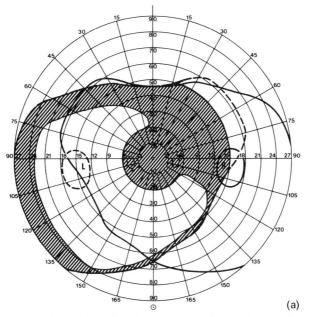

(a)

Fig. 5.6(a). Peripheral field L eye, 10/330 white (vision 7/200).

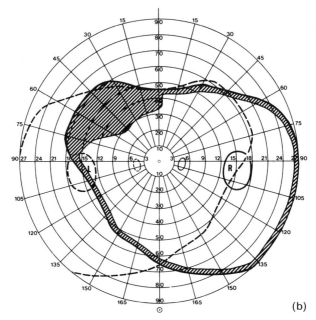

Fig. 5.6(b). Peripheral field R eye, 3/330 white (vision 20/15–1) Optic nerve metastases from adenocarcinoma of the lung (from Susac *et al.* 1973).

Pupils and fundus appearance

By the time of presentation, when vision has already markedly deteriorated, pupillary responses may be absent or sluggish (Fischer-Williams *et al.* 1955; Terry and Dunphy 1933). In less affected cases, an afferent pupillary defect can be detected by appropriate testing (Kamin and Hepler 1972; Susac *et al.* 1973). Fundus abnormalities are common; occasionally tumour tissue may be visible (Cherrington 1961; Gallie *et al.* 1975) but more often the disc appears swollen (Terry and Dunphy 1933; Katz *et al.* 1961) followed by the development of optic atrophy. In some instances, optic atrophy is present from the beginning or develops during the course of observation (Fischer-Williams *et al.* 1955; Kamin and Hepler 1972), and occasionally the optic disc remains normal (Altrocchi and Eckman 1973). Retinal haemorrhages have been described (Katz *et al.* 1961), particularly where tumour tissue is visibly involving the optic nerve head (Cherrington 1961).

Natural history and response to steroids

The visual failure is usually rapidly progressive. Spontaneous remissions are not seen, but a dramatic response to corticosteroid therapy can obscure the correct diagnosis. In a case of solitary plasmacytoma involving the right optic nerve (Kamin and Hepler 1972), repeated courses of corticosteroid therapy produced an improvement in visual acuity, and a similar response to sub-Tenon triamcinolone was encountered for a short period in a case of carcinomatous optic neuropathy (Susac *et al*. 1973).

Other clinical features

Characteristically the ophthalmic symptoms are accompanied by other neurological disturbances, particularly radiculopathy and other cranial nerve palsies, although in Walshe's case (1923) this was limited to a history of difficulty in swallowing and signs of a VI nerve palsy on examination. Neuroradiological investigations are frequently normal, but abnormalities of the cerebrospinal fluid, particularly the presence of tumour cells and a depressed glucose concentration, are frequent and suggest the diagnosis. Gamma globulin concentration may be raised with local tumour infiltration, a level of 35 mg per cent being encountered in the case of plasmacytoma referred to previously.

Leukaemia and the reticuloses

Optic nerve infiltration in the leukaemias is frequently encountered and may similarly be asymptomatic, occurring as an incidental post-mortem finding (Allen and Straatsma 1961). Kraus and O'Rourke (1963) have related the occurrence of optic neuritis to the presence of a reticulosis in two cases. Their first example developed bilateral optic neuritis after an upper respiratory tract infection at the age of 11. In retrospect, the histology of a cervical lymph node removed at the time was compatible with Hodgkin's disease, although this diagnosis was not established until 16 years later. Vision failed to recover. Their second case developed unilateral visual failure 5 years after a diagnosis of lymphosarcoma, based on lymph node biopsy, had been made. The findings of an absent direct light response, decreased visual acuity with a central scotoma and slight disc swelling were felt to establish a diagnosis of optic neuritis and with corticosteroid therapy vision recovered completely. A year before, the patient had developed an acute spinal cord disturbance, with myelographic block but negative exploration, which had also improved. The authors considered that a demyelinating process affecting optic nerve and spinal cord represented a non-metastatic neurological complication of the lymphomatous disease, although clearly, the possibility of a coincident multiple sclerosis cannot be excluded.

Tuberculoma

Optic nerve compression due to tuberculoma may be mistaken for optic neuritis. Patients presenting with visual failure may complain of ocular pain (Lynn 1959) with a paracentral scotoma and impaired colour vision on examination (Werner 1945), although in both these cases, radiological abnormalities suggested the possibility of optic nerve compression. Tuberculous osteomyelitis of the anterior clinoid process may similarly present a picture of unilateral visual loss in association with a central scotoma (Miller and Frenkel 1971).

   In that example, the field defect extended to the periphery over a period of five months with the appearance of optic atrophy and radiological evidence of destruction of the anterior clinoid process and optic foramen. Culture of biopsies from the optic nerve sheath revealed *Myco. tuberculosis* and bone biopsy revealed typical tubercles. Visual disturbances arising in the course of tuberculous meningitis are considered in Chapter 6.

Aneurysm

Aneurysms of the internal carotid, anterior communicating, posterior communicating, and ophthalmic arteries have all been described as causing a visual disturbance as their presenting feature, the clinical features of which are analogous to the syndrome produced by other compressive lesions affecting the optic nerve (Knight *et al.* 1972). Post-mortem examination of the optic nerve in such cases has shown severe loss of fibres (Stern and Ernest 1975).

The character of the visual symptoms

Visual failure may be gradual (Conway 1926; Harris 1928; Walsh and Ford 1940; Meadows 1949; Cunningham and Sewell 1971) or sudden (Jefferson 1937; Walsh and Ford 1940; Rubinstein, Wilson, and Levin 1968; Stern and Ernest 1975). Pain occurs frequently and may be exacerbated by eye movement (Stern and Ernest 1975), when it has been considered due to blood within the optic nerve sheath.

   Visual hallucinations, mentioned by Meadows (1949) have been described in detail in two cases by Jefferson (1937). In one, a ball of yellow light appeared before the affected eye, followed by visual failure on waking the following morning. In the other, glittering lights were present for a brief period in the eye subsequently showing progressive vision loss.

The type of field defect

Meadows (1949) considered that a crossed homonymous defect in the contralateral field with severe ipsilateral central loss was particularly

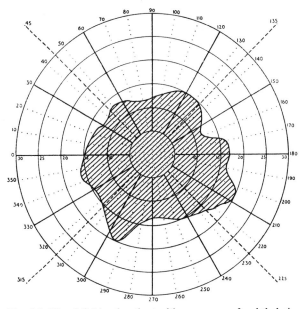

Fig. 5.7. Visual fields of patient with aneurysm of ophthalmic artery (from Rubinstein *et al.* 1968).

suggestive of aneurysmal compression. Various types of visual loss due to aneurysm are described, including unilateral central scotomata (Fig. 5.7). (Jefferson 1937; Rubinstein *et al.* 1968; Knight *et al.* 1972), the defects, however, often extending to the periphery by the time of the first examination (Meadows 1949; Stern and Ernest 1975).

Pupils and fundus appearance

The pupillary responses are frequently depressed or absent or may reveal an afferent defect with the swinging light test (Cunningham and Sewell 1971; Knight *et al.* 1972; Stern and Ernest 1975).

Optic atrophy is the usual fundoscopic finding, sometimes developing late after the onset of visual symptoms. Optic disc swelling with adjacent haemorrhages was seen in one case by Meadows (1949).

Natural history and response to steroids

Spontaneous improvement in the visual defect has been frequently observed (Conway 1926; Harris 1928; Meadows 1949; Rubinstein *et al.* 1968; Cunningham and Sewell 1971). In the case described by Knight *et al.* (1972)

improvement of visual acuity from 20/40 to 20/30 coincided with the use of corticosteroids and cyanocobalamin.

Other clinical features

The development of a bitemporal field defect, the occurrence of ophthalmoplegia ipsilateral to the affected eye or frank subarachnoid haemorrhage will clearly help to establish the correct diagnosis. The presence of an orbital bruit has been accepted as evidence of an aneurysmal basis for visual failure even where subsequent arteriography has failed to demonstrate such a lesion (Meadows 1949). Skull X-rays may reveal bone erosion (Jefferson 1937; Walsh and Ford 1940) but angiography is the definitive investigation.

Cysts of the optic nerve

Two curious examples of cystic lesions of the optic nerve, not thought to be gliomatous in nature, have been described by Holt (1966). In the first, an incongruous homonymous hemianopia was found to be associated with a cystic lesion of the chiasm extending into both optic nerves. Two years later, blurring of vision in one eye occurred in association with pain on eye movement and depression of visual acuity. Subsequent, incomplete recovery occurred and at follow-up 4 years later, no further changes were detected. In the second case, a cystic swelling of the left optic nerve presented with visual disturbance and was found to be associated with gross disc swelling. A cystic lesion arising from the optic nerve sheath, in a patient with neurofibromatosis, failed to produce visual impairment despite causing expansion of the optic foramen (Spencer 1972).

Conclusions

It is apparent that a clinical syndrome embracing unilateral visual loss with ocular pain can be produced by a number of pathological processes causing compression of the optic nerve, although typically these present with insidious visual failure with near normal visual acuity, severely depressed colour vision and an initially normal optic fundus.

Pain on eye movement is not confined to optic neuritis, being described in optic nerve glioma, meningioma, and aneurysm. On occasions, visual loss due to compression is rapid, sometimes appearing overnight, and a tendency for it to accelerate during pregnancy is particularly suggestive of meningioma and, to a lesser degree, craniopharyngioma or pituitary tumour.

Central field defects can occur with tumour but, with time, extend to the periphery. Any of the fundoscopic changes described in optic neuritis may be reproduced by compressive or infiltrative lesions and, paradoxically, spontaneous improvement in vision may occur despite the presence of meningioma, pituitary tumour, craniopharyngioma or aneurysm.

An apparent response of the visual defect, or the ocular pain, to corticosteroid therapy cannot be taken as evidence of a primary demyelinating process in the optic nerve. A similar response is described with optic nerve glioma, pituitary tumour, and plasmacytoma of the optic nerve.

A slowly progressive unilateral visual failure should always suggest the possibility of a compressive aetiology, and, even where the evidence points to separate optic nerve lesions, independent bilateral sheath meningioma need to be considered. Neuroradiological techniques, particularly computerized axial tomography, will usually identify such cases. The role of visual evoked responses in differential diagnosis is considered in Chapter 14.

REFERENCES

Allen, R. A. and Straatsma, B. R. (1961). Ocular involvement in leukaemia and allied disorders. *Archs Ophthal., N.Y.* **66**, 490–508.

Altrocchi, P. H. and Eckman, P. B. (1973). Meningeal carcinomatosis and blindness. *J. Neurol. Neurosurg. Psychiat.* **36**, 206–10.

Bardram, M. and Møller, H. V. (1952). Diagnosis of tumours in anterior and middle cranial fossae. *Acta ophthal.* **30**, 65–96.

Bradley, W. G. (1968). Symptomatic optic neuritis. *Dis. nerv. Syst.* **29**, 668–73.

Burke, W. J. (1968). Optic neuritis. *Proc. Aust. Assoc. Neurol.* **5**, 243–5.

Cherrington, F. J. (1961). Metastatic adenocarcinoma of the optic nerve-head and adjacent retina. *Br. J. Ophthal.* **45**, 227–30.

Conway, J. A. (1926). Two cases of cerebral aneurysm causing ocular symptoms with notes of other cases. *Br. J. Ophthal.* **10**, 78–98.

Condon, J. R. and Rose, F. C. (1967). Optic nerve glioma. *Br. J. Ophthal.* **51**, 703–6.

Cunningham, R. D. and Sewell, J. J. (1971). Aneurysm of the ophthalmic artery with drusen of the optic nerve head. *Am. J. Ophthal.* **72**, 743–5.

Cushing, H. and Walker, C. B. (1915). Distortions of the visual fields in cases of brain tumour. Chiasmal lesions, with especial reference to bitemporal hemianopsia. *Brain* **37**, 341–400.

Dandy, W. E. (1922). Prechiasmal intracranial tumors of the optic nerves. *Am. J. Ophthal.* **5**, 169–88.

De Schweinitz, G. E. (1923). Concerning certain ocular aspects of pituitary body disorders mainly exclusive of the visual central and peripheral hemianopic field defects. *Trans. ophthal. Soc. U.K.* **43**, 12–109.

— and Holloway, T. B. (1912). A clinical communication on certain visual-field defects in hypophysis disease with special reference to scotomas. *J. Am. med. Ass.* **59**, 1041–5.

Ehlers, N. and Malmros, R. (1973). The suprasellar meningioma. A review of the literature and presentation of a series of 31 cases. *Acta ophthal Suppl.* **121**, 1–74.

Enoksson, P., Lundberg, N., Sjöstedt, S. and Skanse, B. (1961). Influence of pregnancy on visual fields in suprasellar tumours. *Acta psychiat. neurol. scand.* **36**, 524–38.

Fischer-Williams, M., Bosanquet, F. D., and Daniel, P. M. (1955). Carcinomatosis of the meninges. A report of three cases. *Brain* **78**, 42–58.

Franceschetti, A. and Blum, J. D. (1951). Néurite rétrobulbaire aiguë transitoire dans un cas de tumeur cerebrale. *Confinia neurol.* **11**, 302–7.

Gallie, B. L., Graham, J. E., and Hunter, W. S. (1975). Optic nerve head metastasis. *Archs. Ophthal., N.Y.* **93**, 983–6.

Garfield, J. and Neil-Dwyer, G. (1975). Delay in diagnosis of optic nerve and chiasmal compression presenting with unilateral failing vision. *Br. med. J.* **1**, 22–5.

Glaser, J. S., Hoyt, W. F., and Corbett, J. (1971). Visual morbidity with chiasmal glioma. *Archs Ophthal., N.Y.* **85**, 3–12.

Goldstein, I. and Wexler, D. (1931). Metastasis in the sheath of the optic nerve from carcinoma of the stomach. *Archs Ophthal., N.Y.* **6**, 414–19.

Hagedoorn, A. (1937). The chiasmal syndrome and retrobulbar neuritis in pregnancy. *Am. J. Ophthal.* **20**, 690–9.

Hamilton, A. M., Garner, A., Tripathi, R. C., and Sanders, M. D. (1973). Malignant optic nerve glioma. Report of a case with electron microscopic study. *Br. J. Ophthal.* **57**, 253–64.

Harris, S. T. (1928). A case of aneurysm of the anterior cerebral artery causing compression of the optic nerves and chiasma. *Br. J. Ophthal.* **12**, 15–22.

Henderson, W. R. (1939). The pituitary adenomata. A follow-up study of the surgical results in 338 cases (Dr. Harvey Cushing's series). *Br. J. Surg.* **26**, 811–921.

Holt, H. (1966). Cysts of the optic nerve. *Am. J. Ophthal.* **61**, 1166–70.

Hoyt, W. F., Meshel, L. G., Lessell, S., Schatz, N. J., and Suckling, R. D. (1973). Malignant optic glioma of adulthood. *Brain* **96**, 121–32.

Hudson, A. C. (1912). Primary tumours of the optic nerve. *Ophthal Hosp. Rep.* **18**, 317–439.

Jane, J. A. and McKissock, W. (1962). Importance of failing vision in early diagnosis of suprasellar meningioma. *Br. med. J.* **2**, 5–7.

Jefferson, G. (1937). Compression of the chiasma, optic nerves, and optic tracts by intracranial aneurysms. *Brain* **60**, 444–97.

Kamin, D. F. and Hepler, R. S. (1972). Solitary intracranial plasmacytoma mistaken for retrobulbar neuritis. *Am. J. Ophthal.* **73**, 584–6.

Katz, J. L., Valsamis, M. P., and Jampel, R. S. (1961). Ocular signs in diffuse carcinomatous meningitis. *Am. J. Ophthal.* **52**, 681–90.

Kelly, R. (1962). Lesions of the optic chiasm due to compression. *Trans. ophthal. Soc. U.K.* **82**, 149–64.

Knight, C. L., Hoyt, W. F., and Wilson, C. B. (1972). Syndrome of incipient prechiasmal optic nerve compression. *Archs Ophthal., N.Y.* **87**, 1–11.

Kraus, A. M. and O'Rourke, J. (1963). Lymphomatous optic neuritis. *Archs Ophthal., N.Y.* **70**, 173–5.

Larsson, S. and Nord, B. (1947). Klinisk bild av retrobulbarnevrit vid intrakraniella tumörer. *Nord. Med.* **34**, 1059–65.

Lillie, W. I. (1934). The clinical significance of retrobulbar and optic neuritis. *Am. J. Ophthal.* **17**, 110–19.

Lloyd, G. A. S. (1971). The radiology of primary orbital meningioma. *Br. J. Radiol.* **44**, 405–11.

Lynn, B. H. (1959). Retrobulbar neuritis. A survey of the present condition of cases occurring over the last fifty-six years. *Trans. ophthal. Soc. U.K.* **79**, 701–16.

Meadows, S. P. (1949). Optic nerve compression and its differential diagnosis. *Proc. R. Soc. Med.* **42**, 1017–34.

— (1954). In Discussion on the neuro-ophthalmological aspects of failure of vision in children. *Proc. R. Soc. Med.* **47**, 494–9.

Miller, B. W. and Frenkel, M. (1971). Report of a case of tuberculous retrobulbar neuritis and osteomyelitis. *Am. J. Ophthal.* **71**, 751–6.

Nettleship, E. (1897). Central amblyopia as an early symptom in tumour at the chiasma. *Trans. ophthal. Soc. U.K.* **17**, 277–89.

Pfaffenbach, D. D., Kearns, T. P., and Hollenhorst, R. W. (1972). An unusual case of optic nerve-chiasmal glioma. *Am. J. Ophthal.* **74**, 523–5.

Rubinstein, M. K., Wilson, G., and Levin, D. C. (1968). Intraorbital aneurysms of the ophthalmic artery. Report of a unique case and review of the literature. *Archs Ophthal., N.Y.* **80**, 42–4.

Rychener, R. O. (1949). Central scotoma due to pituitary tumour. *Am. J. Ophthal.* **32**, 996.

Schlezinger, N. S., Alpers, B. J., and Weiss, B. P. (1946). Suprasellar meningiomas associated with scotomatous field defects. *Archs Ophthal., N.Y.* **35**, 624–42.

Senelick, R. C. and Van Dyk, H. J. L. (1974). Chromophobe adenoma masquerading as corticosteroid-responsive optic neuritis. *Am. J. Ophthal.* **78**, 485–8.

Spencer, W. H. (1972). Primary neoplasms of the optic nerve and its sheaths: clinical features and current concepts of pathogenetic mechanisms. *Trans. Am. ophthal. Soc.* **70**, 490–528.

Stern, W. H. and Ernest, J. T. (1975). Ophthalmic artery aneurysm. *Am. J. Ophthal.* **80**, 203–6.

Susac, J. O., Smith, J. L., and Powell, J. O. (1973). Carcinomatous optic neuropathy. *Am. J. Ophthal.* **76**, 672–9.

Terry, T. L. and Dunphy, E. B. (1933). Metastatic carcinoma in both optic nerves simulating retrobulbar neuritis. *Archs Ophthal., N.Y.* **10**, 611–14.

Traquair, H. M. (1930). Toxic amblyopia, including retrobulbar neuritis. *Trans. ophthal. Soc. U.K.* **50**, 351–85.

Wagener, H. P. and Love, J. G. (1943). Fields of vision in cases of tumor of Rathke's pouch. *Archs Ophthal., N.Y.* **29**, 873–87.

Walsh, F. B. (1956). Tumors of the optic nerves and chiasm: differential diagnosis. *Trans. Am. Acad. Ophthal. Oto-lar.* **60**, 82–93.

—and Ford, F. R. (1940). Central scotomas. Their importance in topical diagnosis. *Archs Ophthal., N.Y.* **24**, 500–32.

Walshe, F. M. R. (1923). A case of secondary carcinomatous infiltration of the pia-arachnoid of the brain presenting exclusively ocular symptoms during life: meningitis carcinomatosa. *Br. J. Ophthal.* **7**, 113–23.

Werner, L. E. (1945). Retro-bulbar neuritis. *Trans. ophthal. Soc. U.K.* **65**, 376–93.

Williamson-Noble, F. A. (1939). The ocular consequences of certain chiasmal lesions. *Trans. ophthal. Soc. U.K.* **59**, 627–81.

Wilson, P. and Falconer, M. A. (1968). Patterns of visual failure with pituitary tumours. Clinical and radiological correlations. *Br. J. Ophthal.* **52**, 94–110.

Woods, A. C. and Rowland, W. M. (1931). An etiologic study of a series of optic neuropathies. *J. Am. med. Ass.* **97**, 375–9.

6 Differential diagnosis: infectious and post-infectious disorders

The role of focal infection in the production of optic neuropathies is not clearly understood (Woods and Rowland 1931).

Iridocyclitis

Uveitis is occasionally associated with a central scotoma (Østerberg 1931), the field defect being attributed to macular detachment, optic neuritis, or a combination of the two (Walsh and Ford 1940). The relationship between optic neuritis and uveitis is considered further in Chapter 12, pp. 221–2.

Sinusitis

Anatomical factors

A close anatomical relationship between the optic nerves and one or both sphenoid sinuses has been reported in some 50 per cent of individuals (Loeb 1909). Rarely, the nerve traverses the sphenoid and posterior ethmoid sinuses, although in most cases the posterior ethmoid cells do not extend to the optic foramen (Syme 1910). Further studies (Syme 1924) established a tendency for the sphenoid sinus to extend above or below the optic foramen, with the bone separating nerve from neuro-periosteum being often thin or absent. Hiatuses in the bone have been found in between 4 (Weille and Vang 1953) and 13 per cent of cases (Young 1924). Prolongation from the posterior ethmoidal or spheno-ethmoidal cells are much rarer, although the former has a close anatomical relationship with the optic nerve after its entry into the orbit. A dehiscence of the bone of the posterior ethmoid cells in close relationship to the optic nerve is uncommon, being found in only two of 171 specimens by Weille and Vang (1953). Extension of purulent sinus disease into the pituitary fossa (Pickworth 1928) or the optic nerve (Van der Hoeve 1922; Doesschate 1928) has been identified at post-mortem examination.

Clinical and radiological evidence

In a series of papers, the aetiology of cases of optic neuropathy collected at the Johns Hopkins Hospital and the Mayo Clinic was considered, including the possible influence of sinus disease. In the first review from the Johns Hopkins (Woods and Rowland 1931), 8 per cent were thought to be due to posterior sinus disease, though in half the association was made because of a prompt improvement of vision following radical drainage of the posterior ethmoid and sphenoid sinuses. A subsequent report gave a figure of 4 per cent, usually on the basis of histological evidence of chronic sinusitis in material removed at operation (Moore 1937), but in the final publication (Bagley 1952) no examples due to sinus disease were found amongst a further 133 cases. Of the 225 cases of retrobulbar neuritis in the first paper from the Mayo Clinic (Benedict 1933), only one was attributed to sinus disease, despite the fact that over 60 per cent had had sinus operations performed elsewhere. Amongst a further 89 patients (Benedict and Koch 1937), one was considered secondary to sinusitis, the diagnosis being based on radiological evidence. Gifford (1931) came to similar conclusions, finding 3 examples amongst 203 patients with retrobulbar neuritis. Walsh and Ford (1940) considered that non-suppurative disease of the accessory sinuses only rarely accounted for retrobulbar neuritis and central scotoma, although Ford (1944) later attributed an improvement of vision in a case of optic neuritis to the onset of nasal catarrh, suggesting that the spontaneous drainage of the sinuses had thereby relieved pressure on the optic nerve. Weille and Vang (1953) found a significant focus of infection in 10 of 38 patients with retrobulbar neuritis, the sinuses being implicated in 4, whilst Bossy and Jéquier (1961) considered that 23 per cent of patients with retrobulbar neuritis or optic atrophy, some of whom had multiple sclerosis, had evidence of sinusitis. In a recent group of 37 cases of optic neuritis in whom sinus exploration was performed (Calvet, Calmettes, and Coll 1967) evidence of sinus pathology was confined to five.

The criteria for making a diagnosis of sinus disease will obviously influence the frequency with which optic neuritis is attributed to this cause. Where perforation of bone by purulent material has occurred, the association is evident, but often less strict criteria have been used, including radiological abnormalities or non-specific histological changes in biopsy specimens. White (1928), previously one of the chief protagonists for an association between sinus pathology and optic nerve disease, stated that the tissue removed from the sphenoid sinus in cases of optic neuritis did not differ significantly from that found in individuals without visual disturbances. This, in turn, stimulated a search for a primary source of infection in other sites, including teeth and tonsils.

Reports of the frequency of radiological abnormalities in the paranasal sinuses in patients with optic neuritis have seldom considered the findings in a control population. In 104 cases of optic neuritis, defined as involvement of the optic nerve by any inflammatory, demyelinating, or degenerative disorder, radiological abnormalities of the paranasal sinuses (either maxillary or ethmoid) were found in 11 per cent (Tarkkanen and Tarkkanen 1971).

The changes were ipsilateral to the affected optic nerve in seven cases, contralateral in one, and bilateral in four. Of the patients with radiological abnormalities, 50 per cent had symptoms attributable to sinus disease, and the same percentage had some evidence of multiple sclerosis. An interesting comparison is afforded by a study in which the frequency of sinus infection (the criteria were not given) in patients with uveitis was compared with a control population (Guyton and Woods 1941). The figures of 12·4 and 13 per cent are almost identical and very similar to the frequency of radiological sinus abnormalities in optic neuritis patients (Tarkkanen and Tarkkanen 1971). Interestingly, their analysis indicates that uveitis had been similarly attributed by previous authors to foci of infection at various sites, with claims of a dramatic response to the removal of such foci. In a recent series of 94 patients with optic neuritis investigated radiologically, 16 (17 per cent) had thickened membranes in the maxillary sinuses and four (4·3 per cent) had maxillary sinusitis (Nikoskelainen and Riekkinen 1974). Of these 20 patients, 15 were subsequently diagnosed as having multiple sclerosis. In only one, with acute rhinitis and bilateral maxillary sinusitis, was the infection considered the basis of the optic neuritis.

In our series, 125 patients had sinus X-rays performed. Abnormalities, confined to the maxillary or frontal sinuses, were encountered in 17 (13·6 per cent) and where unilateral, were ipsilateral to the optic neuritis in six and contralateral in four. There were fluid levels in four cases, opacity of one or more sinuses in five, mucosal thickening in seven and a retention cyst in one. Of nine patients with radiological changes and no evidence of multiple sclerosis who were followed for a minimum period of six months, five (55 per cent) had some evidence of multiple sclerosis subsequently.

The features of optic neuritis alleged to be due to sinus disease

In the past, attempts have been made to define certain clinical features distinguishing the optic neuritis of sinus disease from that due to other causes. The visual disturbance has been considered to begin acutely, often being found on waking (Vail 1931) or to develop gradually over several days (Koch 1946). The incidence of visual field abnormalities in patients with sinusitis has been variously quoted between 2·4 and 70 per cent (Gifford 1931). Traquair (1924) reported a series of 91 cases of sinus disease, examined by an oculist not informed of the diagnosis; three cases had slight concentric constriction, one had a unilateral enlargement of the blind spot, and in another, a left retrobulbar neuritis was found in a patient with a right antral infection and positive serology. Woods and Dunn (1923) also encountered two cases of optic neuropathy, previously attributed to sinus disease, where evidence of neurosyphilis was subsequently obtained.

It is apparent that, whatever the evidence for an occasional association between sinus disease and optic neuritis, there are no clinical features of the latter which allow such an association to be predicted.

The response to therapy

A dramatic improvement in vision following various sinus procedures has often been taken as evidence for a relationship between optic neuritis and sinus disease. In view of the occasional close anatomical relationship between the sphenoid and posterior ethmoid sinuses on the one hand and the optic nerve on the other, a spread of infection from one to the other is conceivable, with a consequent response to treatment aimed at eradicating the infection (Woods and Rowland 1931). For spread from more distant sinuses, the haematogenous route was proposed (White 1928). Alternative explanations for the assumed efficacy of sinus procedures have been advanced, including the concept of antidromic vasodilator impulses from hyperaemic mucosa to an allegedly ischaemic optic nerve (Benedict and Koch 1937; Koch 1946). Alternatively, an allergic phenomenon has been proposed, sensitization of tissues by bacterial invasion of the sinuses in some way leading to the development of optic neuritis.

When the incidence of sinus abnormalities, either clinical or radiological, is assessed critically, it appears no more frequent in patients with optic neuritis than in those with uveitis or with other ophthalmological disorders. The natural history of the condition has almost always been neglected in assessing the results of sinus procedures and, indeed, White's (1928) figures for recovery of vision after sinus exploration (63 per cent returning to normal and 29 per cent improving) are comparable to those encountered in untreated cases. It might have been thought that the eventual development of multiple sclerosis in some of these cases would finally allow dismissal of the influence of sinus disease, though, even then, certain authors have maintained the possibility of an association (Tarkkanen and Tarkkanen 1971).

Syphilis

Syphilis received a prominent place in early accounts of the differential diagnosis of optic neuritis, Nettleship (1884a), for example, considering it responsible for 20 per cent of his cases. In the review of cases from the Johns Hopkins by Woods and Rowland (1931), 23 were attributed to syphilis, the majority showing a primary optic atrophy. They stressed the inadequacy of a blood Wassermann reaction for the diagnosis of such cases, 7 of their patients having a negative reaction in the blood but positive in the cerebro-spinal fluid.

Sloan and Woods (1938) assessed the visual disturbances in 433 patients with neurosyphilis: 103 showed evidence of optic nerve involvement, over

50 per cent having some form of central field defect. Lesions were encountered as frequently in parenchymatous as in meningovascular disease and were generally symmetrical, being attributed to separate bilateral optic nerve involvement. Levin, Trevett, and Greenblatt (1947) were able to collect 34 cases of neurosyphilis in whom gradual loss of vision had been the first manifestation of the disease. Bruetsch (1948) published the post-mortem findings in 12 cases of syphilitic optic atrophy. He concluded that in tabes dorsalis, general paresis, tabo-paresis, and meningovascular disease, chronic low grade inflammatory changes occur in the pia-arachnoid surrounding the nerve and in the nerve septa, with demyelination and atrophy of nerve fibres leading to secondary gliosis. Walsh (1956), in a survey of syphilis of the optic nerve, considered various forms of involvement, including optic neuritis, chorioretinitis, papilloedema, and primary optic atrophy. Optic neuritis was considered to be rare in early syphilis, but frequent in the secondary and tertiary stages. No features distinguished syphilitic optic neuritis from the syndrome occurring in non syphilitic individuals, though it was commonly bilateral with optic disc swelling and pronounced and rapid loss of vision. Primary optic atrophy was associated with peripheral constriction of the visual fields, central vision often being preserved.

The character of the visual symptoms

In Sloan and Woods' experience (1938), visual failure was usually gradual, but could either be progressive or fluctuant. Visual acuity often only became depressed in the later stages of the disease, particularly in those with concentric constriction of the fields. Of five cases recorded by Graveson (1950), four had developed sudden visual failure, three noticing the symptom on waking, but the progression may also be measured in a matter of days (Earl and Zilkha 1964; Lorentzen 1967). The tendency for bilateral involvement was emphasized by Sloan and Woods (1938), and of 250 cases from the Johns Hopkins Hospital (Bruetsch 1948), only 10 had unilateral optic atrophy at the time of the initial examination. Where the initial vision loss is unilateral, involvement of the second eye is usual within a few months and almost invariable within 3 years (Levin *et al.* 1947). Three of five cases described by Graveson (1950) complained of sudden, unilateral visual failure but, in all of them, fundoscopic abnormalities were present in the apparently unaffected eye. Lorentzen (1967) has, however, encountered a case of unilateral visual impairment in whom no abnormalities were detected in the other eye over a follow up period of 20 months.

Bilateral retro-orbital pain (Earl and Zilkha 1964) and supra-orbital pain with tenderness of the globe (Graveson 1950) are described, but pain syndromes are in general uncommon, whilst pain on ocular movement has not been recorded.

The type of field defect and fundus appearance

In their survey, Sloan and Woods (1938) found, on visual field examination of patients with primary optic atrophy, concentric constriction (Fig. 6.1), localized peripheral defects, central or centro-caecal scotomata with normal peripheries (Fig. 6.2), and similar scotomata with peripheral constriction. Several patients in this last category had had nerve-fibre-bundle defects at an earlier stage (Fig. 6.3). In most cases, the fields of the two eyes were similar and defects for red preceded those for blue. Forty-seven per cent of those with parenchymatous syphilis had central scotomata compared with 64 per cent of patients with meningovascular disease. Of three patients with active optic neuritis and associated swelling of the optic disc, visual fields showed either enlargement of the blind spot, central or paracentral scotomata, or nerve-fibre-bundle defects. Amongst the 54 patients described by Levin *et al.* (1947) peripheral constriction was the commonest field defect, and Graveson (1950) considered enlargement of the blind spot and concentric constriction to be the earliest field changes, although in his own cases three had central or paracentral scotomata at the time of examination. He concluded that an impaired visual acuity in the absence of a central scotoma favoured a diagnosis of syphilis. Sloan and Woods (1938) encountered 12 patients with visual field defects in the absence of optic atrophy, but considered that with further follow-up, optic atrophy would probably have developed. All their examples of 'active' optic neuritis had swelling of the optic disc, associated with haemorrhages in one case.

Many authors consider that acute retrobulbar neuritis does not occur with syphilis (Graveson 1950) and though Walsh (1956) claimed that 10 per cent of all optic neuritis cases due to syphilis were retrobulbar, the clinical characteristics of these were not defined.

Natural history and response to steroids

Opinions differ on the natural history of syphilitic optic nerve disease. It has been suggested that an acute optic neuritis tends to recover completely save perhaps for residual enlargement of the blind spot or a minor peripheral defect (Sloan and Woods 1938). Subsequent accounts have always involved treatment with penicillin, concluding that prognosis for recovery of vision is good (Graveson 1950; Walsh 1956; Earl and Zilkha 1964; Lorentzen 1967).

The response of primary optic atrophy is less favourable. According to Hahn (quoted by Earl and Zilkha 1964), corticosteroid therapy alone has no effect on the condition, although Walsh (1956) has stressed the importance of avoiding a Jarisch-Herxheimer reaction when treating such patients. Bagley (1952) found no improvement in vision in any of the cases of syphilitic optic atrophy which he reviewed. Levin *et al.* (1947) observed

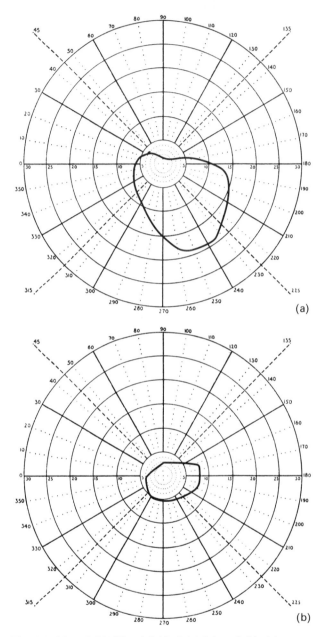

(a)

(b)

Fig. 6.1. (a) and (b). Visual field of (a) left and (b) right eye, showing advanced stage of concentric contraction, with preservation of good central vision in a case of advanced primary atrophy of the optic nerve. Solid line bounds the field for a 1° white test object. Visual acuity for the left eye was 20/30 and for the right 20/15 (from Sloan and Woods 1938).

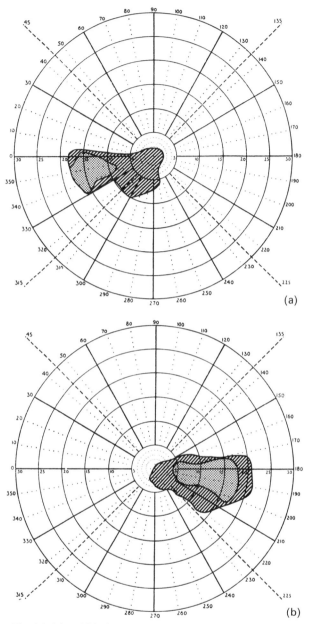

(a)

(b)

Fig. 6.2. (a) and (b). Cecocentral scotomata associated with normal peripheral fields. The central fields (to 30° only) are shown in the figure. (a) and (b) show a scotoma for 1° (dots) and ½° (lines) white test objects in the left and right eye, respectively, in a case of moderate atrophy of the papillomacular bundle. Both peripheral fields for a 1° white test object were normal. Vision for the left eye was 20/200 and for the right 12/200 (from Sloan and Woods 1938).

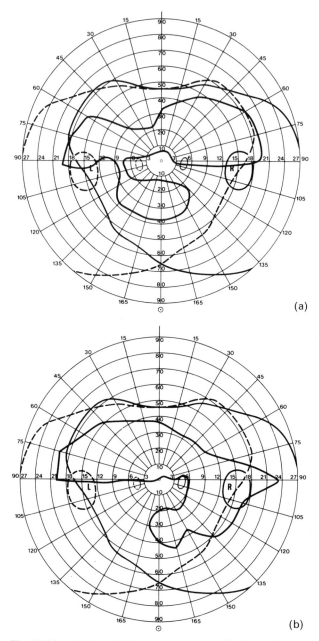

Fig. 6.3(a) and (b). Solid line bounds field for 1° white object in patient with nerve fiber bundle defects (from Sloan and Woods 1938).

improvement in two of 54 cases with optic atrophy and Walsh (1956) has suggested that the response to treatment may depend on the severity of visual loss.

Other clinical features

Optic neuritis is rare in early syphilis, but more common in the later stages, usually as part of a more general neurological disturbance (Walsh 1956). A partial or complete Argyll Robertson pupil occurred in 49 of 54 cases of syphilitic optic atrophy in one series (Levin *et al*. 1947) but, in optic neuritis, a depressed light response may be the sole pupillary abnormality.

Cases with syphilitic optic neuropathy may have negative blood serology (Moore 1937), the percentage reaching 20 in one series (Levin *et al*. 1947).

The significance of the finding of spirocheates in temporal artery sections of a patient with typical cranial arteritis (Smith, Israel, and Harner 1967) is uncertain. This patient had histological changes of temporal arteritis with positive blood serology. Using fluorescein labelled anti-treponemal globulin, spirochaetes were demonstrated in temporal artery sections. In a review of nine other cases of biopsy proven arteritis, of whom four were surviving, two had a positive FTA–ABS, and a positive reaction was known to have been present in one of the deceased. No details were given of the response of these patients to steroid therapy alone and the case described was treated with corticosteroids, penicillin and anticoagulants.

Bacterial infections

Tuberculous meningitis and papillitis

On occasions, tuberculous disease appears confined to the optic papilla and adjacent retina and choroid, without extension posteriorly. Generally such cases present with tumour-like masses arising from the optic disc. In one example, presenting with pain and visual loss on waking (Lamb 1937), examination revealed iritis, posterior synechiae, and a cloudy vitreous with swelling of the disc and peripapillary haemorrhage. Histology of the enucleated eye suggested tuberculous disease, although acid-fast bacilli were not seen. When cases present with unilateral visual failure due to a central scotoma (Fig. 6.4), and show subsequent improvement, problems in diagnosis become considerable (Miller and Frenkel 1971). In this particular patient, the scotoma later broke out into the periphery, and skull X-rays subsequently revealed destruction of the anterior clinoid process and the walls of the optic foramen. Biopsy suggested tuberculous disease and the organism was cultured from the optic nerve sheath. Mooney (1956) has made an extensive study of the ocular sequelae of tuberculous meningitis. Ocular lesions were encountered in 72 per cent of 65 cases, including two

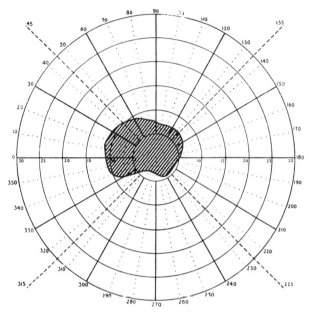

Fig. 6.4. Right visual field showing a central scotoma to a 6 mm/1000 red target (from Miller and Frenkel 1971).

children with retrobulbar neuritis. Optic atrophy, present in 20 per cent, was attributed to an arachnoiditis with a secondary disturbance of vascular supply. Decompression of the optic pathway produced improvement in vision in some patients.

Diphtheria

Two cases of disc swelling developing in the course of diphtheria were given by Bolton (1902) but without details of visual function. The same author found an example in the literature of bilateral visual failure with normal optic fundi and subsequent recovery (Framaget 1900, quoted by Bolton 1902).

Scarlet fever

Fits and bilateral blindness 3 weeks after the onset of scarlet fever have been described in a child of 15 months (Nettleship 1884*b*). Vision failed to improve in one eye, with the subsequent development of optic atrophy.

Pertussis

Between 1870 and 1930, 17 cases of blindness with whooping cough were recorded in the literature (Lazarus and Levine 1934), half having other neurological abnormalities in addition. Most recovered, but one case examined at post-mortem had a haemorrhagic effusion into the optic nerve sheath.

Brucellosis

Visual failure, usually bilateral, has been described in this condition (Green 1939; Wagener 1947), although in many instances the specificity of the bacteriological diagnosis appears open to doubt. Generally ocular involvement consists of choroiditis or iritis, optic nerve disease alone being relatively rare.

Botulism

Experimental studies of the effects of botulinus toxin on the optic nerve reveal focal infiltration by round cells with an increase of neuroglial cells, mirroring clinical descriptions of optic nerve involvement by the disease (Swab and Gerald 1933).

Sub-acute bacterial endocarditis

Although papillitis is recorded in one third of cases (Dienst and Gartner 1944), in many the combination of disc swelling with enlargement of the blind spot but little or no visual impairment suggests papilloedema is the more likely explanation. Four of the five personal cases of Dienst and Gartner (1944) had disc swelling, but details of visual acuity were not given. Histological changes included oedema of the disc head with perivascular cellular infiltration, but sections of the optic nerve were not studied.

Other bacterial infections

Optic nerve involvement has been reported in erysipelas, epidemic meningitis, tularaemia, plague, enteric diseases, and leptospirosis (Henderson 1956). Papilloedema, retinal infiltration (Switz, Casey, and Bogaty 1969) and optic atrophy (Stoupel, Monseu, Pardoe, Hiemann, and Martin 1969) have been seen in Whipple's disease but not, apparently, a typical optic neuritis, although infiltration of the optic nerve by PAS positive material has been seen at post-mortem examination (Switz *et al.* 1969).

Mycotic infections

Aspergillosis

This condition may affect the optic nerve. In one case unilateral then bilateral visual blurring was associated initially with a response to corticosteroid therapy (Goldhammer, Lawton Smith, and Yates 1974). After further vision loss, craniotomy revealed an intrasellar mycotic abscess with diffuse infiltration of the optic nerves and an associated meningo-encephalitis.

Histoplasmosis

Presentation with sudden unilateral visual failure and associated frontal headache occurred in the patient described by Husted and Shock (1975). Fundoscopy revealed a nodular mass arising from the nasal aspect of the disc in one eye, with chorioretinal scarring typical of histoplasmosis in the other. The diagnosis was based on the combination of a positive skin test and the subsequent development of chorioretinal scarring similar to that in the previously affected eye.

Torulosis

Both papilloedema (Rose, Grant, and Jeanes 1958) and optic nerve involvement (Henderson 1956) have been described in this disease.

Parasitic infections

Onchocerciasis

Optic atrophy has been recorded in up to 60 per cent of patients with this disease (Bird, Anderson, and Fuglsang 1976). The majority have choroido-retinal changes typical of the condition and peripheral field constriction is more common than central involvement. In the active stages optic disc swelling is common and arcuate field defects not infrequent.

Nematode optic neuritis

Toxocara canis may present as a tumour-like mass arising from the optic disc, sometimes preceded by optic disc swelling and vitreous haze (Bird, Lawton Smith, and Curtin 1970). Examples of optic nerve involvement by malaria and toxoplasmosis have also been cited (Henderson 1956).

Virus infections and encephalitic illnesses

Lumsden (1972) has discussed in detail the nosological entity of the various forms of post-vaccinial encephalitis and their relation to multiple sclerosis. Encephalitic illnesses following measles, varicella, rubella, and smallpox vaccination are characteristically, although not invariably, of the perivenous demyelinating type. The same histological pattern is shared by post-rabies vaccinal lesions and experimental allergic encephalomyelitis. The similarity of the histological changes of perivenous encephalitis to those of multiple sclerosis has prompted Lumsden to suggest that the initiating mechanism in the two conditions is identical. In the case of pertussis infection, on the other hand, and with scarlatina, Miller, Stanton, and Gibbons (1956) were unable to find examples of clinically typical or histologically proven perivenous encephalomyelitis, whilst mumps meningoencephalitis was considered to be usually a consequence of invasion by living virus. Berliner (1935) reviewed the features of optic nerve involvement in acute disseminated encephalomyelitis, indicating the frequency with which the visual pathway was affected. Optic nerve involvement tended to be bilateral, often with papillitis, conclusions reached previously by McAlpine (1931). Berliner found occasional cases where optic neuritis developed several months after the acute onset of the disease and quoted evidence suggesting that relapses did not exclude the diagnosis of encephalomyelitis, although Lumsden (1972) has suggested that such cases may exemplify a progression from para-infectious encephalomyelitis to multiple sclerosis. Visual failure is a regular feature of the experimental model produced by injection of brain extract with Freund's adjuvant (Kabat, Wolf, and Bezer 1950), and may show a remitting and relapsing course. Rarely the central nervous system involvement in the animal model may be confined almost exclusively to the optic nerves, tracts and lateral geniculate bodies.

A syndrome of bilateral severe visual failure with recovery suggests a primary demyelinating process with relative sparing of axonal function. If this assumption is correct, the syndrome should be more commonly associated with those infections capable of causing perivenous demyelination. Bilateral visual failure with recovery has been recorded in pertussis, a condition not associated with perivenous demyelinating encephalomyelitis (Miller *et al.* 1956), whilst mumps is capable of causing a reversible visual failure, although its associated encephalitis is generally considered due to direct virus invasion. The post-mortem findings in a case of mumps encephalitis with unilateral visual failure have been described (Woodward 1907) though the case was complicated by evidence of increased intraocular pressure in life. Histological examination revealed severe fibre atrophy in the optic nerve with obliteration of small blood vessels. Visual evoked responses may provide useful information in such cases, a markedly delayed response clearly favouring optic nerve demyelination.

Measles

Visual failure is not uncommon in this condition. Walsh and Ford (1940) reported a bilateral case with disc oedema, central scotomata, and subsequent recovery, and similar examples appear in the literature (Berliner 1935; Ström 1953; Tyler 1957; Srivastava and Nema 1963). Optic neuritis may occur in isolation or as part of a generalized encephalomyelitis (Tyler

1957). Prognosis for recovery is good, though Ström (1953), on the finding of fundal arterial narrowing, has argued that the visual disturbance is secondary to a toxic destruction of retinal capillary endothelium.

Rubella

Connolly, Hutchinson, Allen, Lyttle, Swallow, Dermott, and Thomson (1975) have recently discussed a number of neurological disturbances occurring in association with rubella infection. One patient, who recovered completely, had severe visual failure with papillitis but no other neurological abnormalities. Similar examples were found in the literature, some in association with encephalitis or myelitis.

Chicken-pox

Berliner (1935) described bilateral papillitis and other neurological abnormalities in a boy of 6, 2 weeks after the onset of chicken-pox, and examples have been given by others (Walsh and Ford 1940; Hatch 1949; Bagley 1952).

Herpes zoster

Cases of herpes ophthalmicus with ipsilateral visual loss not due to corneal lesions have been published (Paton 1923; Wynne Parry and Laszlo 1943).

Glandular fever

Severe bilateral visual failure has been recorded in this condition by Bonynge and Von Hagen (1952), associated with pain on ocular movement and tenderness of the globe. The cerebrospinal fluid contained 6 cells per mm³, with a protein concentration of 55 mg per cent and mid zone Lange curve. In a similar case reported recently (Pickens and Sangster 1975) recovery was incomplete. The cases of Tanner (1954), one of whom had irido-cyclitis in addition, probably had papilloedema rather than papillitis.

Mumps

There have been several reports of optic neuritis due to mumps, some with incomplete recovery and some unilateral (Woodward 1907; Swab 1938; Strong, Henderson, and Gangitano 1974). A pleocytosis with an elevated globulin content may be found in the cerebrospinal fluid despite a lack of involvement of other parts of the central nervous system (Young 1933).

Influenza

An attack of influenza (grippe) was considered the cause of a subsequent bilateral papillitis associated with a CSF pleocytosis and elevated globulin content (Knapp 1916).

Epidemic encephalitis

In a review of the literature regarding visual disturbances in this condition, Spiller (1923) found examples of optic neuritis and quoted two of his own cases; clinical details were sparse, however, and an adequate distinction from papilloedema not made.

Encephalitis of undetermined origin

On the basis of a preceding flu-like illness, cases of unilateral (Wagener 1952) or bilateral visual failure (Lillie 1934) have been attributed to an encephalitis or encephalomyelitis of undetermined origin.

Post-vaccination

Optic neuritis following anti-rabies inoculation has been observed both in humans and experimental animals. Bilateral papillitis with recovery has followed the use of a sheep vaccine (Cormack and Anderson 1934), and visual disturbances are one of the chief clinical manifestations of the demyelinating encephalomyelitis associated with this procedure (Uchimura and Shiraki 1957). Histologically, well preserved axon cylinders accompany severe demyelination, the combination being thought responsible for the recovery of vision which characteristically occurs. Other forms of vaccination can produce a similar effect, two cases following smallpox vaccination having been examined at post-mortem (Wagener 1952). A predominantly perivenous demyelination coexisted with some axonal destruction. The use of a combined smallpox, tetanus, and diphtheria vaccine led to bilateral visual failure in a 7-year-old child with complete recovery (McReynolds, Havener, and Petrohelos 1953).

Guillain–Barre syndrome

The case of this syndrome with unilateral optic neuritis described by Nikoskelainen and Riekkinen (1972) is unsatisfactory, particularly as an episode of acute myelitis was a prominent feature of the neurological illness. A more satisfactory example described by Behan, Lessell, and Roche (1976) had immunological evidence of hypersensitivity to both central and peripheral myelin.

Cat-scratch disease

A case of cat-scratch disease, diagnosed on the basis of appropriate exposure, positive skin tests, and node biopsies, was associated with unilateral papillitis and median nerve compression by an inflamed lymph node (Sweeney and Drance 1970). Other patients with neurological involvement have been described, possibly on the basis of a post-infectious encephalitis. One of our own series may have had the illness.

N.S.W. aged 38. This patient received a scratch to the right lower lid 6 weeks before the onset of visual symptoms. A 'stye' had subsequently developed and was present on admission. Pain on ocular movement with blurring of vision developed in the right eye.

Examination revealed a right papillitis with vision reduced to counting fingers. In addition, cells and opacities were noted in the vitreous with subsequent cells and flare appearing in the right anterior chamber. CSF protein was 80 mg per cent with a normal cell count. Full recovery of vision occurred and neither at presentation nor at follow-up 16 months later was there any evidence of multiple sclerosis. Tests for cat-scratch disease were not made and the lower lid lesion not biopsied.

Insect stings

The possibility of a hypersensitive reaction to insect stings causing a neurological disturbance has been considered. Goldstein, Rucker, and Woltman (1960) gave several examples including a left papillitis following two weeks after a bee sting in the left temple.

Conclusions

Sinus infection as an aetiological factor in optic neuritis no longer receives the emphasis accorded it in the earlier part of the century. Clinical or radiological evidence of sinus disease is no more frequent in optic neuritis patients than in a control population. Enthusiasm for various sinus procedures in the treatment of the condition has taken no account of the spontaneous recovery which generally occurs.

Syphilis is capable of causing optic nerve disturbances without evidence of generalized central nervous system involvement. More typically progressive visual failure with optic atrophy and constricted fields is seen, but an acute optic neuritis occurs, usually bilateral and often with disc swelling.

The syndrome of optic neuritis has been described in association with a vast number of bacterial, mycotic, and parasitic infections, although in most instances the disturbance only superficially resembles the condition seen in multiple sclerosis. Perivenous demyelinating encephalomyelitis, however, may cause a disturbance of optic nerve function, which clinically and pathologically mirrors exactly that associated with multiple sclerosis, although bilateral involvement is the rule. A visual disturbance of a similar type is encountered in pertussis, despite the contention that perivenous demyelinating encephalomyelitis does not occur in that condition. The implication of this paradox is that either the infection is capable of causing such a reaction, or that a severe, but totally reversible, visual failure may not necessarily be based on optic nerve demyelination.

REFERENCES

Bagley, C. H. (1952). An etiologic study of a series of optic neuropathies. *Am. J. Ophthal.* **35**, 761–72.

Behan, P. O., Lessell, S., and Roche, M. (1976). Optic neuritis in the Landry–Guillain–Barre–Strohl syndrome. *Br. J. Ophthal.* **60**, 58–9.

Benedict, W. L. (1933). Retrobulbar neuritis and disease of the nasal accessory sinuses. *Archs Ophthal., N.Y.* **9**, 893–906.

— and Koch, F. L. P. (1937). Optic neuritis and retrobulbar neuritis: etiology and treatment. *J. Mich. St. med. Soc.* **36**, 946–59.

Berliner, H. L. (1935). Acute optic neuritis in demyelinating diseases of the nervous system. *Archs Ophthal., N.Y.* **13**, 83–98.

Bird, A. C., Lawton-Smith, J., and Curtin, V. T. (1970). Nematode optic neuritis. *Am. J. Ophthal.* **69**, 72–7.

— Anderson, J., and Fuglsang, H. (1976). Morphology of posterior segment lesions of the eye in patients with onchocerciasis. *Br. J. Ophthal.* **69**, 72–7.

Bolton, C. (1902). Notes on two cases of optic neuritis in diphtheria. *Lancet* **2**, 1624.

Bonynge, T. W. and Von Hagen, K. O. (1952). Severe optic neuritis in infectious mononucleosis. Report of a case. *J. Am. med. Ass.* **148**, 933–4.

Bossy, A. and Jéquier, M. (1961). Sinusites, néurites optiques et sclérose en plaques. *Confinia neurol.* **21**, 217–22.

Bruetsch, W. L. (1948). Unilateral syphilitic primary atrophy of the optic nerves. *Archs Ophthal., N.Y.* **39**, 80–8.

Calvet, J., Calmettes, L., and Coll, J. (1967). Le rôle des sinusites dans l'étiologie des néurites optiques rétro-bulbaires. *Revue Oto-Neuro-Ophtal.* **39**, 43–7.

Connolly, J. H., Hutchinson, W. M., Allen, I. V., Lyttle, J. A., Swallow, M. H., Dermott, E., and Thomson, D. (1975). Carotid artery thrombosis, encephalitis, myelitis and optic neuritis associated with rubella virus infections. *Brain* **98**, 583–94.

Cormack, H. S. and Anderson, L. A. P. (1934). Bilateral papillitis following antirabic inoculation: recovery. *Br. J. Ophthal.* **43**, 167–8.

Dienst, E. C. and Gartner, S. (1944). Pathologic changes in the eye associated with subacute bacterial endocarditis. Report of five cases with autopsy. *Archs Ophthal., N.Y.* **31**, 198–206.

*Doesschate, T. (1928). Pathologisch-anatomische befunde bei rhinogenem sehnervenleiden. *Klin. Mbl. Augenheilk.* **80**, 831–2.

Earl, C. J. and Zilkha, K. J. (1964). Syphilitic optic neuritis. *Acta ophthal.* **45**, 769–72.

Ford, R. (1944). Retro-bulbar neuritis. Five cases due to paranasal sinusitis. *Br. J. Ophthal.* **28**, 511–15.

Gifford, S. R. (1931). The relation of the paranasal sinuses to ocular disorders. *Archs Ophthal., N.Y.* **5**, 276–86.

Goldhammer, Y., Lawton-Smith, J., and Yates, B. M. (1974). Mycotic intrasellar abscess. *Am. J. Ophthal.* **78**, 478–84.

Goldstein, N. P., Rucker, C. W., and Woltman, H. W. (1960). Neuritis occurring after insect stings. *J. Am. med. Ass.* **173**, 1727–30.

Graveson, G. S. (1950). Syphilitic optic neuritis. *J. Neurol. Neurosurg. Psychiat.* **13**, 216–24.

Green, J. (1939). Ocular manifestations in undulant fever. *Archs Ophthal., N.Y.* **21**, 51–67.

Guyton, J. S. and Woods, A. C. (1941). Etiology of uveitis. A clinical study of 562 cases. *Archs Ophthal., N.Y.* **26**, 983–1018.

Hatch, H. A. (1949). Bilateral optic neuritis following chicken pox. Report of a case with apparently complete recovery. *J. Pediat.* **34**, 758–9.

112 *Differential diagnosis: infectious and post-infectious disorders*

Henderson, J. W. (1956). Disease secondary to systemic infection. *Trans. Am. Acad. Ophthal. Oto-lar.* **60**, 36–8.

Husted, R. C. and Shock, J. P. (1975). Acute presumed histoplasmosis of the optic nerve head. *Br. J. Ophthal.* **59**, 409–12.

Kabat, E. A., Wolf, A., and Bezer, A. E. (1950). Experimental studies on acute disseminated encephalomyelitis in rhesus monkeys. In *Multiple sclerosis and the demyelinating diseases*. Research Publications of the Association for Research in Nervous and Mental Diseases, Vol. 28. Williams and Wilkins, Baltimore.

Knapp, A. (1916). Optic neuritis after influenza, with changes in the spinal fluid. *Archs Ophthal., N.Y.* **45**, 247–9.

Koch, F. L. P. (1946). The optic neuritides. *Conn. St. med. J.* **10**, 763–5.

Lamb, H. D. (1937). A case of tuberculous papillitis with anatomic finding. *Am. J. Ophthal.* **20**, 390–6.

Lazarus, S. D. and Levine, G. (1934). Blindness in whooping cough. *Am. J. Dis. Child.* **47**, 1310–17.

Levin, S., Trevett, L. D., and Greenblatt, M. (1947). Syphilitic primary optic atrophy. *New Engl. J. Med.* **237**, 769–72.

Lillie, W. I. (1934). The clinical significance of retrobulbar and optic neuritis. *Am. J. Ophthal.* **17**, 110–19.

Loeb, H. W. (1909). A study of the anatomic relations of the optic nerve to the accessory cavities of the nose. *Ann. Otol. Rhinol. Lar.* **18**, 243–73.

Lorentzen, S. E. (1967). Syphilitic optic neuritis. *Acta ophthal.* **45**, 769–72.

Lumsden, C. E. (1972). In *Multiple sclerosis. A reappraisal* (eds D. McAlpine, C. E. Lumsden, and E. C. Acheson) (2nd edn). Churchill Livingstone, Edinburgh and London.

McAlpine, D. (1931). Acute disseminated encephalomyelitis. Its sequelae and its relationship to disseminated sclerosis. *Lancet* **1**, 846–52.

McReynolds, W. U., Havener, W. H., and Petrohelos, M. A. (1953). Bilateral optic neuritis following smallpox vaccination and diphtheria-tetanus toxoid. *Am. J. Dis. Child.* **86**, 601–3.

Miller, B. W. and Frenkel, M. (1971). Report of a case of tuberculous retrobulbar neuritis and osteomyelitis. *Am. J. Ophthal.* **71**, 751–6.

Miller, H. G., Stanton, J. B., and Gibbons, J. L. (1956). Parainfectious encephalomyelitis and related syndromes. A critical review of the neurological complications of certain specific fevers. *Q. Jl. Med.* **25**, 427–505.

Mooney, A. J. (1956). Some ocular sequelae of tuberculous meningitis. *Am. J. Ophthal.* **41**, 753–68.

Moore, J. I. (1937). An etiologic study of a series of optic neuropathies. *Am. J. Ophthal.* **20**, 1099–1108.

Nettleship, E. (1884*a*). On cases of retro-ocular neuritis. *Trans. ophthal. Soc. U.K.* **4**, 186–226.

— (1884*b*). On cases of recovery from amaurosis in young children. *Trans. ophthal. Soc. U.K.* **4**, 243–66.

Nikoskelainen, E. and Riekkinen, P. (1972). Retrobulbar neuritis as an early symptom of Guillain–Barré syndrome. *Acta ophthal.* **50**, 111–15.

— — (1974). Optic neuritis—A sign of multiple sclerosis or other diseases of the central nervous system. A retrospective analysis of 116 patients. *Acta Neurol. Scand.* **50**, 690–718.

Østerberg, G. (1931). Iridocyclitis with central scotoma. *Acta ophthal.* **9**, 310–15.

Paton, L. (1923). Optic atrophy after herpes ophthalmicus. *Proc. R. Soc. Med.* **16**, 27–30.

Pickens, S. and Sangster, G. (1975). Retrobulbar neuritis and infectious mononucleosis. *Br. med. J.* **4**, 729.

Pickworth, F. A. (1928). Perforation of the pituitary fossa by a septic lesion of the sphenoidal sinus associated with recent epilepsy and insanity. *J. Lar. Otol.* **43**, 186–90.

Rose, F. C., Grant, H. C., and Jeanes, A. L. (1958). Torulosis of the central nervous system in Britain. *Brain* **81**, 542–55.

Sloan, L. L. and Woods, A. C. (1938). Perimetric studies in syphilitic optic neuropathies. *Archs Ophthal., N.Y.* **20**, 201–54.

Smith, J. L., Israel, C. W., and Harner, R. E. (1967). Syphilitic temporal arteritis. *Archs Ophthal., N.Y.* **78**, 284–8.

Spiller, W. G. (1923). High grade choked discs in epidemic encephalitis. *J. Am. med. Ass.* **80**, 1843–4.
Srivastava, S. P. and Nema, H. V. (1963). Optic neuritis in measles. *Br. J. Ophthal.* **47**, 180–1.
Stoupel, N., Monseu, G., Pardoe, A., Heimann, R., and Martin, J. J. (1969). Encephalitis with myoclonus in Whipple's disease. *J. Neurol. Neurosurg. Psychiat.* **32**, 338–43.
Ström, T. (1953). Acute blindness as post-measles complication. *Acta paediat. Stockh.* **42**, 60–5.
Strong, L. E., Henderson, J. W., and Gangitano, J. L. (1974). Bilateral retrobulbar neuritis secondary to mumps. *Am. J. Ophthal.* **78**, 331–2.
Swab, C. M. (1938). Encephalitic optic neuritis and atrophy due to mumps. Report of a case. *Archs Ophthal., N.Y.* **19**, 926–9.
— and Gerald, H. F. (1933). The ophthalmic lesions of botulism: additional notes and research. *Br. J. Ophthal.* **17**, 129–44.
Sweeney, V. P. and Drance, S. M. (1970). Optic neuritis and compressive neuropathy associated with cat scratch disease. *Can. med. Ass. J.* **103**, 1380–1.
Switz, D. M., Casey, T. R., and Bogaty, G. V. (1969). Whipple's disease and papilloedema. *Archs intern. Med.* **123**, 74–7.
Syme, W. S. (1910). Chronic sphenoidal sinus disease. *Lancet* **1**, 422–6.
— (1924). The sphenoidal sinus in relation to the optic nerve. *J. Lar. Otol.* **39**, 375–80.
Tanner, O. R. (1954). Ocular manifestations of infectious mononucleosis. *Archs Ophthal., N.Y.* **51**, 229–41.
Tarkkanen, J. and Tarkkanen, A. (1971). Otorhinolaryngological pathology in patients with optic neuritis. *Acta ophthal.* **49**, 649–57.
Traquair, H. M. (1924). The value of visual changes in the diagnosis of optic nerve disease due to latent morbid conditions of the nasal accessory sinuses. *J. Lar. Otol.* **39**, 384–92.
Tyler, H. R. (1957). Neurological complications of rubeola (measles) *Medicine, Baltimore* **36**, 147–67.
Uchimura, I. and Shiraki, H. (1957). A contribution to the classification and the pathogenesis of demyelinating encephalomyelitis with special reference to the central nervous system lesions caused by preventive inoculation against rabies. *J. Neuropath. exp. Neurol.* **16**, 139–208.
Vail, H. H. (1931). Retrobulbar optic neuritis originating in nasal sinuses: New method of demonstrating relation between sphenoid sinus and optic nerve. *Archs Otolar.* **13**, 846–63.
Van Der Hoeve, J. (1922). Optic nerve and accessory sinuses. *Archs Ophthal., N.Y.* **51**, 210–22.
Wagener, H. P. (1947). Ocular lesions in brucellosis. *Am. J. med. Sci.* **214**, 215–19.
— (1952). Edema of the optic disks in cases of encephalitis. *Am. J. med. Sci.* **223**, 205–15.
Walsh, F. B. (1956). Syphilis of the optic nerve. *Trans. Am. Acad. Ophthal. Oto-lar.* **60**, 39–42.
— and Ford, F. R. (1940). Central scotomas. Their importance in topical diagnosis. *Archs Ophthal., N.Y.* **24**, 500–32.
Weille, F. L. and Vang, R. R. (1953). Sinusitis as focus of infection in uveitis, keratitis and retrobulbar neuritis. *Archs Otolar.* **58**, 154–65.
White, L. E. (1928). The location of the focus in optic nerve disturbances from infection. *Ann. Otol. Rhinol. Lar.* **37**, 128–64.
Woods, A. C. and Dunn, J. R. (1923). Etiologic study of a series of optic neuropathies. *J. Am. med. Ass.* **80**, 1113–17.
— and Rowland, W. M. (1931). An etiologic study of a series of optic neuropathies. *J. Am. med. Ass.* **97**, 375–9.
Woodward, J. H. (1907). The ocular complications of mumps. *Ann. Ophthal.* **16**, 7–38.
Wynne-Parry, T. G. and Laszlo, G. C. (1943). Herpes zoster ophthalmicus—two rare manifestations. *Br. J. Ophthal.* **27**, 465–7.
Young, G. (1924). Retrobulbar neuritis of sphenoidal sinus origin. *J. Lar. Otol.* **39**, 381–3.
Young, R. C. (1933). Mumps encephalitis: Report of a case with bilateral optic neuritis, rapid and complete blindness and complete recovery. *New Orl. med. surg. J.* **86**, 25–6.

7 Differential diagnosis: deficiency and toxic disorders

The term 'toxic amblyopia' means, literally, partial blindness due to toxins, but is always used in a restricted sense as referring to loss of vision due to the absorption in one way or another of external poisons (Traquair 1930).

Vitamin deficiency

Nutritional amblyopia is characterized by reduced visual acuity, with a central or paracentral scotoma and, typically, some degree of temporal pallor (Carroll 1956a). Deficiencies of a single vitamin may be responsible, for example, with pellagra (B_6) (Levine 1934) and beri-beri (B_1) (Beam 1947), but, particularly in the visual disturbances of prisoners of war, a more complex pathogenesis operates. In some instances, the onset of visual failure is rapid, developing overnight (Spillane and Scott 1945), and disc swelling may be found in the early stages (Spillane and Scott 1945). Despite the likelihood of a nutritional basis for the amblyopia, response to treatment is variable, since some cases improve (Livingston 1946), whilst others show little change (Spillane and Scott 1945; Carroll 1956a). In a series of 11 prisoners of war, all with visual symptoms in life, four showed degeneration of the papillomacular bundle of the optic nerve on post-mortem examination, with demyelination of the posterior columns in seven (Fisher 1955).

Pernicious anaemia

In early reports of optic neuropathy in association with pernicious anaemia, the visual symptoms were accompanied by evidence of sub-acute combined degeneration of the spinal cord (Hine 1935). With elaboration of the syndrome, it became apparent that the visual symptoms could occur in isolation.

The character of the visual symptoms
Bilateral involvement, though usual, may be asymmetrical (Sharpe and Hyland 1952; Nelson and Weaver 1956; Enoksson and Norden 1960), and, in a single instance, a unilateral visual field defect has been described (Hamilton, Ellis, and Sheets 1959). Though a rapid visual failure has been encountered in two reports, one was complicated by the presence of a macular haemorrhage (Box 1936) and the other almost certainly represented an ischaemic optic neuropathy (Bradley 1968).

The type of field defect

The scotoma may be central (Hine 1935; Talbot 1936; Enoksson and Turner 1960), paracentral (Hamilton *et al.* 1959) or centro-caecal (Turner 1940; Benham 1951; Sharpe and Hyland 1952; Lerman and Feldmahn 1961; Freeman and Heaton 1961; Olivarius and Jensen 1961; Björkenheim 1966) (Figs. 7.1, 7.2). Marked peripheral constriction has been described in two patients (Cohen 1936), but both had considerable impairment of visual acuity, suggesting the presence of central field defects in addition.

The similarity of the scotomata to those encountered in tobacco amblyopia has prompted the suggestion that smoking is of importance in precipitating visual symptoms (Freeman and Heaton 1961).

Pupils and fundus appearance

The pupillary responses are depressed to a varying degree. Abnormalities of the optic disc are confined to atrophy, disc swelling not being recorded.

Natural history

Although spontaneous recovery of the depressed vision has not been recorded, response to B_{12} replacement therapy is usually complete.

Other clinical features

The development of optic neuropathy in pernicious anaemia appears unrelated to the duration of the disease, presence or degree of anaemia, or to evidence of other neurological involvement (Turner 1940). Visual loss has antedated other manifestations of the disease in a third of reported cases (Hamilton *et al.* 1959), whilst 25 per cent of patients will have no anaemia and 16 per cent no evidence of subacute combined degeneration (Freeman and Heaton 1961). A positive Lhermitte's sign (Gautier-Smith 1973) may further the resemblance to multiple sclerosis. Minor changes in the cerebrospinal fluid occur when the optic neuropathy is accompanied by evidence of more widespread neurological involvement (Enoksson and Norden 1960).

Despite the equal sex distribution of pernicious anaemia, the vast majority of those developing optic neuropathy are male. This, and the similarity of the visual field defect to that encountered in tobacco amblyopia, has stimulated an analysis of the possible influence of cigarette smoking on the development of the condition (Freeman and Heaton 1961). Isolated cases occur in non-smokers (Enoksson and Norden 1960; Björkenheim 1966), but in all other reports where tobacco consumption has been detailed, the patients were smokers. It has been shown that mean B_{12} levels are lower in patients with tobacco amblyopia and, indeed, Foulds, Chisholm, Stewart, and Wilson

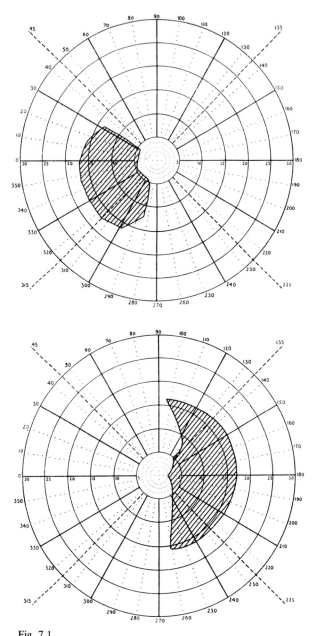

Fig. 7.1.
L and R
Centrocaecal scotomata as the presenting sign in pernicious
anaemia V.A. (corrected) 20/80 R. 20/80+ L.
Tangent screen 1 metre
Test object 3 mm white 5 mm blue and red.
(From Lerman and Feldmahn 1961.)

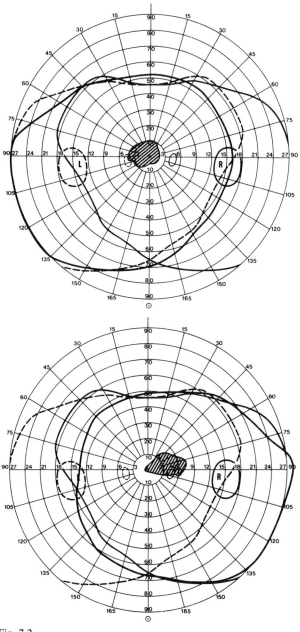

Fig. 7.2.
L and R
Bilateral retrobulbar neuritis in pernicious anaemia with subacute
degeneration of the spinal cord.
VA 2/80 R 1/60 L
Scotoma 4/2000 Periphery 3/2000
(From Traquair 1957.)

(1969) have suggested that the diagnoses of tobacco amblyopia and the optic neuropathy of pernicious anaemia are interchangeable. Furthermore, the histological changes encountered in the two conditions are similar (Freeman and Heaton 1961; Duke-Elder and Scott 1971a).

Tobacco–alcohol amblyopia

This condition has become less common since Traquair (1930) was able to collect 1088 cases from the Royal Infirmary, Edinburgh, between 1913 and 1926. This condition represented 6·1 per cent of the 506 cases of optic neuropathy collected at the Johns Hopkins Hospital between 1923 and 1952 (Bagley 1952).

The character of the visual symptoms

Symptoms are usually confined to males and begin in a later age group than that associated with the majority of cases of optic neuritis (Fig. 7.3). The involvement, though generally bilateral, may be asymmetrical, and Traquair (1930) claimed that field defects were always detectable in the less affected eye, even with normal visual acuity. Unilateral cases are rarely reported and not often fully substantiated, one case, for example, being complicated by the presence of a pituitary tumour (Lillie 1934). Visual failure is usually of gradual onset and may be more noticeable in bright light (Traquair 1930; Lillie 1934).

The type of field defect

The field defect consists of a centrocaecal scotoma, beginning nasally to the blind spot and gradually extending towards, and into, fixation. Within the scotoma, islands of denser loss are detectable around the horizontal meridian, particularly adjacent to the blind spot and to fixation (Traquair 1930). With further extension, an irregular temporal hemianopia for red may appear, or all perception of red may be lost. The edges of the scotoma are sloping and poorly defined and never extend far into the nasal field. During recovery the sequence is reversed. Peripheral defects, hemianopic and nerve-fibre bundle defects, do not occur. Other authors have considered a relative or absolute central scotoma, indistinguishable from those encountered in other conditions (Lillie 1934), to be more typical but further experience has supported Traquair's contention.

Pupils and fundus appearance

The optic disc may show little change and, even in severe cases, fails to develop the degree of pallor associated with demyelination (Traquair 1930).

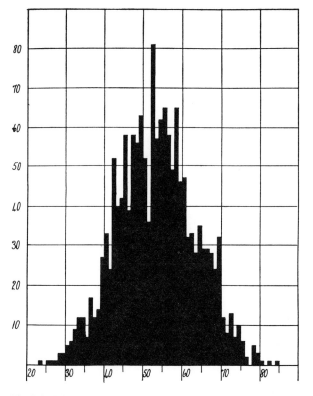

Fig. 7.3. Tobacco amblyopia. Ages of 1525 patients, 1913–1929 (ordinate axis: number of patients; abscissa axis: age of patients) (from Traquair 1930).

Natural history

Spontaneous visual improvement does not occur whilst exposure to tobacco continues. Recovery is usual when smoking has stopped, but may be delayed for several weeks or months. Treatment with hydroxy-cobalamin accelerates the process, even when smoking continues (Foulds, Chisholm, and Pettigrew 1974) and vitamin B complex may exert a similar therapeutic effect.

Other clinical features

The role of alcohol in these cases has received greater emphasis in the United States than elsewhere. Traquair (1930) dismissed its role but some American authors have considered it more relevant, even, on occasions, in isolation (Victor 1963). The role of cyanide intoxication in this condition has been emphasized by Foulds *et al.* (1974). An inability to detoxify cyanide to thiocyanate has been postulated, improvement being achieved with the use of cystine, acting as a source of organic sulphur. The importance of B_{12} deficiency in precipitating visual symptoms is established. Achlorhydria is a common finding (Leishman 1951), and mean B_{12} levels are lower than in a control population (Heaton, McCormick, and Freeman 1958). Evidence of defective absorption of the vitamin can be found in some 40 per cent of cases of tobacco amblyopia (Foulds *et al.* 1974).

In one series, average tobacco consumption was 3 oz/week, no cases being seen when intake fell below 1 oz/week (Traquair 1930). Although most examples have been due to the smoking of tobacco, it has also followed exposure through chewing, sniffing, or eating. Both the papillomacular bundle within the optic nerve and the retinal ganglion cells have been considered the major site of pathological involvement. The histological changes in the optic nerve are analogous to those observed in pernicious anaemia (Freeman and Heaton 1961) with degeneration, neuroglial proliferation, and round cell infiltration (Duke-Elder and Scott 1971*b*).

Tropical amblyopia

Visual disorders may figure prominently in the various neurological syndromes described under the general title of Jamaican neuropathy. A slowly progressive, bilateral visual syndrome is usual, remissions being encountered rarely, but, on occasion, a sudden visual failure has been noted on waking (Osuntokun 1968). The disorder begins in an age group similar to optic neuritis (Crews 1963) and affects predominantly central vision (Fig. 7.4) (Crews 1963; Montgomery, Cruickshank, Robertson, and McMenemey 1964), although more bizarre field defects may be encountered (MacKenzie and Phillips 1968). Marked abnormalities of the cerebrospinal fluid can occur with abnormal colloidal gold curves and elevated concentrations of gamma globulin. Demyelination is a prominent feature in the optic nerves examined.

Dietary cyanide has been implicated in the causation of some forms of this syndrome, cassava (the tuber of manoic), being implicated in the Nigerian cases (Osuntokun 1968); the method of cooking cassava in Nigeria is not likely, however, to lead to cyanide intake, since the source of the cyanide is peeled from the root before cooking (Tuboku-Metzger 1969).

Drugs and toxic agents

Grant (1974) lists 42 substances reported to cause optic neuritis (defined as impaired visual acuity with an abnormal optic disc) and 40 causing

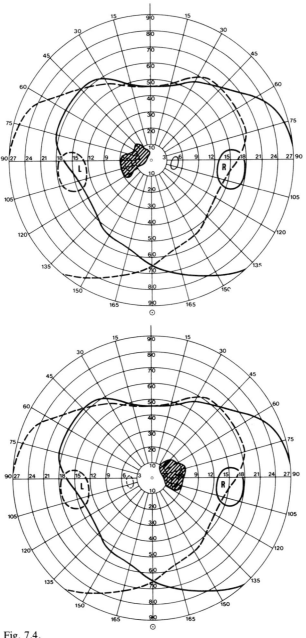

Fig. 7.4.
L and R
Outer limit of peripheral fields and paracentral scotomata to 2 mm
white object at $\frac{1}{3}$ metre.
V.A. 6/36 R 6/18 L
(From Mackenzie and Phillips 1968.)

retrobulbar neuritis (impaired vision with normal optic discs). Carroll (1956*b*) detailed 50 causes of toxic amblyopia, including substances having a primary effect on the retina. In many of these, the association has been based on a single case report or the implicated drug has long since been withdrawn from the market. Long-term follow-up of these cases has seldom been undertaken or, if it has, development of multiple sclerosis in some has indicated the irrelevance of the original association (Lynn 1959). Ideally, to establish a connection, re-exposure to the drug should cause fresh visual disturbance but, for ethical reasons, this policy has seldom been pursued. The following description generally concentrates on those drugs or agents where the association seems more definite.

Aniline dyes

Exposure to these substances, once used in hair dyes, has been reported to cause unilateral retrobulbar neuritis (Berger 1909) or bilateral papillitis (Keschner and Rosen 1941). The numbers reported are few, however, and the association not established.

Organic arsenical compounds

Administration of these substances to experimental animals produces a depletion of retinal ganglion cells with glial cell proliferation and optic nerve demyelination (Longley, Clausen, and Tatum 1942). Tryparsamide has caused severe visual failure, usually recovering on withdrawal of the drug (Moore 1937).

Aspidium (male fern)

This agent, used as an anthelmintic, characteristically produces a visual loss, sometimes with hallucinations, associated with deep orbital pain or pain on eye movement. Symptoms may be noted on waking and, although generally bilateral, are frequently asymmetrical and occasionally confined to one eye. Recovery occurs in the majority of cases, often with residual optic atrophy. In an outbreak in cattle, optic nerve examination of one specimen showed axonal fallout with myelin depletion and lymphocytic infiltration (Rosen, Edgar, and Smith 1969).

Binitrotoluene

In a single case (Hamilton and Nixon 1918) a remitting and relapsing peripheral neuropathy, attributed to intermittent exposure to binitro-toluene, was followed by the development of bilateral central scotomata with optic atrophy. With cessation of exposure (in a munitions factory) partial recovery occurred.

Bromisovalum

This drug, introduced as an hypnotic, is no longer available in Great Britain. Although occasional cases of visual disturbance were attributed to its use, in a series of 8 patients addicted to it, the clinical picture was dominated by a cerebello-bulbar syndrome (Harenko 1967).

Broxyquinoline

A combination of ataxia, peripheral sensory impairment, and unilateral optic atrophy in a 12-year-old boy followed exposure to this agent, introduced as an amoebocide in the early 1960s. The visual impairment progressed to bilateral optic atrophy, but long-term follow-up was not reported (Strandvik and Zetterström 1968).

Cafergot

Bilateral papillitis was reported in a 21-year-old female after ingestion of 40 cafergot tablets over 7 days (Gupta and Strobus 1972). Intake finally reached 104 tablets, with further visual failure. Cerebrospinal fluid examination was normal and recovery complete. In this instance the drug had been used for headache, but in another case a similar syndrome followed when ergot extract was used as an abortifacient (Kravitz 1935). The fundal vessels were not described in either example, and neither appears to have shown evidence of the type of peripheral vascular disturbance encountered with ergot intoxication (Perkin 1974).

Carbon dioxide

In two patients, exposure to high CO_2 concentrations led to the development of an ophthalmoplegia with constricted visual fields and enlarged blind spots but preserved visual acuities. Damage to the retinal ganglion cells, suggested by abnormalities of the EOG, was confirmed at post-mortem examination in one of the cases (Freedman and Sevel 1966).

Carbon disulphide

Severe, chronic poisoning with this agent may lead to impaired vision with central scotomata and depressed red/green discrimination. The changes are uncommon, being encountered in only 2 of 100 cases of intoxication in workers in a yarn and staple fibre factory (Vigliani 1950).

Carbon tetrachloride

Exposure has led to visual failure, often with constricted visual fields, and sometimes accompanied by other signs of intoxication, including headache, nausea, cramps, and impairment of memory (Smith 1950).

Carbromal

The hypnotic carbrital contains a combination of phenobarbitone and carbromal. Copas, Kay, and Longman (1959) reported intoxication in five patients, one of whom had an ill-defined blurring of the optic discs and another a temporal constriction of the visual fields. Although the evidence for visual impairment in this series is unconvincing, there are other reports in the literature suggesting occasional peripheral or central field defects, sometimes with optic atrophy.

Cephaloridine

This drug has been implicated as the cause of visual failure with disc swelling and peripheral pigmentation in one patient (Ballingall and Turpie 1967) but the case was a complicated one, with staphylococcal septicaemia, renal failure, and concurrent exposure to cloxacillin and fusidic acid.

Chloramphenicol

Joy, Scalettar, and Sodee (1960) found five cases in the literature where optic nerve involvement followed the use of this drug, three of them with associated peripheral neuropathy. The authors' own case, with visual blurring, showed optic disc swelling and congestion of retinal veins. Dosage usually exceeds 100 g over a period longer than 6 weeks before symptoms arise, and the complication is more common in children. Post-mortem examination shows optic atrophy with demyelination and degeneration of retinal ganglion cells (Grant 1974).

Chlorodinitrobenzene

Once used in munitions factories, this substance has similar effects to dinitrobenzene, with gradual visual loss due to central scotomata and constricted fields. In some instances, a peripheral neuropathy has accompanied the visual symptoms.

Chlorpropamide

The ability of this drug to affect vision is uncertain. In one instance, amaurosis appeared only after 6 months' exposure, and the picture of bilateral centro-caecal scotomata may have been more related to the patient's smoking habits, since, although visual improvement coincided with drug withdrawal, the patient was also treated with vitamins B_1 and B_{12} (Givner 1961). In a more convincing example, bilateral visual failure in a non-smoker was attributed to the drug, even though symptoms had commenced within two days of its use (George 1963). The drug had been used in the treatment of diabetes in both cases, neither of whom had any evidence of peripheral neuropathy.

Digitalis

Toxic effects develop in 7 per cent of patients receiving digitalis, a quarter of whom will manifest visual symptoms. Disturbances of colour vision and visual hallucinations are common, particularly with exposure to digitoxin. Central scotomata may occur and fundoscopy occasionally reveals narrowing of retinal arterioles (Robertson, Hollenhorst, and Callahan 1966*a*). Thresholds to dark adaptation change in digitalized subjects, implying a toxic effect on retinal receptor cells (Robertson, Hollenhorst and Callahan 1966*b*).

Disulfiram

This drug was implicated in the development of visual blurring in an alcoholic, who was not drinking at the time symptoms appeared (Norton and Walsh 1972). Vision improved with drug withdrawal, and similar examples, quoted from the French literature, included one patient in whom fresh visual symptoms and signs appeared on further exposure to the drug.

Dynamite

Visual failure following exposure to the atmosphere formed after dynamite explosion has been described. Carbon dioxide was considered the agent responsible in a man with permanent visual loss associated with optic atrophy (Brose 1899).

Ethambutol

The relationship of this drug to optic nerve disease is established, with axial and periaxial forms of toxicity (Liebold 1966). The former produce reduced visual acuity with central scotomata and marked impairment of green discrimination, the latter, peripheral field defects with near normal acuities and preserved red/green awareness. In one series, toxic effects of both types occurred with a mean daily dose of 43–7 mg/kg, the mean duration to onset of symptoms being 188 days for axial and 125 days for periaxial cases. After onset, signs progressed for a further 3 to 4 weeks despite withdrawal of the drug, the axial group averaging 6½ months to recovery, with occasional cases showing residual signs (Liebold 1966). Visual impairment with a daily dosage of 25 mg/kg, of up to 2 years' duration, occurred in 6 per cent of patients, but with a negligible frequency when intake was restricted to 15 mg/kg/day (Citron 1969). On occasions the initial visual disturbance is unilateral, but it generally involves the other eye within a month.

Ethchlorvynol

This drug, marketed as Placidyl, has been used as a non-barbiturate hypnotic. In a patient exposed to both alcohol and tobacco, bilateral central scotomata and a peripheral neuropathy developed after prolonged intake at high dosage (Brown and Meyer 1969). Vision improved on withdrawal of the drug combined with administration of thiamine, pyridoxine, and hydroxycobalamin.

Sodium fluoride

One case of bilateral macular oedema and unilateral papillitis has been attributed to sodium fluoride. Vision remained impaired in the more severely affected eye (Geall and Beilin 1964).

Insecticides and fungicides

Campbell (1952) recorded seven patients with neurological complications considered secondary to the use of insecticides, 2 showing a retrobulbar neuritis. Either DDT or pentachlorophenol was considered the responsible agent. DDT has been implicated in the causation of bilateral papillitis (Silverman and Laval 1963) and a preparation containing dieldrin and pentachlorophenol in a syndrome of bilateral visual failure with central scotomata (Jindal 1968). In a case of bilateral optic neuritis thought to be due to parathion intoxication (Brihaye, Graff, and Smulders, 1962) demyelination of the retrobulbar optic nerve was found, with lymphocytic infiltration, maximal at the site of penetration of central vessels. In an outbreak of poisoning by the fungicide, ethyl mercury toluene sulphonanilide (Jalici and Abbasi 1961), a number of neurological complications developed, including dysarthria, ataxia, pyramidal signs and, infrequently, constriction of the visual fields with subsequent optic atrophy.

Halogenated oxyquinoline derivatives

Tsubaki, Honma, and Hoshi (1971) observed neurological symptoms in 35·4 per cent of patients taking clioquinol for more than 14 days. In 16 patients that they examined personally, a syndrome was found resembling sub-acute myelo-optico-neuropathy (S.M.O.N.). In one series, 96 per cent of patients with S.M.O.N. gave a history of clioquinol intake prior to the onset of neurological symptoms. The role of a virus infection was considered in one report of 113 patients, though of those with an adequate drug history, 78·8 per cent had taken the drug before symptoms began (Shimada and Tsuji 1971). The possible significance of clioquinol in these cases was suggested by the finding of green urine, due to a chelate of the drug, in two patients (Igata 1971). By 1973, a total of 1839 cases of S.M.O.N. had been collected and, of these, 75 per cent had received clioquinol (Nakae, Yamamoto, Shigematsu, and Kono 1973).

Outside Japan, the association has only rarely been made (Steinitz 1971; Rose 1978) and Diodoquin, a related drug used as an amoebicide in the United States, does not give rise to neurological symptoms (Marsden and Knight 1971). Although most authors have cautiously accepted an association, cases of S.M.O.N. have occurred apparently in the absence of ingestion of the drug. Furthermore, there is a poor correlation between dosage and severity of neurological disease, and there is a paucity of cases reported outside Japan (Baumgartner *et al*. 1979). Oakley (1973), however, considered the association established and referred to case reports from Australia, Switzerland, Sweden, Denmark, Holland, Great Britain, and the United States.

Several cases of optic atrophy have been reported in children on long-term dosage for acrodermatitis enteropathica (Baumgartner *et al*. 1979). A further relationship to isolated optic nerve disease is raised by the case of a 12-year-old girl taking clioquinol as part of the treatment for ulcerative colitis. Bilateral paracentral scotomata appeared, improved on drug withdrawal but returned within 2 days of restoring the drug (Reich and Billson 1973). Further improvement in vision followed cessation of the drug, and no subsequent spontaneous relapses were seen.

Hexamethonium

Bilateral blindness has followed intramuscular hexamethonium associated with a fall in systolic blood pressure from 270 to 180 mm (Bruce 1955). Attenuation of retinal arterioles and slight retinal oedema were observed. Vision failed to recover and bilateral optic atrophy followed. The syndrome was compared to that seen with systemic collapse or exsanguination.

Iodoform

Various reports in the German literature implicated this topical antiseptic in the causation of visual disturbance, but it is no longer available.

Iophendylate

In a 29-year-old woman having myelography following a cervical flexion/extension injury, pain and warmth appeared around the right eye (contrast had entered the cranium), associated with scintillations (Tabaddor 1973). The symptoms subsided rapidly but 1 month later, further pain occurred with the development of a central scotoma in the right eye. Skull X-ray revealed the presence of myodil droplets in the region of the optic nerve, the cerebrospinal fluid showing a mildly elevated protein concentration with a normal electrophoretic pattern; recovery was rapid. A vascular aetiology was considered the cause of the immediate reaction, the later disturbance being attributed to an arachnoiditis, in spite of the rapidity with which the symptoms improved.

Isoniazid

Because of the known propensity for tuberculous meningitis to cause visual disturbances (pp. 103–4), optic neuropathy attributable to isoniazid depends on its occurrence in tuberculous cases without central nervous system infection. Peripheral neuropathy is a recognized complication of the drug, the effect being dose-dependent and reversible by pyridoxine therapy. Three patients with optic atrophy have been reported; all received 200 mg of isoniazid daily and none had evidence of a peripheral neuropathy (Sutton and Beattie 1955; Keeping and Searle 1955). The combination of optic atrophy and peripheral neuropathy has been seen (Dixon, Roberts, and Tyrell 1956; Kass, Mandel, Cohen, and Dressler 1957) as has a syndrome resembling neuromyelitis optica. Post-mortem examination in the latter case revealed demyelination of the optic tracts with extensive softening of the grey matter of the spinal cord maximal in the mid-dorsal region (Dixon *et al.* 1956). The peripheral nerves were not examined. Tuberculous disease was confined to the lungs. In another case with post-mortem examination (Kass *et al.* 1957) sections of the optic nerve were considered unremarkable despite the history of bilateral papillitis with severe visual failure and subsequent optic atrophy. Hughes and Mair (1977) have recently reported three cases of acute myelopathy in patients with pulmonary tuberculosis, one patient having, in addition, bilateral retrobulbar neuritis. This patient, and one other, had been treated with isoniazid but the authors preferred to consider the possibility of an abnormality of cell mediated immunity as the precipitating factor.

Lead

Lead has long been considered an occasional cause of optic neuritis. An early example (Loewe 1906) had a history of exposure and developed signs of generalized intoxication, with colic, anorexia, and a gingival line, in addition to bilateral visual failure; and a similar case was recorded in the Mayo Clinic material (Lillie 1934). Loewe (1906) reviewed the literature, finding over 60 cases. Any type of fundal change is seen and the amaurosis is frequently evanescent with complete recovery. Gibson (1931) believed that ocular manifestations in children reflected raised intracranial pressure, with papilloedema and sixth nerve palsies, and recommended therapeutic lumbar puncture. It seems certain, however, that a genuine optic neuropathy occurs, exemplified by more recent cases (Carroll 1952; Baghdassarian 1968). It has been suggested that ocular involvement may rarely be the initial or early manifestation of intoxication. In one patient the combination of visual failure and ocular pain suggested an optic neuritis (Baghdassarian 1968), signs of generalized toxicity being restricted to the demonstration of basophilic stippling. Lead has even been implicated in the causation of multiple sclerosis (Cone, Russell, and Harwood 1934). The patient in question developed a combination of optic neuritis and transverse myelitis, with grossly abnormal cerebrospinal fluid, and a histological pattern resembling Devic's disease. Exposure to lead had been confined to lunch-time painting sessions for 2 years but the findings of lead in bone, liver, brain, and spinal cord was considered sufficient explanation for the clinical disturbance.

Methyl alcohol

This substance, a constituent of wood alcohol, is recognized to cause an acute optic neuropathy. Three examples have been given by Woods and Rowland (1931).

Methyl ethyl ketone

Following exposure to this solvent for $1\frac{1}{2}$ hours, an 18-year-old seaman developed sudden visual failure with slight ataxia (Berg 1971). Field testing was unsatisfactory but suggested arcuate scotomata with enlargement of the blind spots. Cortico steroids and B complex vitamins were given, vision eventually recovering completely. Although both methanol and formaldehyde were found in blood specimens, neither was thought responsible for the amaurosis.

Mono-amine-oxidase inhibitors

Pheniprazine, once used in the treatment of hypertension, occasionally produced a syndrome of optic neuropathy with central scotoma and early impairment of red/green colour discrimination (Jones 1961). Histological examination reveals areas of degeneration and inflammatory cell infiltration with associated demyelination. Optic nerve involvement from other mono-amine-oxidase inhibitors has not been recorded.

Oral contraceptives

Walsh, Clark, Thompson, and Nicholson (1965) collected eight cases of optic neuritis which had been attributed to the use of oral contraceptives. The very variable features, including recovery in some despite continuing the drug, and progression in others despite its withdrawal, cast doubt on the significance of the association.

Penicillamine

In a patient with Wilson's disease (Goldstein, Hollenhorst, Randall, and Gross 1966) treatment with penicillamine led to visual blurring 12 months later. Subsequently arteriolar sheathing and obstruction of macular arterioles were seen. With reduction of dosage (1500 to 750 mg daily) vision recovered, leaving residual optic atrophy. This patient had received pyridox-ine therapy throughout, tending to refute the suggestion (Tu, Blackwell, and Lee 1963) that the visual disturbance is due to an induced pyridoxine deficiency.

Phenothiazines

A pigmentary retinopathy develops in some individuals given phenothiazines in high dosage (Weekley, Potts, Reboton, and May 1960). Appelbaum (1963) discussed a number of ocular disturbances arising during thioridazine therapy, but terms such as 'optic neuritis' and 'neuro-retinitis' were not defined and the association not established.

Quinine

Objective ophthalmoscopic signs may be minimal and systemic disturbances lacking in cases of quinine amblyopia. An action on retinal ganglion cells with a possible secondary vascular component is accepted (Bard and Gills 1964). Peripheral constriction of the visual fields is usual and pigmentary abnormalities may follow (Moore 1937).

Streptomycin

It has been suggested (Thomas 1950) that streptomycin causes upper tem-poral arcuate scotomata for red, generally following doses of 1–2 g daily over a period of 12–37 days. In many of these cases, however, fields were done after the drug had been discontinued, in one instance the interval being 6 months. The changes were unilateral or bilateral and were seldom re-assessed. Sykowski (1951) implicated streptomycin as the cause of bilateral retrobulbar neuritis, the drug having been given in large doses for pyelitis. Recovery of vision followed withdrawal of the drug, but long-term follow-up was not undertaken.

Sulfanilamide

Bilateral papillitis in association with methaemoglobinaemia has been described after large doses, with recovery on cessation of the drug (Bucy 1937).

Thallium

Many cases of intoxication by this agent in the 1930s arose from its presence in a proprietary preparation for hair removal. The optic neuropathy was usually accompanied by a peripheral neuropathy and often by hair loss (Lillie and Parker 1932; Mahoney 1932). The accidental substitution of thallium for common salt, and its subsequent use in cooking, led to an outbreak in a family (Carroll 1952). Manschot (1969) has reviewed the subject in detail. In a single, personal case, post-mortem examination showed a complete loss of retinal ganglion cells with atrophy of the corresponding nerve fibre layer. Atrophic changes were present in the optic nerves, olives, and parts of the cerebellum.

Trichlorethylene

This agent occasionally causes optic nerve damage, usually in association with signs of other cranial nerve involvement (Buxton and Hayward 1967; Feldman and Mayer 1968).

Vinyl benzene (Styrene)

This substance is used in the glass fibre industry. In one report, bilateral centro-caecal scotomata occurred, the patient being a cigarette smoker and moderate drinker. B complex vitamins and cortico steroids were given and vision recovered (Pratt-Johnson 1964). As with other, isolated, reports of an association between a toxic agent and visual disturbance, the possibility of another disease process being present cannot be excluded. Grant (1974) cites a case of central scotoma following exposure. Further examination, and a study of the patient's family revealed the correct diagnosis of Leber's optic atrophy.

Conclusions

A number of vitamin deficiencies may produce visual disturbances, the best studied being the syndrome associated with pernicious anaemia, where a characteristic bilateral centro-caecal scotoma develops, not necessarily associated with anaemia or other neurological disturbance. There is a close similarity between the optic neuropathy of pernicious anaemia and that of tobacco–alcohol amblyopia, both conditions responding to hydroxy-cobalamin, even if smoking continues.

The syndrome of tropical amblyopia is not well defined and its relationship to intoxication by dietary cyanide has not, as yet, been confirmed.

Although a number of drugs and toxic agents can clearly influence optic nerve or retinal function, the association in other instances rests on single case reports. The best established examples are with ethambutol, isoniazid, lead, methyl alcohol, phenothiazines, quinine, thallium, organic arsenical compounds, aspidium, carbon disulphide, carbon tetrachloride, chloramphenicol, and digitalis. In many instances the overlap of the visual syndrome with that due to optic neuritis is minimal. Peripheral constriction of the fields is as common as central involvement and ocular pain is conspicuously absent, with the well documented exception of aspidium. The development of multiple sclerosis has refuted a drug cause of the presenting optic neuritis in some instances, but with two substances, isoniazid and lead, a syndrome resembling Devic's disease has been attributed to intoxication. Most toxic optic neuropathies are bilateral, and unilateral cases should cast suspicion on the diagnosis.

REFERENCES

Appelbaum, A. (1963). An ophthalmoscopic study of patients under treatment with thioridazine. *Archs Ophthal., N.Y.* **69**, 578–80.
Baghdassarian, S. A. (1968). Optic neuropathy due to lead poisoning. *Archs Ophthal., N.Y.* **80**, 721–3.
Bagley, C. H. (1952). An etiologic study of a series of optic neuropathies. *Am. J. Ophthal.* **35**, 761–72.
Ballingall, D. L. K. and Turpie, A. G. G. (1967). Cephaloridine toxicity. *Lancet* **2**, 835–6.
Bard, L. A. and Gills, J. P. (1964). Quinine amblyopia. *Archs Ophthal., N.Y.* **72**, 328–31.
Baumgartner, G., Gawel, M. J., Kaeser, H. E., Pallis, C. A., Rose, F. C., Schaumberg, H. H., Thomas, P. K., and Wadia, N. H. (1979). Neurotoxicity due to halogenated hydroxy-oxyquinolines: A clinical analysis of cases reported outside Japan (in press).
Beam, A. D. (1947). Amblyopia due to dietary deficiency. *Am. J. Ophthal.* **30**, 66–70.
Benham, G. H. H. (1951). The visual field defects in subacute combined degeneration of the spinal cord. *J. Neurol. Neurosurg. Psychiat.* **14**, 40–6.
Berg, E. F. (1971). Retrobulbar neuritis. A case report of presumed solvent toxicity. *Ann. Ophthal.* **3**, 1351–3.
Berger, E. (1909). Visual disturbances due to the use of hair dye containing anilin. *Archs Ophthal., N.Y.* **38**, 397–400.
Björkenheim, B. (1966). Optic neuropathy caused by vitamin-B_{12} deficiency in carriers of the fish tapeworm, diphyllobothrium latum. *Lancet* **1**, 688–90.
Box, C. R. (1936). Amaurosis in pernicious anaemia. *Lancet* **2**, 1269.
Bradley, W. G. (1968). Symptomatic optic neuritis. *Dis. nerv. Syst.* **29**, 668–73.
Brihaye, M. Graff, E., and Smulders, J. (1962). Retrobulbar optic neuritis: anatomical and clinical study (poisoning by parathion ?) *Mult. Scler. Abstr.* **7**, 17.
Brose, L. D. (1899). Amaurosis following the entrance of a well after the use of dynamite. *Archs Ophthal., N.Y.* **28**, 402–6.
Brown, E. and Meyer, G. G. (1969). Toxic amblyopia and peripheral neuropathy with ethchlorvynol abuse. *Am. J. Psychiat.* **126**, 882–4.
Bruce, G. M. (1955). Permanent bilateral blindness following the use of hexamethonium chloride. *Archs Ophthal., N.Y.* **54**, 422–4.
Bucy, P. C. (1937). Toxic optic neuritis resulting from sulfanilamide. *J. Am. med. Ass.* **109**, 1007–8.
Buxton, P. H. and Hayward, M. (1967). Polyneuritis cranialis associated with industrial trichlorethylene poisoning. *J. Neurol. Neurosurg. Psychiat.* **30**, 511–18.
Campbell, A. M. G. (1952). Neurological complications associated with insecticides and fungicides. *Br. med. J.* **2**, 415–17.
Carroll, F. D. (1952). Optic neuritis. A 15-year study. *Am. J. Ophthal.* **35**, 75–82.
——(1956a). Nutritional amblyopia. *Trans. Am. Acad. Ophthal. Oto-lar.* **60**, 71–3.
——(1956b). Toxic amblyopia. *Trans. Am. Acad. Ophthal. Oto-lar.* **60**, 74–82.
Citron. K. M. (1969). Ethambutol—A review with special reference to ocular toxicity. *Tubercle, Lond.* Vol. 50 (Supplement), 32–6.
Cohen, H. (1936). Optic atrophy as the presenting sign in pernicious anaemia. *Lancet* **2**, 1202–3.
Cone, W., Russell, C., and Harwood, R. U. (1934). Lead as a possible cause of multiple sclerosis. *Archs Neurol. Psychiat., Chicago* **31**, 236–69.

Copas, D. E., Kay, W. W., and Longman, U. H. (1959). Carbromal intoxication. *Lancet* 1, 703–5.

Crews, S. J. (1963). Bilateral amblyopia in West Indians. *Trans. ophthal. Soc. U.K.* 83, 653–67.

Dixon, G. J., Roberts, G. B. S., and Tyrell, W. F. (1956). The relationship of neuropathy to the treatment of tuberculosis. *Scott. med. J.* 1, 350–4.

Duke-Elder, S. and Scott, G. I. (1971a). *System of ophthalmology*, Vol. XII, *Neuro-ophthalmology*, p. 151. Henry Kimpton, London.

————. (1971b) *System of Ophthalmology*, Vol XII, *Neuro-ophthalmology*, p. 152. Henry Kimpton, London.

Enoksson, P. and Norden, A. (1960). Vitamin B_{12} deficiency affecting the optic nerve. *Acta med. scand.* 167, 199–208.

Feldman, R. G. and Mayer, R. F. (1968). Studies of trichlorethylene intoxication in man. *Neurology, Minneap.* 18, 309.

Fisher, M. (1955). Residual neuropathological changes in Canadians held prisoners of war by the Japanese. *Can. Serv. med. J.* 11, 157–99.

Foulds, W. S., Chisholm I. A., and Pettigrew, A. R. (1974). The toxic optic neuropathies. *Br. J. Ophthal.* 58, 386–90.

————Stewart, J. B., and Wilson, T. M. (1969). The optic nerve neuropathy of pernicious anaemia. *Archs Ophthal., N.Y.* 82, 427–32.

Freedman, A. and Sevel, D. (1966). The cerebro-ocular effects of carbon dioxide poisoning. *Archs Ophthal., N.Y.* 76, 59–65.

Freeman, A. G. and Heaton, J. M. (1961). The aetiology of retrobulbar neuritis in Addisonian pernicious anaemia. *Lancet* 1, 908–11.

Gautier-Smith, P. C. (1973). Lhermitte's sign in subacute combined degeneration of the cord. *J. Neurol. Neurosurg. Psychiat.* 36, 861–3.

Geall, M. G. and Beilin, L. J. (1964). Sodium fluoride and optic neuritis. *Br. med. J.* 2, 355–6.

George, C. W. (1963). Central scotoma due to chlorpropamide (Diabenese). *Archs Ophthal., N.Y.* 69, 773.

Gibson, J. L. (1931). Ocular plumbism in children. *Br. J. Ophthal.* 15, 637–42.

Givner, I. (1961). Centrocecal scotomas due to chlorpropamide. *Archs Ophthal., N.Y.* 66, 64.

Goldstein, N. P., Hollenhorst, R. W., Randall, R. V., and Gross, J. B. (1966). Possible relationship of optic neuritis, Wilson's disease and DL-Penicillamine therapy. *J. Am. med. Ass.* 196, 734–5.

Grant, W. M. (1974). *Toxicology of the eye.* Charles C. Thomas, Springfield, Illinois.

Gupta, D. R. and Strobus, R. J. (1972). Bilateral papillitis associated with cafergot therapy. *Neurology, Minneap.* 22, 793–7.

Hamilton, A. S. and Nixon, C. E. (1918). Optic atrophy and multiple peripheral neuritis developed in the manufacture of explosives (Binitrotoluene). *J. Am. med. Ass.* 70, 2004–6.

Hamilton, H. E., Ellis, P. P., and Sheets, R. F. (1959). Visual impairment due to optic neuropathy in pernicious anaemia. Report of a case and review of the literature. *Blood* 14, 378–85.

Harenko, A. (1967). Irreversible cerebello-bulbar syndrome as the sequela of bromisovalum poisoning. *Annls. Med. intern. Fenn.* 56, 29–36.

Heaton, J. M., McCormick. A. J. A., and Freeman, A. G. (1958). Tobacco amblyopia: A clinical manifestation of vitamin-B_{12} deficiency. *Lancet* 2, 286–90.

Hine, M. L. (1935). Subacute combined degeneration of cord in pernicious anaemia with retrobulbar neuritis. *Proc. R. Soc. Med.* 29, 386.

Hughes, R. A. C. and Mair, W. G. P. (1977). Acute necrotic myelopathy with pulmonary tuberculosis. *Brain* 100, 223–38.

Igata, A. (1971). Halogenated oxyquinoline derivatives and neurological syndromes. *Lancet* 2, 42–3.

Jalici, M. A. and Abbasi, A. H. (1961). Poisoning by ethyl mercury toluene and sulphonanilide. *Br. J. ind. Med.* 18, 303–8.

Jindal, H. R. (1968). Bilateral retrobulbar neuritis due to insecticides. *Post-grad. med. J.* 44, 341–2.

Jones, III, O. W. (1961). Toxic amblyopia caused by pheniprazine hydrochloride (JB-516, Catron). *Archs Ophthal., N.Y.* **66**, 29–36.

Joy, R. J. T., Scalettar, R., and Sodee, D.B. (1960). Optic and peripheral neuritis. *J. Am. med. Ass.* **173**, 1731–4.

Kass, K., Mandel, W., Cohen, H. and Dressler, S.H. (1957). Isoniazid as a cause of optic neuritis and atrophy. *J. Am. med. Ass.* **164**, 1740–3.

Keeping, J. A. and Searle, C. W. A. (1955). Optic neuritis following isoniazid therapy. *Lancet* **2**, 278.

Keschner, M. and Rosen, V. H. (1941). Optic neuritis caused by a coal tar hair dye. *Archs Ophthal., N.Y.* **25**, 1020–4.

Kravitz, D. (1935). Neuro-retinitis associated with symptoms of ergot poisoning. *Archs Ophthal., N.Y.* **13**, 201–6.

Leishman, R. (1951). Gastric function in tobacco amblyopia. *Trans. ophthal. Soc. U.K.* **71**, 319–26.

Lerman, S. and Feldmahn, A. L. (1961). Centrocaecal scotoma as the presenting sign in pernicious anaemia. *Archs Ophthal., N.Y.* **65**, 381–5.

Levine, J. (1934). Pellagra as a cause of optic neuritis. *Archs Ophthal., N.Y.* **12**, 902–9.

Liebold, J. E. (1966). The ocular toxicity of ethambutol and its relation to dose. *Ann. N.Y. Acad. Sci.* **135**, 904–9.

Lillie, W. I. (1934). The clinical significance of retrobulbar and optic neuritis. *Am. J. Ophthal.* **17**, 110–19.

— and Parker, H. L. (1932). Retrobulbar neuritis due to thallium poisoning. *J. Am. med. Ass.* **98**, 1347–9.

Livingston, P. C. (1946). Ocular disturbances associated with malnutrition. *Trans. ophthal. Soc. U.K.* **66**, 19–44.

Loewe, O. (1906). A case of transient lead amaurosis. *Archs Ophthal., N.Y.* **35**, 164–71.

Longley, B. J., Clausen, N. M., and Tatum, A. L. (1942). The experimental production of primary optic atrophy in monkeys by administration of organic arsenical compounds. *J. Pharmac. exp. Ther.* **76**, 202–6.

Lynn, B. H. (1959). Retrobulbar neuritis. A survey of the present condition of cases occurring over the last fifty-six years. *Trans ophthal. Soc. U.K.* **79**, 701–16.

Mackenzie, A. D. and Phillips, C. I. (1968). West Indian amblyopia. *Brain* **91**, 249–60.

Mahoney, W. (1932). Retrobulbar neuritis due to thallium poisoning from depilatory cream. Report of 3 cases. *J. Am. med. Ass.* **98**, 618–20.

Manschot, W. A. (1969). Ophthalmic pathological findings in a case of thallium poisoning. In *Occupational and medicative hazards in ophthalmology* (Ed. J. François,). pp. 348–9. S. Karger, Basel and New York.

Marsden, P. D. and Knight, R. (1971). Halogenated oxyquinoline derivatives. *Lancet* **1**, 854.

Montgomery, R. D., Cruickshank, E. K., Robertson, W. B., and McMenemey, W. H. (1964). Clinical and pathological observations on Jamaican neuropathy. *Brain* **87**, 425–62.

Moore, J. I. (1937). An etiologic study of a series of optic neuropathies. *Am. J. Ophthal.* **20**, 1099–1108.

Nakae, K., Yamamoto, S., Shigematsu, I., and Kono, R. (1973). Relation between subacute myelo-optic neuropathy (S.M.O.N.) and clioquinol: nationwide survey. *Lancet* **1**, 171–3.

Nelson, M. G. and Weaver, J. A. (1956). A case of Addisonian pernicious anaemia presenting with optic atrophy, iron-deficiency anaemia and pigmentation of the skin. *Ir. J. med. Sci.* **6**, 229–33.

Norton, A. L. and Walsh, F. B. (1972). Disulfiram-induced optic neuritis. *Trans. Am. Acad. Ophthal. Oto-lar.* **76**, 1263–5.

Oakley, Jnr, G. P. (1973). The neurotoxicity of the halogenated hydroxyquinolines. *J. Am. med. Ass.* **225**, 395–7.

Olivarus, B. De F. and Jensen, L. (1961). Retrobulbar neuritis and optic atrophy in pernicious anaemia. *Acta ophthal.* **39**, 190–7.

Osuntokun, B. O. (1968). An ataxic neuropathy in Nigeria. A clinical, biochemical and electrophysiological study. *Brain* **91**, 215–48.

Perkin, G. D. (1974). Ischaemic lateral popliteal nerve palsy due to ergot intoxication. *J. Neurol. Neurosurg. Psychiat.* **37**, 1389–91.

Pratt-Johnson, J. A. (1964). Retrobulbar neuritis following exposure to vinyl benzene (styrene). *Can. med. Ass. J.* **90**, 975–7.

Reich, J. A. and Billson, F.A. (1973). Toxic optic neuritis. Clioquinol ingestion in a child. *Med. J. Aust.* **2**, 593–5.

Robertson, D. M., Hollenhorst, R. W., and Callahan, J. A. (1966*a*). A discussion and report of three cases of central scotomas. *Archs Ophthal., N.Y.* **76**, 640–5.

—— (1966*b*). Receptor function in digitalis therapy. *Archs Ophthal, N.Y.* **76**, 852–7.

Rose, F. C. (1978). On the diagnosis of subacute myelo-optaic neuropathy (S.M.O.N) outside Japan. In *Epidemiological issues in reported drug-induced illnesses—S.M.O.N. and other examples* (ed. M. Geur and I. Shigematsu), pp. 271–82. McMaster University Library Press. Hamilton, Ontario, Canada.

Rosen, E. S., Edgar, J. T., and Smith, J. L. S. (1969). Male fern retrobulbar neuropathy in cattle. *Trans. ophthal. Soc. U.K.* **89**, 285–99.

Sharpe, V. J. H. and Hyland. H. H. (1952). Optic nerve degeneration in pernicious anaemia. *Can. med. Ass. J.* **67**, 660–5.

Shimada, Y. and Tsuji, T. (1971). Halogenated oxyquinoline derivatives and neurological syndromes. *Lancet* **2**, 41–2.

Silverman, S.M. and Laval, J. (1963). Bilateral simultaneous retrobulbar neuritis. *Am. J. Ophthal.* **55**, 1020–3.

Smith, A.R. (1950). Optic atrophy following inhalation of carbon tetrachloride. *Archs ind. Hyg.* **1**, 348–51.

Spillane, J. D. and Scott, G.I. (1945). Obscure neuropathy in the Middle East. *Lancet* **2**, 261–4.

Steinitz, H. (1971). Halogenated oxyquinoline derivatives and neurological syndromes. *Lancet* **2**, 43.

Strandvik, B. and Zetterström, R. (1968). Amaurosis after broxyquinoline. *Lancet* **1**, 922–3.

Sutton, P. H. and Beattie, P. H. (1955). Optic atrophy after administration of isoniazid with P.A.S. *Lancet* **1**, 650–1.

Sykowski, P. (1951). Streptomycin causing retrobulbar optic neuritis. *Am. J. Ophthal.* **34**, 1446.

Tabaddor, K. (1973). Unusual complications of iophendylate injection myelography. *Archs Neurol., Chicago* **29**, 435–6.

Talbot, G. (1936). Pernicious anaemia with retro-bulbar neuritis. *Br. J. Ophthal.* **20**, 619–21.

Thomas, E.B. (1950). Scotomas in conjunction with streptomycin therapy. Report of eleven cases. *Archs Ophthal., N.Y.* **43**, 729–41.

Traquair, H. M. (1930). Toxic amblyopia, including retrobulbar neuritis. *Trans. ophthal. Soc. U.K.* **50**, 351–85.

— (1957). *Clinical perimetry* (7th ed.)(ed. G. I. Scott). Henry Kimpton, London.

Tsubaki, T., Honma, Y., and Hoshi, M. (1971). Neurological syndrome associated with clioquinol. *Lancet* **1**, 696–7.

Tu, J., Blackwell, R. Q., and Lee, P. (1963). DL-Penicillamine as a cause of optic axial neuritis. *J. Am. med. Ass.* **185**, 83–6.

Tuboku-Metzger, A.F. (1969). Diet and neuropathy. *Br. med. J.* **4**, 239.

Turner, J. W. A. (1940). Optic atrophy associated with pernicious anaemia. *Brain* **63**, 225–36.

Victor, M. (1963). Tobacco-alcohol amblyopia. *Archs Ophthal., N.Y.* **70**, 313–18.

Vigliani, E. C. (1950). Clinical observations on carbon disulfide intoxication in Italy. *Ind. Med. Surg.* **19**, 240–2.

Walsh, F. B., Clark, D. B., Thompson, R. S., and Nicholson, D. H. (1965). Oral contraceptives and neuro-ophthalmological interest. *Archs Ophthal., N.Y.* **74**, 628–40.

Weekley, R. D., Potts, A. M., Reboton, J., and May, R. H. (1960). Pigmentary retinopathy in patients receiving high doses of a new phenothiazine. *Archs Ophthal. N.Y.* **64**, 65–76.

Woods, A. C. and Rowland, W. M. (1931). An etiologic study of a series of optic neuropathies. *J. Am. med. Ass.* **97**, 375–9.

8 Differential diagnosis: hereditary and other disorders

That the phenomena of the disease resemble the picture of bulbar or retrobulbar neuritis is beyond dispute. (Wilson 1954).

Hereditary

The majority of cases of familial optic neuropathy are unlikely to cause diagnostic confusion with optic neuritis. A classification of these disorders has been proposed by Waardenburg (1963):
1. Autosomal, recessive types of congenital and early infantile optic atrophy.
2. Optic atrophy and spastic paraplegia—dominant and sex-linked.
3. Behr's infantile optic atrophy.
4. Autosomal dominant optic atrophy:
    a moderate, benign type—early infantile or congenital ?stationary;
    b severe infantile type.
5. Leber's disease.

Recessive, congenital type

The condition presents at, or shortly after, birth, vision loss is profound and other neurological manifestations exceptional.

Optic atrophy and spastic paraplegia

Optic atrophy occurs less commonly in hereditary spastic paraplegia than in the hereditary ataxias. In a typical family described by Bickerstaff (1950), two children of the fourth generation developed visual symptoms in association with disc swelling. Vision loss (bilateral in one) was profound, though some recovery occurred. One of the children subsequently developed a mild spastic paraparesis (Bickerstaff, personal communication), but visual disturbances were absent in those members of the family with a typical paraplegia. No information is available on subsequent generations.

Visual loss in Friedreich's ataxia has been reported in between 9 and 12 per cent of patients (Greenfield 1963). In the family described by Sanger Brown (1892), where the ataxia was associated with considerable spinocerebellar degeneration (Meyer 1897), visual failure was sometimes of late onset and, initially, unilateral. An exacerbation of the visual disturbance by bright light, and of the ataxia by exertion, was noted in some individuals. A diagnosis of multiple sclerosis has been entertained in some cases of hereditary ataxia (Ferguson and Critchley 1929), but remissions were conspicuously absent and visual failure, when present, slowly progressive. Leeuwen and Van Bogaert (1949) have recorded a case of ataxia with optic atrophy, thought to be on a hereditary basis, though a positive family history was lacking. Sudden vision loss occurred in this case, coincidental with progression of a pre-existing ataxia. Post-mortem examination showed degeneration of both papillomacular bundles. Three types of optic atrophy in association with the hereditary ataxias have been distinguished (Leeuwen and Van Bogaert 1949). In the first, visual failure is considerable but incomplete, central field defects predominating. With the second type, visual failure is more rapid and profound, beginning at a younger age and associated with severe optic atrophy. The final group is distinguished by a combination of marked impairment of visual acuity with peripheral constriction of the visual fields, though this category appears less well defined than the other two.

Behr's infantile optic atrophy

This condition, beginning in early childhood, and usually transmitted as a recessive, combines optic atrophy with ataxia and pyramidal signs. The clinical overlap with optic neuritis is slight but in one family (Leeuwen and Van Bogaert 1949) the appearance of the complete syndrome in the fourth generation had been preceded by an isolated mild optic atrophy in three earlier generations.

Autosomal dominant optic atrophy

The condition is either congenital or usually develops within the first few years of life (Kok-Van Alphen 1960). The severity of visual loss varies and is sometimes asymmetrical (Lodberg and Lund 1950). Central scotoma, peripheral constriction, or a combination of the two have all been described. Some cases, initially classified as Leber's disease, have shown dominant transmission through males (Thompson and Cashell 1935), and are best included in this group. In one family, with dominant transmission (Norris 1882), onset was as late as 48 years, with subsequent severe visual failure and optic atrophy.

Leber's optic atrophy

This is the particular hereditary disorder (as the chapter epigraph indicates) affecting optic nerve function most likely to cause diagnostic confusion with optic neuritis, both from certain characteristics of the visual failure, and from a tendency for a more generalized neurological disorder to develop with features resembling multiple sclerosis. The criteria for diagnosis have been clouded by the inclusion, in Bell's monograph (1931) of cases without the typical transmission (e.g. Norris, 1882, 1884), or with features more suggestive of retinitis pigmentosa (Griscom 1921).

The character of the visual symptoms

Sudden visual failure, sometimes discovered on waking (Bedell 1934; Bruyn and Went 1964), may occur, but the majority of cases reach a maximum disability within 2 months of the onset, progression beyond 6 months being rare. Bilateral, simultaneous involvement is usual but intervals of 3 and 8 years (Mathieu 1901) and 3½ years (Taylor and Holmes 1913) have been recorded, as has apparent unilateral loss alone (Guzmann 1913). The mean age of European male cases is 23 years and of females 25 years (Bell 1931), though onset in young children and in individuals over the age of 50 years is recorded.

Pain is uncommon, but dull frontal (Taylor 1892), orbital (Storey 1885), or retro-orbital pains have been described, the last exacerbated by eye movement (Lawton Smith, Hoyt, and Susac 1973). A history of migraine, not necessarily coinciding with vision loss, is not uncommon (Taylor and Holmes 1913).

The type of field defect

Central scotomata predominate in both males (88 per cent) and females (82 per cent) (Fig. 8.1), though often with some degree of peripheral constriction in addition (42·5 and 62 per cent respectively (Bell 1931)). Norris (1884) postulated a characteristic scotoma extending between 5 and 10° from fixation whilst Wilson (1954) had stressed an absolute central scotoma with irregular edges in the chronic stages. Paracentral and even annular scotomata (Hancock 1908) have been encountered.

Pupils and fundus appearance

Lawton Smith *et al*. (1973) have recently emphasized the possibly unique fundal changes in the acute stages, including blurred disc margins, glistening opacity of the peripapillary nerve fibre layer, tortuous retinal vessels, and an irregular telangiectatic dilatation of capillaries in the peripapillary and pre-papillary networks. Fluorescein angiography showed no evidence of abnormal vascular permeability. Bell (1931) concluded that 'the appearance of the fundus may vary from complete normality to that indicative of an acute inflammatory reaction—with reddening of the nerve head, blurring of its margins, dilatation and tortuosity of the vessels and perhaps some small haemorrhages'. Norris (1884) observed retinal striations extending from the disc margin, macular oedema, and subsequent vascular sheathing in some instances, the last confirmed by Taylor (1892). Batten (1909) described symmetrical retinal haemorrhages and macular oedema in a case seen three

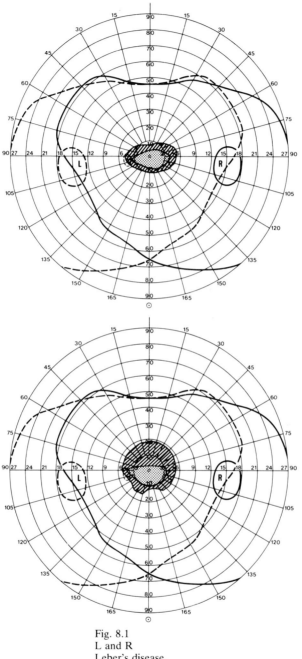

Fig. 8.1
L and R
Leber's disease.
V.A. R. C.F. L. C.F. at 1 metre
Scotoma 1, 20/330
(From Traquair 1923.)

weeks after the onset of visual symptoms. A similar account of these changes was given by Van Heuven (1924).

Natural history and response to steroids

Slight visual recovery may occur but on occasions has been virtually complete, either in one (Taylor 1892; Taylor and Holmes 1913) or both eyes (Leber 1871; Nettleship 1903; Hancock 1908; Bruyn *et al*, 1964), sometimes several years after onset. Recurrences of visual failure are rare (Guzman, 1913; Bruyn and Went 1964; Wallace 1970). ACTH therapy has been proposed (Lees, MacDonald, and Turner 1964), though there is no evidence for its value.

Other clinical features

In one series (Bell 1931) of 661 cases, 86·7 per cent were male, though a higher female incidence has been recorded in Japanese patients. Diagnostic problems can arise when a more generalized neurological disturbance coincides with, or follows, vision loss. After the onset of symptoms, some patients notice an exacerbation of visual blurring by various factors, of the type encountered by individuals with multiple sclerosis (Uhthoff 1890). Precipitating factors have included exercise (Norris 1884; Lawton Smith *et al*. 1973), emotional stress (Taylor and Holmes 1913), hot baths, or drinking warm fluids (Lawton Smith *et al*. 1973).

Limb cramps and paraesthesiae have long been noted in association with the optic atrophy (Taylor 1892; Batten 1909) and may be accompanied by sphincter disturbances and depressed limb reflexes (Taylor and Holmes 1913). Spasticity with exaggerated reflexes and extensor plantar responses is described, sometimes with athetosis of the limbs (Bruyn and Went 1964). Short-lived confusional episodes occur, as can a more florid encephalitic syndrome embracing headache, disturbance of consciousness, epilepsy, disorders of respiratory rhythm, and pyramidal dysfunction (Wallace 1970). Some patients show the picture of a progressive dementia (Wilson 1963; Adams, Blackwood, and Wilson 1966).

The associated neurological symptoms may resemble multiple sclerosis to the extent that a second diagnosis has been considered (Lees *et al*. 1964; Bruyn and Went 1964). One patient, for example, developed a hemiparesis shortly after the onset of bilateral visual failure, whilst another showed a progressive limb spasticity with sensory and sphincter disturbances. Bruyn and Went (1964) considered multiple sclerosis the more likely diagnosis in the only female in their family who presented with diplopia followed by visual failure, limb spasticity, and sensory disturbance with incontinence, particularly as cerebrospinal fluid examination revealed an abnormal cell count and paretic Lange curve.

Although the cerebrospinal fluid is usually normal in patients with Leber's optic atrophy, even in the pressure of more generalized neurological disturbance (Lees *et al*. 1964), abnormalities have been encountered. In one case, a mildly elevated cell count and protein concentration were accompanied by a considerable increase in the relative concentration of gamma globulin (Wilson 1963).

The presence of an optico-chiasmatic arachnoiditis in the acute stages of visual failure has been stressed by some authors, and considered a possible pathogenic factor for the visual symptoms (Bruyn and Went 1964). On the, admittedly limited, pathological evidence available, this view seems unlikely.

Despite the considerable symptomatic overlap between the two conditions therefore, a careful recording of the pattern of familial involvement and the clinical features should normally facilitate their separation.

Vascular disorders

Ischaemic optic neuropathy

In its typical form, this condition is unlikely to cause problems in differential diagnosis. The basic lesion in anterior ischaemic optic neuropathy is occlusion of the posterior ciliary arteries (Hayreh 1974*a*) leading to infarction of the optic nerve head and retrobulbar zone.

The character of the visual symptoms

Sudden visual loss is usual, preceded in some cases by short-lived episodes of a similar nature (Eagling, Sanders, and Miller 1974). Pain is infrequent in the absence of temporal arteritis, and is only rarely affected by eye movement (Sanders 1971). Peak age for development of symptoms lies between 55 and 64 years (Ellenberger, Keltner, and Burde 1973), but is higher in cases of temporal arteritis (median 71 years in one series). Involvement of the second eye is common in anterior ischaemic optic neuropathy, either from the beginning or during the follow-up period, but rarely develops in temporal arteritis after 2 months have elapsed from the initial presentation.

The type of field defect

Although the visual loss in temporal arteritis is often complete, it is rather less profound in 'arteriosclerotic' cases, 50 per cent having an acuity of 6/12 or better in one series (Eagling *et al*. 1974). Arcuate and altitudinal field defects are common (Fig. 8.2) constituting 60 per cent of the changes in one group of 40 cases (Eagling *et al*. 1974).

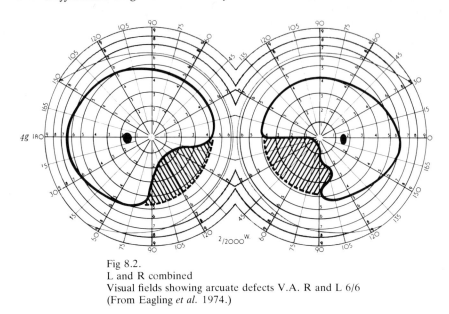

Fig 8.2.
L and R combined
Visual fields showing arcuate defects V.A. R and L 6/6
(From Eagling *et al.* 1974.)

Pupils and fundus appearance

An afferent pupillary defect is common. The optic disc is always abnormal in anterior ischaemic optic neuropathy, showing either swelling or atrophy according to the interval between onset and examination (Hayreh 1974*b*). Evidence of disc swelling is often accompanied by small, linear or flame-shaped haemorrhages.

Natural history and response to steroids

Approximately half the patients with temporal arteritis will develop vision loss, but rarely when 10 or more months have elapsed from presentation. Improvement of vision is recorded in approximately one third of cases of anterior ischaemic optic neuropathy, and further vision loss in a previously affected eye is unusual.

Corticosteroid therapy prevents involvement of the second eye in temporal arteritis. Its role in the treatment of anterior ischaemic optic neuropathy, though favoured by some authors (Hayreh 1974*c*), remains controversial (Eagling *et al*. 1974). Some patients with temporal arteritis and continuing high ESR, despite steroid therapy, will have repeat negative arterial biopsies and it is suggested can discontinue therapy with impunity. Such a reliance on histological changes is probably not warranted, however, and it is well recognized that the typical abnormalities are often patchily distributed along the vessel.

Other clinical features

The ESR is almost invariably raised in temporal arteritis, but may be normal, either in patients with a typical history (Eagling *et al*. 1974), or in patients with vision loss in the absence of systemic symptoms (Simmons and Cogan 1962; Cullen 1963). Such cases may have a superficial resemblance to optic neuritis, but the age of onset, lack of ocular pain and poor recovery in untreated cases should suggest the diagnosis. The majority of patients with temporal arteritis have systemic symptoms, including 10 per cent with polymyalgia rheumatica. Arterial tenderness is common, and in addition to an elevated ESR, a low grade anaemia with leucocytosis and increased γ_2 globulin levels are frequent.

In some patients with anterior ischaemic optic neuropathy, evidence of ipsilateral carotid artery disease may be suggested by the presence of hemispheric ischaemia or cholesterol emboli on fundus examination.

Fluorescein angiography shows reduced and delayed choroidal filling by posterior ciliary arteries in the initial stages, associated with abnormal staining of the optic discs, sometimes sectorally. It has been suggested (Hayreh 1974*b*) that the appearances are distinguishable from other causes of optic disc swelling, but a typical pattern has been observed in a patient who subsequently developed evidence of multiple sclerosis (Eagling *et al*. 1974).

Diabetes mellitus

Disturbances of vision in diabetic patients, unrelated to retinopathy or refractive changes, were recognized by Foster Moore (1920). It has been suggested (Skillern and Lockhart 1959) that a specific optic neuropathy occurs in uncontrolled diabetes, but an appraisal of the characterisitics of the visual disorder reveals similarities with acute ischaemic optic neuropathy. In the majority of patients visual failure is rapid, though the contribution of optic nerve damage in such cases may be complicated by the coexistence of macular oedema, vitreous haemorrhage, or diabetic retinopathy (Lubow and Makley 1971).

In some cases previous transient episodes of visual impairment have occurred, and occasionally ipsilateral orbital pain has coincided with vision loss. Disc oedema is common in the early stages, and bilateral involvement frequent. Central field defects predominate, sometimes with an arcuate component and, in general, prognosis for recovery of vision is poor (Freund, Carmon and Cohen 1965). In many patients, the presence of diabetes will not have previously been suspected, though evidence of diabetic retinopathy or peripheral neuropathy is found frequently (Yanko, Ticho, and Ivry 1972). A vasculopathy affecting the posterior ciliary arteries has been suggested as the most likely aetiological factor (Lubow and Makley 1971) and, despite the ingravescent course of some cases (Skillern and Lockhart 1959), an ischaemic optic neuropathy appears the best explanation for the reported examples.

Juvenile diabetes mellitus may be associated with a form of familial optic atrophy, inherited as an autosomal recessive (Rose, Fraser, Friedmann and Kohner 1966). The onset of visual symptoms in these cases averages 11–12 years, and the syndrome is therefore, distinct from that described as congenital, autosomal recessive optic atrophy.

Systemic lupus erythematosus

Optic nerve lesions may occur in this condition, sometimes as the sole, or early manifestation of the disease (Hackett, Martinez, and Larson 1974). In the reported cases, the onset of vision loss, sometimes accompanied by pain, has been sudden with relatively little subsequent recovery. Abnormalities of the cerebrospinal fluid, including raised cell counts and protein concentration, and abnormal Lange curves, have been encountered, though in some instances they have only appeared with evidence of more widespread neurological disease. Post-mortem examination of an affected optic nerve has shown fibrinoid necrosis of the arterioles with myelin and axonal loss.

Polyarteritis nodosa

Ocular involvement is relatively common in this condition, ranging from episcleritis and retinopathy to vascular lesions of the optic radiation. Sudden vision loss, with disc oedema initially, has been attributed to ischaemic optic neuropathy (Kimbrell and Wheliss 1967), a concept supported by pathological evidence of severe involvement of the posterior ciliary arteries in a patient with visual symptoms (Goldstein and Wexler 1937).

Dysproteinaemia

Recurrent cranial nerve palsies, including optic nerve involvement, have been described in association with dysproteinaemia (Kreindler and Macouei-Patrichi 1968). The neurological manifestations may be associated with hepatosplenomegaly and were accompanied in all cases by abnormal serum proteins.

Arachnoiditis

The concept of a localized arachnoiditis confined to optic nerves and chiasm as a cause of visual failure receives less emphasis now than previously. The phenomenon has been attributed to a variety of causes, including trauma, syphilis, tuberculosis, rheumatic fever, and so on. A case with sudden onset of visual disturbance, with partial recovery, but further episodes affecting each eye separately was found to have a dense localized arachnoiditis at exploration (Rychener 1948). The condition has been stated to produce virtually any type of field defect, central scotomata being usually bilateral and associated with early impairment of visual acuity. Optic atrophy is more common than disc swelling. Air encephalography may fail to reveal an abnormality and the cerebrospinal fluid is usually normal. Surgical decompression produced visual improvement in 28 per cent of one series of 66 cases (Hartmann 1945).

A chiasmal arachnoiditis has been described as a prominent feature in some cases of Leber's optic atrophy where exploration has been undertaken in the acute stages of the disease (Bruyn and Went 1964), though decompression had no effect on the visual symptoms.

Sarcoidosis

The optic nerve is the second commonest cranial nerve to be involved by this disease (Colover 1948). Papillitis, papilloedema, optic neuritis, and optic atrophy have all been described, though often without clear definitions of the terms (Gould and Kaufman 1961; Matthews 1965). Sudden visual failure, simulating acute optic neuritis, may be due to vitreous haemorrhage (Jefferson 1957) and transient amaurosis to papilloedema (Jefferson 1957).

Problems in diagnosis are particularly likely when the disease appears confined to the central nervous system (Douglas and Maloney 1973) or where sarcoid tissue causes optic nerve compression. The latter may present with sudden visual failure (Frisén, Lindgren, MacGregor, and Stattin 1977), the diagnosis only being established by examination of tissue removed at operation. Careful search may fail to reveal evidence of sarcoid tissue in other organs, even during prolonged follow-up. Examination of the cerebrospinal fluid may be unhelpful, since changes similar to those seen in multiple sclerosis are encountered, including abnormal gamma-globulin levels.

Behçet's disease

Though periodic attacks of ocular pain and vision loss can occur in this condition (Sezer 1956), a florid uveitis is the typical ocular disturbance found on examination, sometimes associated with retinal oedema and vascular sheathing.

Vogt-Harada-Koyanagi syndrome

Papillitis with severe vision loss is described in this condition (Hague 1944), but the other clinical features such as iritis, poliosis, and deafness, though sometimes delayed, establish the diagnosis.

Thyroid disease

Central field defects (Fig. 8.3 a–d) may develop in patients with thyrotoxicosis (Goldzieher M. A., McGauack, Peterson, Goldzieher J. W., and Miller 1951), disappearing with its control. The defects are usually unilateral, and commonly associated with exophthalmos (Igersheimer 1955). Central, paracentral, or arcuate field defects may be associated with a normal optic disc, optic atrophy, or papillitis. On occasions, such field defects may appear when the patient appears clinically euthyroid.

Parathyroid disease

Unilateral visual failure has been described in a patient with post thyroidectomy hypoparathyroidism associated with an afferent pupillary defect and a centrocaecal scotoma. The presence of disc oedema, retinal swelling, and arteriolar narrowing suggests a diagnosis of ischaemic optic neuropathy, the association with parathyroid disease probably being a chance one (Bajandas and Lawton-Smith 1976).

Non-metastatic optic neuropathy

Most cases described under this heading have been shown to have tumour invasion at post-mortem examination. In a case of multiple myeloma (Langdon 1939) bilateral sixth nerve palsies were followed by unilateral vision loss with central scotoma. In the absence of post-mortem examination, the possibility of optic nerve compression cannot be excluded. Bilateral optic neuritis has been described in association with carcinoma of the breast (Rudge 1973), though the clinical features included macular oedema, anterior uveitis, and a prominent cerebrospinal pleocytosis. Following excision of the breast tumour, vision improved from 6/24 to 6/6, though a fluctuating uveitis remained.

Trauma

In some instances, an acute optic neuritis following trauma subsequently progresses to a typical picture of multiple sclerosis (Mackay 1953; Miller

Fig. 8.3 (a)–(d)
Retrobulbar neuritis associated with hyperthyroidism. Visual fields
of R eye at 1 year intervals for 3/1000 white (from Goldzieher *et al.*
1951).

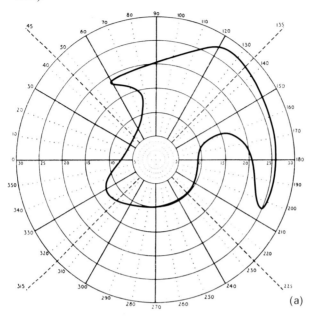

(a)

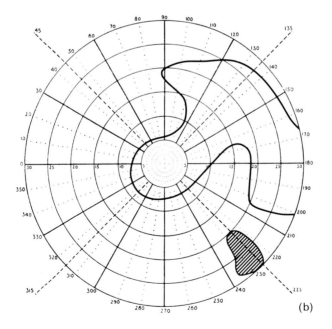

(b)

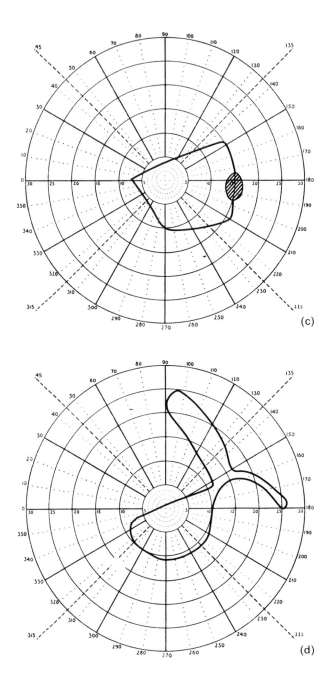

(c)

(d)

1964). Cases of apparent isolated optic neuritis following trauma have generally been followed for insufficient periods to exclude the possibility of multiple sclerosis (Ticho and Feinsod 1973). An acute optic neuritis may follow cataract extraction (O'Keefe and Choudhury 1966), with disc swelling progressing to optic atrophy, probably on an ischaemic basis.

Drusen

Field defects have been described in association with Drusen of the optic nerve, in the form of peripheral constriction or arcuate scotoma with enlargement of the blind spot. A case of transient vision loss with recovery has been described in a patient with bilateral Drusen (Meyer, Gdal-On, and Zonis 1973), and was probably due to a coincidental optic neuritis.

Macular lesions

These are seldom likely to be mistaken for optic neuritis. Central serous retinopathy affects a similar age group to that associated with optic neuritis, but predominates in males. Transient visual blurring may antedate the development of central field defects, but pain is absent, the patient often complains of micropsia and the condition has a characteristic fundus appearance. The prognosis is generally good.

Conclusions

Many of the conditions described in this chapter bear only a superficial resemblance to the optic neuritis of multiple sclerosis. Of the hereditary disorders, Leber's optic atrophy may sometimes cause diagnostic problems, both from the characteristics of the visual failure, and from the more generalized neurological disorders which may be associated with it. The characteristic family history and certain clinical features, such as the usual absence of pain and tendency to bilaterality should distinguish such cases.

The various vascular optic neuropathies generally affect a different age group from optic neuritis and tend to have a poor prognosis. There seems no reason to distinguish a distinct optic neuropathy occurring in diabetes.

In the other conditions considered, diagnostic difficulties are unlikely, and indeed in some instances the syndromes described have probably been due to a coincident optic neuritis or ischaemic optic neuropathy.

REFERENCES

Adams, J. H., Blackwood, W., and Wilson, J. (1966). Further clinical pathological observations on Leber's optic atrophy. *Brain* **89**, 15–26.
Bajandas, F. J. and Lawton Smith, J. (1976) Optic neuritis in hypoparathyroidism. *Neurology, Minneap.* **26**, 451–4.
Batten, R. D. (1909). Two cases of hereditary optic atrophy in a family with recovery in one case. *Trans ophthal. Soc. U.K.* **29**, 144–50.
Bedell, A. J. (1934). Hereditary optic atrophy (Leber's disease). *Am. J. Ophthal.* **17**, 195–204.
Bell, J. (1931). *The treasury of human inheritance* (Ed. K. Pearson), Vol. 2, Part 4. Cambridge University Press.
Bickerstaff, E. R. (1950). Hereditary spastic paraplegia. *J. Neurol. Neurosurg. Psychiat.* **13**, 134–45.
Brown, S. (1892). On hereditary ataxy, with a series of twenty-one cases. *Brain* **20**, 276–89.
Bruyn, G. W. and Went, L. N. (1964). A sex linked heredo-degenerative neurological disorder, associated with Leber's optic atrophy. Part 1. Clinical studies. *J. Neurol. Sci.* **1**, 59–80.
Colover, J. (1948). Sarcoidosis with involvement of the nervous system. *Brain* **71**, 451–75.
Cullen, J. F. (1963). Occult temporal arteritis. *Trans. ophthal. Soc. U.K.* **83**, 725–36.
Douglas, A. C. and Maloney, A. F. J. (1973). Sarcoidosis of the central nervous system. *J. Neurol. Neurosurg. Psychiat.* **36**, 1024–33.
Eagling, E. M., Sanders, M. D., and Miller, S. J. H. (1974). Ischaemic papillopathy, clinical and fluorescein angiographic review. *Br. J. Ophthal.* **58**, 990–1008.
Ellenberger, C. Jr., Keltner, J. L., and Burde, R. M. (1973). Acute optic neuropathy in older patients. *Archs Neurol. Chicago* **28**, 182–5.
Ferguson, F. R. and Critchley, M. (1929). A clinical study of an heredo-familial disease resembling disseminated sclerosis. *Brain* **52**, 203–25.
Foster Moore, R. (1920). Diabetes in relation to diseases of the eye. *Trans. ophthal. Soc. U.K.* **40**, 15–24.
Freund, M., Carmon, A., and Cohen, A. M. (1965). Papilloedema and papillitis in diabetes. *Am. J. Ophthal.* **60**, 18–20.
Frisén, L., Lindgren, S., MacGregor, B. J. L., and Stattin, S. (1977). Sarcoid-like disorder of the intracranial optic nerve. *J. Neurol. Neurosurg. Psychiat.* **40**, 702–7.
Goldstein, I. and Wexler, D. (1937). Bilateral atrophy of the optic nerve in periarteritis nodosa. *Archs Ophthal., N.Y.* **18**, 767–73.
Goldzieher, M. A., McGauack, T. H., Peterson, C. A., Goldzieher, J. W., and Miller, H. R. (1951). Retrobulbar neuritis associated with hyperthyroidism. *Archs Neurol., Chicago* **65**, 189–96.
Gould, H. and Kaufman, H. E. (1961). Sarcoid of the fundus. *Archs Ophthal., N.Y.* **65**, 453–6.
Greenfield, J. G. (1963). In *Greenfield's Neuropathology*, (ed. W. Blackwood, W. H. McMenemey, A. Meyer, R. M. Norman, and D. S. Russell,) 2nd edn, pp. 586. Edward Arnold, London.
Griscom, J. M. (1921). Hereditary optic atrophy. *Am J. Ophthal.* **4**, 347–52.
*Guzman, E. (1913). Ueber hereditäre familiäre sehnervenatrophie. *Wien. klin. Wschr.* **26**, 139–41.
Hackett, E. R., Martinez, R. D., and Larson, P. F. (1974). Optic neuritis in S. L. E. *Archs Neurol. Chicago* **31**, 9–11.
Hague, E. B. (1944). Uveitis; dysacousia; alopecia; poliosis and vitiligo. *Archs Ophthal. N.Y.* **31**, 520–38.
Hancock, W. I. (1908). Hereditary optic atrophy (Leber's disease). *R. Lond. ophthal. Hosp. Rep.* **17**, 167–77.
Hartmann, E. (1945). Optochiasmic arachnoiditis. *Archs Ophthal., N.Y.* **33**, 68–77.
Hayreh, S. S. (1974a). Anterior ischaemic optic neuropathy, terminology and pathogenesis. *Br. J. Ophthal.* **58**, 955–63.
—(1974b). Anterior ischaemic optic neuropathy. II. Fundus on ophthalmoscopy and fluorescein angiography. *Br. J. Ophthal.* **58**, 964–80.

—(1974c) Anterior ischaemic optic neuropathy. III. Treatment, prophylaxis and differential diagnosis. *Br. J. Ophthal.* **58**, 981–9.

Igersheimer, J. (1955). Visual changes in progressive exophthalmos. *Archs Ophthal., N.Y.* **53**, 94–104.

Jefferson, M. (1957). Sarcoidosis of the nervous system. *Brain* **80**, 540–59.

Kimbrell, O. C. and Wheliss, J. A. (1967). Polyarteritis nodosa complicated by bilateral optic neuropathy. *J. Am. med. Ass.* **201**, 61–2.

Kok-Van Alphen, C. C. (1960). A family with the dominant infantile form of optical atrophy. *Acta ophthal.* **38**, 675–85.

Kreindler, A. and Macouei-Patrichi, M. (1968). Recurrent cranial nerve palsies of dysglobulinaemic origin. *J. Neurol. Sci.* **6**, 117–23.

Langdon, H. M. (1939). Multiple myeloma with bilateral sixth nerve paralysis and left retrobulbar neuritis. *Trans. Am. ophthal. Soc.* **37**, 223–8.

Lawton Smith, J., Hoyt, W. F., and Susac, J. O. (1973). Ocular fundus in acute Leber optic neuropathy. *Archs Ophthal., N.Y.* **90**, 349–54.

*Leber, T. (1871). Ueber hereditare und congenital—angelegte sehnervenleiden. *Albrecht v. Graefes Arch. Ophthal.* **17**, 249–91.

Lees, F., MacDonald, A. M. E., and Turner, J. W. A. (1964). Leber's disease with symptoms resembling disseminated sclerosis. *J. Neurol. Neurosurg. Psychiat.* **27**, 415–21.

Leeuwen, M. A.-V. and Van Bogaert, L. (1949). Hereditary ataxia with optic atrophy of the retrobulbar neuritis type, and latent pallido-luysian degeneration. *Brain* **72**, 340–63.

Lodberg, C. V. and Lund, A. (1950). Hereditary optic atrophy with dominant transmission—three Danish families. *Acta ophthal.* **28**, 437–68.

Lubow, M. and Makley, Jr., T. A. (1971). Pseudopapilloedema of juvenile diabetes mellitus. *Archs Ophthal., N.Y.* **85**, 417–22.

Mackay, R. P. (1953). Multiple sclerosis: its onset and duration. A clinical study of 309 private patients. *Med. Clins. N. Am.* **37**, 511–21.

*Mathieu, J. (1901). Contribution a l'etude de la neurite optique retrobulbaire hereditaire. *These de Paris* No. 117, p. 51.

Matthews, W. B. (1965). Sarcoidosis of the nervous system. *J. Neurol. Neurosurg. Psychiat.* **28**, 23–9.

Meyer, A. (1897). The morbid anatomy of a case of hereditary ataxy. *Brain* **20**, 276–89.

Meyer, E., Gdal-On, M., and Zonis, S. (1973). Transient monocular blindness in a case of Drusen of the optic disc. *Ophthalmologica, Basel* **166**, 321–6.

Miller, H. (1964). Trauma and multiple sclerosis. *Lancet* **1**, 848–50.

Nettleship, E. (1903). A case of family optic neuritis (Leber's disease) in which perfect recovery of sight took place. *Trans. ophthal. Soc. U.K.* **23**, 108–10.

Norris, W. F. (1882). Hereditary atrophy of the optic nerves. *Trans. Am. ophthal. Soc.* **3**, 355–9.

—(1884). Hereditary atrophy of the optic nerves. *Trans. Am. ophthal. Soc.* **3**, 662–78.

O'Keefe, D. and Choudhury, K. C. (1966). Bilateral optic neuritis following cataract extraction. *Br. J. Ophthal.* **50**, 608–9.

Rose, F. C., Fraser, G. R., Friedmann, A. I., and Kohner, E. M. (1966). The association of juvenile diabetes mellitus and optic atrophy: clinical and genetical aspects. *Q. Jl. Med.* **35**, 385–405.

Rudge, P. (1973). Optic neuritis as a complication of carcinoma of the breast. *Proc. R. Soc. Med.* **66**, 1106–7.

Rychener, R. O. (1948). Recurrent retrobulbar neuritis, chiasmal arachnoiditis. *Am. J. Ophthal.* **31**, 867.

Sanders, M. D. (1971). Ischaemic papillopathy. *Trans. ophthal. Soc. U.K.* **91**, 369–86.

Sezer, N. (1956). Further investigations on the virus of Behçet's disease. *Am. J. Ophthal.* **41**, 41–55.

Simmons, R. J. and Cogan, D. G. (1962). Occult temporal arteritis. *Archs Ophthal. N.Y.* **68**, 8–18.

Skillern, D. G. and Lockhart III, G. (1959). Optic neuritis and uncontrolled diabetes mellitus in 14 patients. *Ann intern. Med.* **51**, 468–75.

Storey, J. B. (1885). Hereditary amaurosis. *Ophthal. Rev.* **4**, 33–8.

Taylor, J. and Holmes, G.M. (1913). Two families, with several members in each suffering from optic atrophy. *Trans. ophthal. Soc. U.K.* **33**, 95–115.
Taylor, S. J. (1892). Hereditary optic atrophy. *Trans. ophthal. Soc. U.K.* **12**, 146–56.
Thompson, A. H. and Cashell, G. T. W. (1935). A pedigree of congenital optic atrophy embracing sixteen affected cases in six generations. *Proc. R. Soc. Med.* **28**, 1415–25.
Ticho, U. and Feinsod, M. (1973). Traumatic optic neuritis. *Ann. Ophthal.* **5**, 430–2.
Traquair, H. M. (1932). The Doyne Memorial Lecture: The differential characters of scotomata and their interpretation. *Trans. ophthal. Soc. U.K.* **43**, 480–533.
Uhthoff, W. (1890). Untersuchungen uber die bei der multiplen herdsklerose vorkommenden augenstorungen. *Arch. Psychiat. NervKrankh.* **21**, 55–116, 303–410.
*Van Heuven, G. J. (1924). Die diagnose der hereditären leberschen sehnervenatrophie. *Klin. Mbl. Augenheilk.* **73**, 252–3.
Waardenburg, P. J. (1963). In *Genetics and Ophthalmology*, Vol. 2, pp. 1617–73. Blackwell Scientific Publications Ltd., Oxford.
Wallace, D. C. (1970). A new manifestation of Leber's disease and a new explanation for the agency responsible for its unusual pattern of inheritance. *Brain* **93**, 121–32.
Wilson, J. (1963). Leber's hereditary optic atrophy. Some clinical and aetiological considerations. *Brain* **86**, 347–62.
Wilson, S. A. K. (1954). *Neurology* (2nd ed.) (Ed. A. N. Bruce), Vol. 2, p. 1065. Butterworth, London.
Yanko, L., Ticho, U., and Ivry, M. (1972). Optic nerve involvement in diabetes. *Acta ophthal.* **50**, 556–64.

9 CSF and other investigations

Scheid reports that isolated acute retrobulbar neuritis rarely leads to changes in the cerebrospinal fluid (Marshall 1950).

Although an extensive literature exists on the abnormalities of the cerebro-spinal fluid (CSF) in multiple sclerosis, less information is available on the findings in isolated optic neuritis.

Results in our series

The methods used for CSF examination have been detailed in Chapter 2 (pp. 21). Figs. 9.1 and 9.2 give the distribution of protein concentrations found in patients with optic neuritis alone, and in patients with evidence of multiple sclerosis, respectively. Table 9.1 analyses the findings for protein concentration and abnormal cell counts in the two groups of patients, according to the interval between the onset of neurological symptoms and the time of CSF examination. Patients with evidence of multiple sclerosis had a slightly higher mean protein concentration, and were more likely to have levels above 50 mg/100 ml than patients with optic neuritis alone. On the other hand, cell counts above 5/mm^3 were as frequent amongst those with optic neuritis alone as amongst those with evidence of multiple sclerosis.

A colloidal gold test was carried out in 160 patients and found to be abnormal in four. Two of these were 'first-zone' and two 'mid-zone' patterns. One of the four had an elevated white cell count (12/mm^3). Of the four patients, three had evidence of multiple sclerosis at the time of the CSF examination.

CSF findings in the literature

Multiple sclerosis

In a comprehensive review of the literature, Müller (1951) found that an elevated protein content had been reported in 15–75 per cent, pleocytosis in 30–70 per cent, and a positive Lange curve in approximately two-thirds of cases. His own findings, and those of some other authors are summarized in Table 9.2.

Gamma-globulin concentration (Table 9.3)

Kabat, Moore, and Landon (1942) studied gamma-globulin concentrations in the CSF in a number of conditions and found elevated levels in some

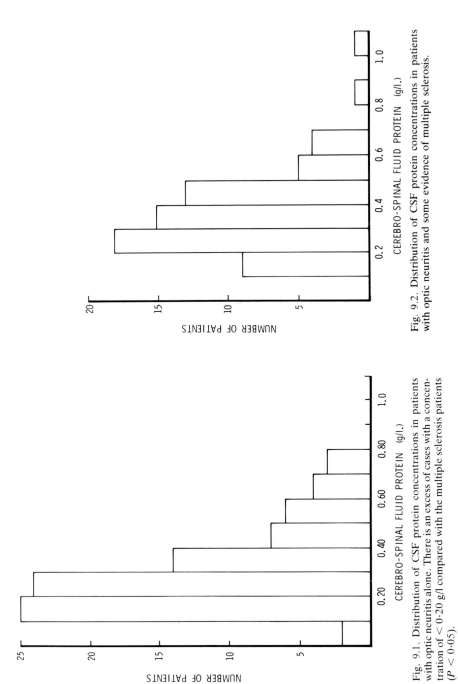

Fig. 9.1. Distribution of CSF protein concentrations in patients with optic neuritis alone. There is an excess of cases with a concentration of < 0·20 g/l compared with the multiple sclerosis patients (*P* < 0·05).

Fig. 9.2. Distribution of CSF protein concentrations in patients with optic neuritis and some evidence of multiple sclerosis.

Table 9.1 Cell counts and protein concentrations (g/l) in patients with optic neuritis

	Number of cell counts* performed	
	Optic neuritis alone: 78	Evidence of multiple sclerosis:† 69
Percentage exceeding 5 cells/mm³		
Overall	15.4	13.0
Of those examined 0–14 days	22.7	15.4
15–28 days	21.4	12.1
after 28 days	0	13.0
	Mean protein concentration: number performed	
	Optic neuritis alone: 77	Evidence of multiple sclerosis: 67
Overall mean g/l	0.32	0.38
Of those examined 0–28 days	0.32	0.38
after 28 days	0.34	0.36
Percentage with protein concentration exceeding 0.5 g/l		
Overall	11.7	19.4
Of those examined 0–28 days	10.9	20.4
after 28 days	13.6	17.4

* Specimens containing more than 10 R.B.C./mm³ have been excluded.
† Patients with a history of fresh neurological symptoms, other than visual, in the month prior to CSF examination have been excluded.

Table 9.2 Cerebrospinal fluid findings in multiple sclerosis

Author	No. of patients	Elevated protein concentration (per cent)	Pleocytosis (per cent)	Abnormal Lange (per cent)	Any abnormality (per cent)
Marshall (1950)	725	11.2		13.7	75
Freedman and Merritt (1950)	2881*	33	35	58	78
Müller (1951)	360		26	50	
Yahr *et al.* (1954)	207			35.7	
Ivers *et al.* (1961)	144	34		33	
Ackerman *et al.* (1975)	349		48	76	

* 252 personal.

Table 9.3 The relative concentration of gamma-globulin to total protein in the cerebrospinal fluid in patients with various neurological disorders

Author	No. of patients	Mean ± SD mg/100 ml	Upper limit	Frequency of abnormal levels		
				MS per cent	Infectious disorders per cent	Other CNS disorders per cent
Kabat *et al.* (1948)	14	3.4±1.1*		57	94 (Syphilis)	
Kabat *et al.* (1950)	100	9.3±1.8	12.9	80		
Freedman and Merritt (1950)	81			80		
Yahr *et al.* (1954)	244		13	66.5		
Ivers *et al.* (1961)	144	10.7±2.8	16	72		
Greenhouse and Speck (1964)	15			80		
Prineas *et al.* (1966)	167	12.0±8.5	29	44	90 (Syphilis)	
Schneck and Claman (1969)	54			14	56	
Kolar *et al.* (1970)	64		12	79.3		
Link and Müller (1971)	64		10.5	73	36	16
Savory and Heintges (1973)	16		10.8	88	58	
Ackerman *et al.* (1975)				54	40	18 (Tumours) 9 (Vascular disorders)

* Refers to absolute concentrations of gamma-globulin.

patients with multiple sclerosis. In subsequent papers (Kabat, Glusman, and Knaub 1948; Kabat, Freedman, Murray, and Knaub 1950), the normal concentration and its standard deviation were established. An increased concentration was found with other conditions, including post-vaccinial encephalomyelitis, collagen vascular disease, and metastatic involvement of the central nervous system. An analysis of the CSF protein suggested that part of its origin might be from within the central nervous system. A comparable frequency of abnormal gamma-globulin concentrations in multiple sclerosis was found by Freedman and Merritt (1950) and Yahr, Goldensohn, and Kabat (1954). In the latter's experience, if cases of neurosyphilis and patients with abnormal serum levels of gamma globulin were excluded, elevated CSF gamma-globulin concentrations were found in less than 3 per cent of patients with neurological disorders other than multiple sclerosis.

Using paper electrophoresis, Ivers, McKenzie, McGuckin, and Goldstein

(1961) found abnormal concentrations in 72 per cent of 144 cases of clinically definite multiple sclerosis. The lower figure obtained by Prineas, Teasdale, Latner, and Miller (1966) is probably explicable on a different methodology, and a large standard deviation encountered in the control population. The authors found that the total protein and relative gamma-globulin concentrations were unaffected by red cell contamination of the cerebrospinal fluid not exceeding 650 cells/c mm. Five patients, without a stated diagnosis, had repeat lumbar puncture carried out within 1 week and, in all, gamma-globulin concentrations had fallen. Where levels were repeated 1 year after myelography, no consistent pattern of change could be detected.

More recent studies (Kolar, Ross, and Herman 1970; Link and Müller 1971) have found elevated concentrations in 70 to 80 per cent of patients with multiple sclerosis. The concept of synthesis of IgG within the central nervous system, stated by Kabat *et al*. (1950) has been supported by Link and Müller (1971).

To some extent, the differing frequencies with which this abnormality has been reported in patients with multiple sclerosis reflect the method used (Thompson 1977). Although absolute gamma-globulin concentrations are more frequently abnormal than relative concentrations (Ackermann, Reider, and Wüthrich 1975) the former is less specific, and indeed correlates significantly with total protein concentration.

Variations in diagnostic criteria are also of importance since the proportion of patients with an abnormal concentration rises as the diagnostic certainty increases (Laterre, Callewaert, Heremans, and Sfaello 1970). As alternatives to the relative concentration of gamma-globulin to total protein, ratios to albumin concentration have been used to obtain a better discrimination from other neurological disorders (Tourtellotte, Tavolato, Parker, and Comiso 1971). Although this ratio is abnormal in 88 per cent of patients with multiple sclerosis (Thompson 1977) it remains of less value as a diagnostic procedure than a study of electrophoretic patterns.

A correlation exists between the cell count in the CSF and the gamma-globulin concentration (Yahr *et al*. 1954; Prineas *et al*. 1966; Laterre *et al*. 1970; Tourtellotte 1970), although the trend has not always reached significance (Olsson and Link 1973).

Abnormal electrophoretic patterns

Link (1967) made an extensive study of various protein fractions in the CSF, in both a control population and in 50 patients with multiple sclerosis. In the normal population, electrophoresis revealed, in the gamma range, four or five distinct fractions, designated gamma 1–5. In patients with multiple sclerosis, two to four narrow fractions were found between γ_3 and γ_5

instead of a relatively broad, homogeneous γ_4 fraction. Evidence was obtained to show that the subfractionation in the γ_4 range was due to IgG. Of eight patients showing a normal gamma-globulin concentration five had evidence of abnormal fractions in the γ_4 range on electrophoresis. In 831 patients with other neurological disorders, abnormal fractions were found in 2·3 per cent (consisting of chronic myelopathy, neurosyphilis, focal epilepsy, lumbosacral root syndrome, acute myelitis, polyneuropathy, and subarachnoid haemorrhage with methaemoglobinaemia).

Laterre *et al.* (1970), using agar gel electrophoresis, studied 2043 patients, including 323 with possible, probable, or definite multiple sclerosis. The percentage of patients with the abnormality increased as the diagnostic certainty rose with, for all cases, a figure of 76·8 per cent. The same morphological change (described as oligoclonal IgG) was found in other conditions, particularly neurosyphilis.

By 1971, Link and Müller were able to report at least two discrete IgG bands in 94 per cent of 64 cases of multiple sclerosis, and concluded that the demonstration of oligoclonal IgG in the CSF was a more reliable and useful finding in multiple sclerosis than the presence of an elevated relative IgG concentration. Oligoclonal IgG was described in 39 per cent of patients with infection of the CNS, and 3 per cent of patients with other neurological disorders. Using agarose electrophoresis, Olsson and Link (1973) concluded that the number and mobility of the discrete gamma bands found in patients with multiple sclerosis remained constant during the course of the disease.

Kappa–lambda ratio

Link and Müller (1971) found an increased ratio of kappa to lambda light chains in the IgG of the CSF in 53 per cent of 64 patients with multiple sclerosis, all of whom had normal serum ratios. The abnormality was considered to be due to an exaggerated synthesis of IgG molecules with light chains of type kappa, within the CNS. The finding of a normal ratio, however, did not exclude the presence of oligoclonal immunoglobulins (Olsson and Link 1973). The abnormality was found in only one of 80 patients with other neurological disorders (a case of polyneuropathy) and was not encountered in infectious disorders of the CNS.

Other proteins

Various other protein fractions have been studied in the CSF, including IgA, IgM, complement factors, transferrin, and β and γ trace proteins. Slightly increased levels of IgA or IgM may be found in multiple sclerosis and in other neurological diseases (Link and Müller 1971; Savory and Heintges 1973).

Relative concentrations of IgA, complement factors C3 and C4, and transferrin tend to increase with exacerbations of multiple sclerosis, as does the absolute concentration of β trace protein, whilst absolute concentrations of γ trace protein appear unchanged (Olsson and Link 1973).

The effect of recent exacerbations

Total protein concentration

Link and Müller (1971) recorded elevated protein concentrations as frequently during the first month after an exacerbation as later, confirming an impression obtained by Müller (1951) from a search of the literature. Using serial estimations in the same patient, during exacerbations and remissions, Olsson *et al.* (1973) corroborated the earlier observations.

Cell count

Freedman and Merritt (1950) found a pleocytosis to be more likely immediately following an exacerbation of multiple sclerosis, as did Müller (1951). Link and Müller (1971) confirmed this trend and found it to be significant in a later study (Olsson and Link 1973). Other workers (Tourtellotte 1970) have failed to find such an association.

Gamma-globulin concentration

Kabat *et al.* (1948) found no correlation between the phase of the disease and the gamma-globulin concentration, a view shared by Yahr *et al.* (1954) and Prineas *et al.* (1966). Link (1967) found the relative IgG concentration to generally rise in exacerbations, but also found cases in which levels fell, and cases where levels rose in some exacerbations but fell in others. Further work by this author (Link and Müller 1971; Olsson and Link 1973) confirmed these findings, indicating that the usual, but not inevitable, type of immunological response during exacerbations is an increased IgG synthesis within the central nervous system.

Electrophoretic pattern

Using agarose electrophoresis, Olsson and Link (1973) found the number and mobility of the gamma bands remained constant during the course of the disease, though the intensity of the bands varied.

Kappa–lambda ratio

Link (1973) has reported variations in the absolute concentrations of kappa and lambda light chain determinants during exacerbations and remissions, indicating the synthesis within the CNS of oligoclonal immunoglobulin with varying light chain type during different phases of the disease.

The influence of the clinical course, degree of disability, and certainty of diagnosis

Total protein concentration

Freedman and Merritt (1950) found no relationship between the course of multiple sclerosis and the protein concentration. No consistent pattern of protein response to course, disability, or type of disease was found by Müller (1951) from an extensive search of the literature, but Olsson, Link, and Müller (1976) found the total protein content to be increased more often in severely disabled patients.

Cell count

Link and Müller (1971) found a significantly lower frequency of pleocytosis in older patients, in patients with the longest duration of their disease, and in those with a higher degree of disability.

Gamma-globulin concentration

Yahr *et al*. (1954) found that the gamma-globulin concentration was unrelated to the mode of onset of the disease, whether it pursued a progressive or remitting and relapsing course, or the total duration. Patients with multiple attacks were more likely to have an elevated concentration, as were those with evidence of a number of separate lesions. Prineas *et al*. (1966) found a correlation with the extent of neurological involvement, assessed clinically, but they, like Link and Müller (1971), found no correlation with the total duration of the disease. Recently, Olsson *et al*. (1976) have found the most elevated values in patients with severe disability, irrespective of the duration of the disease, but only for cases with onset of the disease below the age of 25.

Electrophoretic pattern

No correlation between the electrophoretic pattern and the duration of disease, or its patterns of development, was found by Laterre *et al*. (1970), but there did appear to be an association with the degree of disability and with the certainty of the diagnosis.

Kappa–lambda ratio

Lower ratios have been found in patients without disability but with illness exceeding 10 years in duration compared with patients with severe disability and a similar length of history (Olsson *et al*. 1976).

Other proteins

Relative concentrations of IgA have not been found to correlate with any of the clinical parameters studied by Olsson *et al*. (1976).

Optic neuritis (Table 9.4)

Watkins (1939) examined the CSF of 40 patients with optic neuritis. Multiple sclerosis was diagnosed in 27 per cent, and in some was manifest when the optic neuritis developed.

Table 9.4 Abnormal cell counts and protein concentrations in patients with optic neuritis alone

Author	No. of patients	Percentage with cell count exceeding 4/mm³	Percentage with protein concentration exceeding 0.45 g/l
Sandberg and Bynke (1973)	25	48	24
Link *et al.* (1973)	41	44	49
Nikoskelainen *et al.* (1975*a*)	30	33*	27†
Sandberg-Wollheim (1975)	61	51*	41
Present series		15*	12†

* Refers to counts exceeding 5/mm³.
† Refers to protein concentrations exceeding 0.50 g/l.

A distinction between those with or without multiple sclerosis with respect to the CSF changes was not made. Of 25 patients with optic neuritis alone examined by Sandberg and Bynke (1973), 48 per cent had 5 or more cells per mm³, and 24 per cent had a protein concentration exceeding 0·45 g/l. (One of these cases, incidentally, was subsequently shown to have a meningioma.) Link, Norrby, and Olsson (1973) found, amongst 41 patients with optic neuritis alone, that 44 per cent had a cell count exceeding 4 per mm³ and 49 per cent had a protein concentration exceeding 0·45 g/l. Both abnormalities were more likely in the presence of oligoclonal IgG. In some cases, the examination was made more than 1 month after the onset of symptoms. Nikoskelainen, Irjala, and Salmi (1975*a*) studied 30 patients with idiopathic optic neuritis. Thirty-three per cent had a cell count exceeding 5/mm³ and 27 per cent had a protein concentration exceeding 0·50 g/l. The duration of symptoms prior to CSF examination was not stated.

Of 61 cases recorded by Sandberg-Wollheim (1975) 51 per cent had a cell count exceeding 5/mm³ (maximum 60·5) and 41 per cent had a protein concentration exceeding 0·45 g/l.

Colloidal gold reaction

Watkins (1939) found that 28 per cent of 40 patients with optic neuritis had an abnormal Lange curve, usually in the first zone, though some of these cases had evidence of multiple sclerosis at the time of the examination. It was noted that the presence of an abnormal curve, in patients with optic neuritis alone, did not necessarily presage the development of multiple sclerosis during the period of follow-up. With the subsequent introduction of more sophisticated analytical methods for CSF protein, colloidal gold reactions have not generally been examined in recent series.

Gamma-globulin concentration (Table 9.5)

Yahr *et al.* (1954) failed to find elevated gamma-globulin levels in any of six patients with retrobulbar neuritis, but ten years later Hallett *et al.* (1964) recorded elevated levels of α_2 and γ globulin in some cases. The findings of more recent investigators are summarized in Table 9.5.

Table 9.5 The frequency of elevated relative gamma globulin (IgG) concentration and oligoclonal IgG in patients with optic neuritis alone

Author	No. of patients	Percentage with elevated IgG	Percentage with oligoclonal IgG
Yahr *et al.* (1954)	6		
Schneck and Claman (1969)	5	20	
Laterre *et al.* (1970)	13		23
Sandberg and Bynke (1973)	25	16	24
Link *et al.* (1973)	41	34	51
Nikoskelainen *et al.* (1975*a*)	30	40	17
Sandberg-Wollheim (1975)	61	18	41
Stendahl *et al.* (1976)	30		37

Overall, for a combined total of 168 patients, 25 per cent had elevated levels, a figure approximately one-third of that encountered in multiple sclerosis.

Abnormal electrophoretic patterns

Amongst 13 patients with optic neuritis or neuromyelitis optica, Laterre *et al.* (1970) found three with oligoclonal IgG. The findings from five other recent publications are summarized in Table 9.5.

   Again, the figures are considerably lower than those found in a group of patients with multiple sclerosis. Stendahl, Link, Möller, and Norrby (1976) found a correlation between the presence of oligoclonal IgG and a pleocytosis, as did Link *et al.* (1973).

   Similar correlations have been found with an elevated relative IgG concentration (Sandberg and Bynke 1973; Link *et al.* 1973) and total protein concentration (Link *et al.* 1973).

Kappa–lambda ratio

Link *et al.* (1973) found this in 27 per cent of cases, but later, with others (Stendahl *et al.* 1976) recorded a lower figure of 17 per cent. In both series, a correlation with oligoclonal IgG was found.

The effect of recent onset

Serial examinations of the CSF in uncomplicated optic neuritis have generally not been undertaken, a single specimen usually being obtained soon after the onset of symptoms. From an analogy with the effects on the CSF of recent exacerbations of multiple sclerosis, it might be anticipated that a pleocytosis would be more likely if the examination was performed within 1 month of the onset. An examination of our own results (Table 9.1) confirms this supposition when patients with optic neuritis alone are considered, but not in the group where evidence of multiple sclerosis was apparent.

The possible significance of certain abnormalities in the CSF in uncomplicated optic neuritis, in terms of the prediction of subsequent multiple sclerosis, is considered in Chapter 13.

Measles and other virus antibodies

(a) Measles

Multiple sclerosis

Serum. Abnormally high titres of various measles antibodies have been found in the serum of patients with multiple sclerosis (Fraser 1975). Although some authors (Arnason, Fuller, Lehrich, and Wray 1974; Vandvik and Degre 1975) have failed to find a significant elevation of haemagglutination inhibition antibodies in either serum or CSF, this may reflect the use of relatively insensitive systems (Hutchinson and Haire 1976). Both IgG and IgM antibodies have been detected in the serum, the latter being taken as evidence of persistence of virus antigen in the patient (Haire 1977). The IgM response appears relatively specific for measles virus, with lower titres being found against the related canine distemper and rinderpest viruses. Recent work however (Fraser 1978) suggests that measles virus specific IgM may represent a rheumatoid factor like protein giving a spurious virus specificity by binding to the measles virus specific anti HL.

Cerebrospinal fluid. A similar increase in measles antibody titres in patients with multiple sclerosis has been recorded compared with neurological controls (Brown, Cathala, Gajdusek, and Gibbs 1971). Measles-virus-specific IgG has been found in the CSF of some 60 per cent of patients with multiple sclerosis (Haire, Millar, and Merrett 1974), and alterations in the ratio of serum/CSF antibody titres have been taken as indicative of local production in the central nervous system of antibody against measles virus (Norrby, Link, Olsson, Panelius, Salmi, and Vandvik 1974; Vandvik and Degre 1975). The electrophoretic mobility of the measles antibodies appears to correspond to some, but not all, of the oligoclonal IgG bands, suggesting that some of the latter may represent antibody to other virus agents (Vandvik and Degre 1975).

Optic neuritis

Serum. Link *et al.* (1973) found a marked increase in haemolysis-inhibiting antibody titres to measles in those patients with optic neuritis and oligoclonal IgG, but not in those without. Arnason *et al.* (1974) were unable to find any difference in titres of haemagglutination-inhibiting antibody in patients with optic neuritis, compared with a control population, but Nikoskelainen, Nikoskelainen, Salmi, and Halonen (1975*b*) studying both types of antibody, found significant elevation of both in 33 patients with optic neuritis of unknown cause, though the significance was dependent on the method used for the analysis.

The titres remained stable during the follow-up period. In a study of measles-virus-specific IgG, significantly higher titres were found in patients progressing from optic neuritis to multiple sclerosis than in those with a history of optic neuritis alone (Hutchinson and Haire 1976). These authors suggested that the antibody titres were related to the extent of demyelination in the central nervous system, though this would not explain the findings of Link *et al.* (1973) nor indeed the apparent lack of correlation between the antibody titres and the clinical state in multiple sclerosis (Vandvik and Degre 1975).

Cerebrospinal fluid. In one series of patients with optic neuritis, the finding of measurable haemolysis-inhibiting antibody was dependent on the presence of oligoclonal IgG (Link *et al.* 1973). Similarly, of 30 patients with optic neuritis studied by Stendahl *et al.* (1976), the 5 with reduced serum/CSF measles virus antibody ratio all had oligoclonal IgG. Using three separate antibody techniques, Nikoskelainen, Nikoskelainen, Salmi, and Halonen (1975*c*) found elevated titres in a group of patients with optic neuritis of unknown cause, with 62 per cent of patients with any type of optic neuritis having antibody of at least one type in the CSF. Fifty-three per cent of 17 patients with acute optic neuritis had measles-virus-specific IgG in the CSF, the abnormality being particularly frequent in those with bilateral or recurrent attacks (Hutchinson and Haire 1976).

Other viruses

Multiple sclerosis

Serum. In a group of 97 patients with multiple sclerosis, elevated antibody titres to type C influenza, herpes simplex, parainfluenza 3, mumps, and varicella-zoster were found (Brody, Sever, and Henson 1971), though the titres did not differ significantly from those found in the siblings of the patients, matched for age and sex. A statistical analysis did not show that the increased titre was significantly higher than in a control population though, in an earlier report (Ross, Lenman, and Rutter 1965), the titre for varicella-zoster had been significantly higher than in controls. Virus-specific IgG against a number of viral agents was studied by Haire, Fraser, and Millar (1973*a*) and a significant elevation in titre to herpes simplex found, and marginally to vaccinia, but not to mumps, varicella-zoster, or rubella. In a later survey by the same author, however, no significant difference of the mean IgG antibody titres between multiple sclerosis and a control population was found, for cytomegalovirus, varicella-zoster, herpes simplex, and EB viruses (Haire 1977).

Cerebrospinal fluid. Initial reports of an increased frequency of antibody to vaccinia virus in patients with multiple sclerosis have not been confirmed, but Haire, Fraser, and Millar (1973*b*) found herpes simplex and rubella IgG in 37 and 33 per cent of multiple sclerosis patients respectively, compared with 23 and 10 per cent of those with other neurological diseases and 7 and 6 per cent of normal controls. Depressed serum/CSF antibody ratios for rubella, mumps, herpes simplex, and parainfluenza type 1 virus have been interpreted as indicating local production of antibody in the central nervous system to these agents in some patients with multiple sclerosis (Norrby *et al*. 1974).

Optic neuritis

Serum. Virus antibody levels other than to measles have seldom been studied. Levels to varicella-zoster, mumps, coxsackie B5 and A3, polio 3, echo 6, cytomegalovirus, parainfluenza 1, Epstein-Barr virus, influenza A and B, adenovirus, and herpes simplex were studied by Nikoskelainen *et al*. (1975*b*). No significant differences in titres were found between the patients with optic neuritis and a control population, or a population with other neurological disorders. Serial estimations in 17 patients with optic neuritis followed over a period of several months failed to find any changes in titre.

Cerebrospinal fluid. In a group of 30 patients with isolated optic neuritis, 33 per cent had detectable rubella antibody and 40 per cent Epstein–Barr antibodies. In the former case, the frequency was significantly higher than in the control population studied (Nikoskelainen *et al*. 1975*c*). Elevated titres to parainfluenza 1 virus were no more frequent than in the controls.

Histocompatibility antigens

Multiple sclerosis

An analysis of 1000 patients with multiple sclerosis showed an increased incidence of HLA-A3 and HLA-B7 compared with controls (Bertrams,

Von Fisenne, Höher, and Kuwert 1973). No association between high measles antibody titres in the serum and these histocompatibility types was found by these authors, though an association with HLA-A3, HLA-B7, and W18 was claimed by Jersild, Ammitzbøll, Clausen, and Fog (1973*a*). Arnason *et al*. (1974) confirmed a significant increase in the incidence of HLA-A3 and HLA-B7 in a group of 56 patients with multiple sclerosis. Using a mixed lymphocyte culture test, Jersild, Fog, Hansen, Thomsen, Svejgaard, and Dupont (1973*b*) described the presence of the determinant LD-7A (DW 2) in 70 per cent of 28 patients compared with 16 per cent of a control group. All 13 patients with HL-A7 (HLA-B7) had the determinant and the progress of the disease appeared more rapid in those with it. By 1975, Jersild, Dupont, Fog, Platz, and Svejgaard were able to review the distribution of HLA determinants in 1465 patients; a significant increase in HLA-A3 and HLA-B7 coexisted with a significantly reduced risk for HLA-A12, HLA-A2, and W15. Combining the figures from three separate surveys, LD-7a was found in 56 per cent of 105 patients, compared with 19 per cent of 192 controls. The association of this determinant with a rapidly progressing form of the disease was confirmed.

Recently determinants for B lymphocyte antigens have been analysed. Antigens BT 101, 104, and 106 have been found with increasing frequency, the first being present in 83 per cent of 59 patients with definite multiple sclerosis, compared with 33 per cent of 30 control subjects (Compston, Batchelor, and McDonald 1976). No attempt has been made to determine whether the presence of the antigen affects the clinical course of the disease, and the question of the association between these antigens and the HLA system remains undecided. Interestingly, in a group of Arab patients with multiple sclerosis, a different determinant, BT 102, has been implicated, being present in 88 per cent of the patients compared with 35 per cent of controls (Kurdi, Ayesh, Abdallat, Maayta, McDonald, Compston, and Batchelor 1977).

Optic neuritis

Platz, Ryder, Nielsen, Svejgaard, Thomsen, and Wolheim (1975) analysed the distribution of HLA determinants in 54 patients with optic neuritis, clinical details of which were not given. HLA-A3 was found in 33 per cent (compared with 35 per cent of 233 patients with multiple sclerosis) and the analogous figures for HLA-B7 were 39 per cent and 39 per cent respectively. Fifty per cent of the optic neuritis cases were positive for LD-7a (DW 2) compared with 60 per cent of the multiple sclerosis patients—the difference was not significant.

Such a close comparability between optic neuritis and multiple sclerosis was not found by Arnason *et al*. (1974). These authors included cases over the age of 50, and half of their 30 patients had bilateral involvement. Neither HLA-A3 nor HLA-B7 was encountered more frequently in these cases than in the control population studied. Using a haemagglutination inhibition test to detect measles antibody, no significant difference for the geometric mean titre was found between patients with multiple sclerosis, with optic neuritis, and a control group, though individuals possessing the HLA-A3 antigen were found to have a higher titre of measles antibody, whether or not they suffered from multiple sclerosis. Stendahl *et al*. (1976) have attempted to divide the population of patients with optic neuritis into two groups, according to the presence or absence of oligoclonal IgG. Thirty patients were included, with an age range of 11 to 48 years. Overall, the percentage of patients with HLA-A3, HLA-B7, and LD-7a fell between the figures for the control group and for the patients with multiple sclerosis. Eleven patients were found to have oligoclonal IgG. All had depressed serum/CSF measles virus antibody ratios. The distribution of the determinants HLA-A3 and HLA-B7 appeared uninfluenced by the presence of oligo-clonal IgG, but 50 per cent of those with this pattern were positive for LD-7a, compared with 28 per cent of those without it. The authors observed that the frequency for LD-7a in the patients with oligoclonal IgG was little different from the frequency encountered in multiple sclerosis, though the mean follow-up in their study (1·9 years) was insufficient to determine whether these differences would influence the subsequent development of the disease. Sandberg-Wollheim, Platz, Ryder, Nielsen, and Thomsen (1975) on the other hand found that the presence of oligoclonal IgG in patients with optic neuritis correlated only with higher frequencies of HLA-A3, the determinants HLA-B7 and LD-7a being no more frequent in those with the abnormality than in those without. They concluded that HL-A and MLC typing did not appear to offer any prognostic information as to the subsequent development of multiple sclerosis.

Amongst 146 patients presenting with optic neuritis, BT101 was found in 68 per cent (Compston, Batchelor, Earl, and McDonald 1978), the figure rising to 84 per cent in those with subsequent evidence of multiple sclerosis and differing significantly from the incidence of 58 per cent in those patients without neurological sequelae.

Conclusions

The CSF findings in multiple sclerosis have been documented on numerous occasions, though considerable variability exists between the published series, probably explicable by differing methodology and patient selection. Elevated relative concentrations of IgG are found in 60–80 per cent of cases, and abnormal banding of the γ_4 range on electrophoresis (oligoclonal IgG) in up to 95 per cent. An abnormal ratio of kappa to lambda light chains in the CSF IgG is a better discriminant for multiple sclerosis, but is found in only approximately half the cases.

Recent exacerbations tend to elevate the white cell count and the relative IgG concentration, though less predictably with the latter, but have no effect on total protein concentration or the oligoclonal pattern. Abnormal cell counts lessen with increasing duration of the disease, but both the oligoclonal pattern and an abnormal IgG concentration are more frequent in those with evidence of extensive neurological involvement.

In our own series of patients with optic neuritis alone, abnormal cell counts were encountered in 15·4 per cent and protein concentrations exceeding 0·50 g/l in 11·7 per cent of cases. These figures are somewhat lower than in the other recent series quoted. Abnormal relative IgG concentrations, an oligoclonal IgG pattern and an abnormal kappa/lambda light chain ratio all occur in patients with optic neuritis, but with considerably lesser frequency than they do in patients with multiple sclerosis.

The oligoclonal IgG pattern appears to correlate with a pleocytosis, the total protein concentration and an elevated relative IgG concentration. Our own figures indicate that a pleocytosis in uncomplicated optic neuritis is confined to the first month from the onset of symptoms, whilst abnormal protein concentrations are found as frequently in specimens examined at a later time.

Elevated levels of measles antibody have been demonstrated in both the serum and CSF of patients with multiple sclerosis, with an electrophoretic mobility corresponding to some but not all of the oligoclonal IgG bands. The titres show no correlation with the clinical state. In optic neuritis, the presence of haemolysis-inhibiting antibody to measles in either the serum or CSF appears dependent on the occurrence of oligoclonal IgG.

Antibody titres to other viruses have been examined in both multiple sclerosis and optic neuritis. No consistent pattern has emerged from these studies, though in multiple sclerosis titres to herpes simplex and rubella have been most frequently identified as abnormal. Few observations have been made in patients with optic neuritis—in one series, rubella antibody was detected more frequently in the CSF than in a control population.

The histocompatibility status of patients with multiple sclerosis differs from that of the general population, with an increased incidence of HLA-A3 and HLA-B7. Using a mixed lymphocyte culture test, the determinant LD-7a (DW 2) has been found in over half the cases of multiple sclerosis studied, its presence appearing to correlate with a rapidly progressive form of the disease. In patients with optic neuritis and oligoclonal IgG (and depressed serum/CSF measles virus antibody ratios), LD-7a (DW 2) is encountered as frequently as in multiple sclerosis patients.

Recently B lymphocyte antigenic determinants have been studied, BT 101 being found in 83 per cent of 59 multiple sclerosis patients. The corresponding figure in 146 patients presenting with optic neuritis was 68 per cent, rising to 84 per cent in those with subsequent evidence of multiple sclerosis.

The influence of various CSF abnormalities and histocompatibility status in patients with optic neuritis on the subsequent development of multiple sclerosis is considered in Chapter 13.

REFERENCES

Ackerman, H. P., Rieder, H. P., and Wüthrich, R. (1975). Absolute or relative values in CSF electrophoresis—an evaluation of the γ-globulins in multiple sclerosis and other neurological diseases. *Eur. Neurol.* **13**, 131–43.

Arnason, B. G. W., Fuller, T. C., Lehrich, J. R., and Wray, S. H. (1974). Histocompatibility types and measles antibodies in multiple sclerosis and optic neuritis. *J. Neurol. Sci.* **22**, 419–28.

Bertrams, J., Von Fisenne, E., Höher, P. G., and Kuwert, E. (1973). Lack of association between HL-A antigens and measles antibody in multiple sclerosis. *Lancet* **2**, 441.

Brody, J. A., Sever, J. L., and Henson, T. E. (1971). Virus antibody titres in multiple sclerosis patients, siblings and controls. *J. Am. med. Ass.* **216**, 1441–6.

Brown, P., Cathala, F., Gajdusek, D. C., and Gibbs, C. J. Jr. (1971). Measles antibodies in the cerebrospinal fluid of patients with multiple sclerosis. *Proc. Soc. exp. Biol. Med.* **137**, 956–61.

Compston, D. A. S., Batchelor, J. R., and McDonald, W. I. (1976). B-lymphocyte alloantigens associated with multiple sclerosis. *Lancet* **2**, 1261–5.

Compston, D. A. S., Batchelor, J. R., Earl, C. J., and McDonald, W. I. (1978). Factors influencing the risk of multiple sclerosis developing in patients with optic neuritis. *Brain* **101**, 495–511.

Fraser, K. B. (1975). In *Multiple sclerosis research: Proceedings of a Joint Conference held by the Medical Research Council and the Multiple Sclerosis Society of Great Britain and Northern Ireland* (ed. A. N. Davison, J. H. Humphrey, A. L. Liversedge, W. I. McDonald, and J. S. Porterfield), pp. 53–79. HMSO, London.

— (1978). False-positive measles-specific IgM in multiple sclerosis. *Lancet* **1**, 91–2.

Freedman, D. A. and Merritt, H. M. (1950). The cerebro-spinal fluid in multiple sclerosis. *Res. Publs. Ass. Res. nerv. ment. Dis.* **28**, 428–39.

Greenhouse, A. H. and Speck, L. B. (1964). The electrophoresis of spinal fluid proteins. *Am. J. med. Sci.* **248**, 333–40.

Haire, M. (1977). Significance of virus antibodies in multiple sclerosis. *Br. med. Bull.* **33**, 40–4.

— Fraser, K. B., and Millar, J. H. D. (1973a). Virus-specific immunoglobulins in multiple sclerosis. *Clin. Exp. Immunol.* **14**, 409–16.

— — (1973b). Measles and other virus-specific immunoglobulins in multiple sclerosis. *Br. med. J.* **3**, 612–15.

— Millar, J. H. D., and Merrett, J. D. (1974). Measles-virus specific IgG in cerebrospinal fluid in multiple sclerosis. *Br. med. J.* **4**, 192–3.

Hallett, J. W., Wolkowicz, M. I., Leopold, I. H., and Wijewski, E. (1964). CSF electrophoretigrams in optic neuritis. *Archs Ophthal., N.Y.* **72**, 68–70.

Hutchinson, W. M. and Haire, M. (1976). Measles-virus-specific IgG in optic neuritis and in multiple sclerosis after optic neuritis. *Br. med. J.* **1**, 64–5.

Ivers, R. R., McKenzie, B. F., McGuckin, W. F., and Goldstein, N. P. (1961). Spinal fluid gamma globulin in multiple sclerosis and other neurologic diseases. Electrophoretic patterns in 606 patients. *J. Am. med. Ass.* **176**, 515–19.

Jersild, C., Ammitzbøll, T., Clausen, J., and Fog, T. (1973*a*). Association between HL-A antigens and measles antibody in multiple sclerosis. *Lancet* **1**, 151–2.
— Dupont, B., Fog, T., Platz, P. J., and Svejgaard, A. (1975). Histocompatibility determinants in multiple sclerosis. *Transplant Rev.* **22**, 148–63.
— Fog, T., Hansen, G. S., Thomsen, M., Svejgaard, A., and Dupont, B. (1973*b*). Histocompatibility determinants in multiple sclerosis with special reference to clinical course. *Lancet* **2**, 1221–5.
Kabat, E. A., Freedman, D. A., Murray, J. P., and Knaub, V. (1950). A study of the crystalline albumin, gamma globulin and total protein in the cerebrospinal fluid of one hundred cases of multiple sclerosis and in other diseases. *Am. J. med. Sci.* **219**, 55–64.
— Glusman, M., and Knaub, V. (1948). Quantitative estimation of the albumin and gamma globulin in normal and pathological cerebrospinal fluid by immunochemical methods. *Am. J. Med.* **4**, 653–62.
— Moore, D. H., and Landon, H. (1942). An electrophoretic study of the protein components in cerebrospinal fluid and their relationship to the serum proteins. *J. clin. Invest.* **21**, 571–7.
Kolar, O. J., Ross, A. T., and Herman, J. T. (1970). Serum and cerebrospinal fluid immunoglobulins in multiple sclerosis. *Neurology, Minneap.* **20**, 1052–61.
Kurdi, A., Ayesh, I., Abdallat, A., Maayta, U., McDonald, W. I., Compston, D. A. S., and Batchelor, J. R. (1977). Different B-lymphocyte alloantigens associated with multiple sclerosis in Arabs and Northern Europeans. *Lancet* **1**, 1123–5.
Laterre, E. C., Callewaert, A., Heremans, J. F., and Sfaello, Z. (1970). Electrophoretic morphology of gamma globulins in cerebrospinal fluid of multiple sclerosis and other diseases of the nervous system. *Neurology, Minneap.* **20**, 982–90.
Link, H. (1967). Immunoglobulin G and low molecular weight proteins in human cerebrospinal fluid. *Acta Neurol. Scand.* [Suppl] **28** (Vol. 43).
— (1973). Immunoglobulin abnormalities in multiple sclerosis. *Ann. Clin. Res.* **5**, 330–6.
— and Müller, R. (1971). Immunoglobulins in multiple sclerosis and infections of the nervous system. *Archs Neurol., Chicago* **25**, 326–44.
— Norrby, E., and Olsson, J. E. (1973). Immunoglobulins and measles antibodies in optic neuritis. *New Engl. J. Med.* **289**, 1103–7.
Marshall, D. (1950). Ocular manifestations of multiple sclerosis and relationship to retrobulbar neuritis. *Trans. Am. ophthal. Soc.* **48**, 487–525.
Müller, R. (1951). The correlation between the state of the cerebrospinal fluid and the clinical picture in disseminated sclerosis. *Acta med. scand.* **139**, 153–63.
Nikoskelainen, E., Irjala, K., and Salmi, T. T. (1975*a*). Cerebrospinal fluid findings in patients with optic neuritis. *Acta ophthal.* **53**, 105–19.
— Nikoskelainen, J., Salmi, A. A., and Halonen, P. E. (1975*b*). Virus antibody levels in serum specimens from patients with optic neuritis and from matched controls. *Acta Neurol. Scand.* **51**, 333–46.
— — — — (1975*c*). Virus antibody levels in the cerebrospinal fluid from patients with optic neuritis. *Acta Neurol. Scand.* **51**, 347–64.
Norrby, E., Link, H., Olsson, J. E., Panelius, M., Salmi, A., and Vandvik, B. (1974). Comparison of antibodies against different viruses in cerebrospinal fluid and serum samples from patients with multiple sclerosis. *Infect. Immun.* **10**, 688–94.
Olsson, J. E. and Link, H. (1973). Immunoglobulin abnormalities in multiple sclerosis. *Archs Neurol. Chicago* **28**, 392–9.
— — and Müller, R. (1976). Immunoglobulin abnormalities in multiple sclerosis. Relation to clinical parameters: disability, duration and age of onset. *J. Neurol. Sci.* **27**, 233–45.
Platz, P., Ryder, L. P., Nielsen, L. S., Svejgaard, A., Thomsen, M., and Wolheim, M. S. (1975). HL-A and idiopathic optic neuritis. *Lancet* **1**, 520–1.
Prineas, J., Teasdale, G., Latner, A. L., and Miller, H. (1966). Spinal-fluid gamma globulin and multiple sclerosis. *Br. med. J.* **2**, 922–4.
Ross, C. A. C., Lenman, J. A. R., and Rutter, C. (1965). Infective agents and multiple sclerosis. *Br. med. J.* **1**, 226–9.
Sandberg, M. and Bynke, H. (1973). Cerebrospinal fluid in 25 cases of optic neuritis. *Acta Neurol. Scand.* **49**, 442–52.

Sandberg-Wollheim, M. (1975). Optic neuritis: studies on the cerebrospinal fluid in relation to clinical course in 61 patients. *Acta Neurol. Scand.* **52**, 167–78.

— Platz, P., Ryder, L. P., Nielsen, L. S., and Thomsen, M. (1975). HL-A histocompatibility antigens in optic neuritis. *Acta Neurol. Scand.* **52**, 161–6.

Savory, J. and Heintges, M. G. (1973). CSF levels of IgG, IgA, and IgM in neurologic diseases. *Neurology, Minneap.* **23**, 953–8.

Schneck, S. A. and Claman, H. N. (1969). CSF immunoglobulins in multiple sclerosis and other neurologic diseases. *Archs Neurol., Chicago* **20**, 132–9.

Stendahl, L., Link, H., Moller, E., and Norrby, E. (1976). Relation between genetic markers and oligoclonal IgG in CSF in optic neuritis. *J. Neurol. Sci.* **27**, 93–8.

Thompson, E. J. (1977). Laboratory diagnosis of multiple sclerosis: immunological and biochemical aspects. *Br. med. Bull.* **33**, 28–33.

Tourtellotte, W. W. (1970). Cerebrospinal fluid in multiple sclerosis. In *Handbook of clinical neurology 9.* (ed. P. J. Vinken and G. W. Bruyn), Chapter 11, pp. 234–8. North Holland, Amsterdam.

— Tavolato, B., Parker, J. A., and Comiso, P. (1971). Cerebrospinal fluid electroimmunodiffusion. An easy, rapid, sensitive, reliable, and valid method for the simultaneous determination of immunoglobulin-G and albumin. *Archs Neurol., Chicago* **25**, 345–50.

Vandvik, B. and Degre, M. (1975). Measles virus antibodies in serum and cerebrospinal fluid in patients with multiple sclerosis and other neurological disorders, with special reference to measles antibody synthesis within the central nervous system. *J. Neurol. Sci.* **24**, 201–19.

Watkins, A. L. (1939). The cerebrospinal fluid in cases of optic neuritis, toxic amblyopia and tumours producing central scotomas. *Archs Neurol., Chicago* **41**, 418–22.

Yahr, M. D., Goldensohn, S. S., and Kabat, E. A. (1954). Further studies on the gamma globulin content of cerebro-spinal fluid in multiple sclerosis and other neurological diseases. *Ann. N.Y. Acad. Sci.* **58**, 613–24.

10 Treatment

It may interest you to know that Dr. George Derby's treatment for retrobulbar neuritis, when no definite focus is found, is to put the patient in bed, sweat him, and flush out his kidneys and intestinal tract (White 1928).

It might be thought nihilistic to suggest that, nearly 50 years after Dr. Derby's recommendation, his treatment is as likely to succeed as any of the more modern therapeutic approaches. The tendency for optic neuritis to improve spontaneously and the often heterogeneous material included in earlier surveys has bedevilled attempts to assess the value of various therapeutic regimes. The results, when assessed from properly controlled studies, have not been impressive.

Any assessment must take account of such clinical features of the original attack that can be shown to have an effect on the degree of visual recovery. Factors implicated by earlier authors included pain (Nettleship 1884; Swanzy 1897) particularly if deep-seated (Gunn 1904); the severity and duration of visual loss (Traquair 1930); the presence of optic disc swelling (Lillie 1934); age at onset (Earl and Martin 1967; Bradley and Whitty 1967), and laterality (Bradley and Whitty 1967).

Hyllested and Moller (1961), however, could find no evidence that either the degree of visual impairment at onset, or the presence of optic disc swelling influenced the final degree of recovery, and Bradley and Whitty (1967) similarly found no influence from the fundal appearance, the presence of pain, or the sex of the patient. In our own series, the visual outcome was unrelated to age at onset, sex, laterality, the presence of pain—irrespective of its site—or the fundal appearance. Both Lynn (1959) and Hutchinson (1976) found that multiple attacks conferred a worse prognosis.

White (1924,1925) believed that the outcome of any optic neuropathy was related to the diameter of the optic foramen, as determined radiologically. This concept has never been subjected to critical analysis, although operative decompression of the optic nerve within the foramen has been recommended as a therapeutic measure (Miyazaki 1952).

Early approaches to the treatment of optic neuritis centred on the search for a focus of infection, and concentrated on disease of the paranasal sinuses, teeth, and tonsils. In a group of patients who had had a variety of operative procedures directed at these organs (White 1928), 63 per cent obtained normal vision, 20 per cent improved, and in 17 per cent (the more chronic cases) further visual loss was prevented. The similarity of these figures to those obtained in the natural history of the condition needs no emphasis.

Subsequently, the value of operative procedures on the paranasal sinuses became largely discredited, although occasional authors (Calvet, Calmettes, and Coll 1967) have continued with their use. In order to explain the apparent benefit of surgical exploration where no evidence of infection had been found, it was suggested that the procedure had led to hyperaemia of the sinus mucous membranes, and thereby improved the blood supply to an allegedly ischaemic optic nerve (Koch 1946). As an alternative means for producing such hyperaemic congestion, local applications of cocaine were recommended.

Typhoid vaccine therapy, introduced in multiple sclerosis on the basis that the disease was related to an intestinal infection (Young and Bennett 1927), was suggested by Benedict (1933) and Lillie (1934) as a treatment for optic neuritis. Others regarded the fever and vasodilatation produced by such treatment as more relevant in explaining its possible beneficial effects, and advocated, as a means of producing the latter, the use of oral erythrol tetranitrate (Ravin 1943), inhalation of sodium nitrite (Leinfelder 1950; Marshall 1950) or intravenous histamine (Leinfelder 1950).

The introduction of corticosteroids led to the publication of a number of papers describing uncontrolled trials of the drug in the treatment of optic neuritis. Glaser and Merritt (1952) studied the effect of corticotrophin in a variety of neurological disorders and, in their group of patients with multiple sclerosis, included three with acute optic neuritis. All were thought to have responded, though in varying degree, but little benefit was observed in a group of 11 patients with a more chronic visual disturbance. This report, as well as later ones, was generally based on patients treated with a fixed dose of corticosteroids but Quinn and Wolfson (1952) recommended a titration of the dosage of corticotrophin according to the clinical response. By this means, they described improvement in patients with both optic neuritis and more chronic visual failure secondary to multiple sclerosis, in some of whom long-term therapy was undertaken. A closer analysis of their nine cases with acute optic neuritis reveals that five, or 55 per cent, recovered normal vision, a percentage lower than that generally obtained in a group of untreated cases.

Kazdan and Kennedy (1955) considered the effect of typhoid bacilli injections to be due to the production of a stressful response with a consequent increase in endogenous steroid output, and compared such treatment with a corticotrophin-cortisone regime in 22 patients with acute optic neuritis of unknown aetiology. Approximately 50 per cent of the patients in each treatment group failed to show any improvement in visual acuity, and this, taken with the high mean age of the patients studied, suggests that, in many of the cases, the visual failure was on an ischaemic basis.

Contrary to the initial enthusiasm for the use of corticosteroids reflected by these early papers, Rucker (1956) regarded the treatment as worthless both in acute optic neuritis and multiple sclerosis. Despite this criticism, further uncontrolled trials of the drug were published.

Dhir, Sofat, and Nahata's (1959) series of five cases is too small to allow any conclusions to be drawn, but Giles and Isaacson (1961) examined, retrospectively, a much larger group of 80 cases of acute optic neuritis, spanning a period of 12 years. They assigned the patients to three groups, according to whether they had been treated with corticosteroids (with or without other forms of therapy), vasodilators or typhoid antigen (with or without vasodilators). Most of the patients received vitamin therapy in addition. The numbers in each group were 48, 23, and eight respectively, and therapeutic success (defined as a return to a visual acuity of 20/40 or better) was achieved in 75 per cent, 78 per cent, and 100 per cent. Whatever the treatment, patients in the sixth and seventh decades of life fared less well than their juniors, but the appearance of the optic disc and the type of field defect had no influence on the degree of response. The authors concluded that none of the three regimes appeared to offer a significant advantage over the others.

Support for the use of corticosteroids continued, sometimes on the basis of the response seen in a single patient (Miller 1961), and the idea of a critical dosage necessary to achieve a response was furthered by Alexander and Cass (1963).

The results of the first controlled trial of corticotrophin in acute optic neuritis were published by Rawson, Liversedge, and Goldfarb (1966). Fifty patients with a history of visual symptoms for less than 10 days were entered, and pain, a central scotoma, and a defect of colour vision were made prerequisites for inclusion. More than half the patients had optic disc swelling. The trial was double blind, either corticotrophin gel (40 U daily) or an inert gel being injected for 30 days. Visual acuity (Jaeger), scotoma size, and colour vision were assessed, but only visual acuity was considered in analysis of the results. The authors found that corticotrophin both shortened the duration of pain and accelerated the speed of recovery, as assessed by the proportion of cases reading J1 or 2 after 30 days. Further analysis, one year after the onset of treatment (Rawson and Liversedge 1969), no longer showed a significant benefit for the treated as opposed to the control group, in terms of the proportion of cases having a normal visual acuity (J1 or 2).

Wray (1972) reported a double blind trial using corticotrophin in optic neuritis and multiple sclerosis (personal communication to the author). The drug was thought to be effective in shortening the period of visual loss and in relieving eye pain. Its use was recommended in situations where ocular pain occurred in the absence of visual failure, on the assumption that it would prevent visual loss developing.

Lubow and Adams (1972) recommended doses of prednisone reaching 200 mg in the first 24 hours as shortening the interval to improvement, but had studied only 10 patients in an uncontrolled fashion, comparing their results with patients seen in earlier years and treated less intensively.

Bowden A. N., Bowden, P. M. A., Friedmann, Perkin, and Rose (1974) carried out a trial on 54 patients, half of whom received 40 U of corticotrophin daily for 30 days, the remainder being given an inactive gel. The cases chosen had unilateral visual failure with a central or paracentral scotoma and impaired colour vision, and no evidence of a vascular or compressive lesion as the responsible agent. Progress was assessed by measurement of visual acuity (Snellen), visual fields and macular threshold (using the Friedmann analyser), and colour vision (with Hardy–Rand–Rittler pseudoisochromatic plates). A somewhat longer history was obtained in this series as compared with that of Rawson *et al*. (1966), as the mean duration of visual loss prior to treatment being started was 16·7 days in the treated and 18·5 days in the control group. Treatment appeared to have no influence on either the final visual outcome (assessed by acuity, field index, macular threshold, and colour vision), the incidence of optic atrophy, or the development of further episodes of optic neuritis. Its effect on the duration of ocular pain was not considered. The mean follow-up of the 54 patients was 12·2 months. In a separate analysis, those patients who were treated within 2 weeks of the onset of visual deterioration were considered. Again, no differences were detected between the treated and untreated groups.

Sub-Tenon injection of steroid has been advocated for the treatment of optic neuritis, in view of the high local concentration achievable without systemic side effects. Lawton-Smith, McCrary, Bird, Kurstin, Kelvin, Skilling, Acers, and Coston (1970) considered two injections at fortnightly intervals were capable of controlling cases of optic neuritis that had not improved with oral doses of prednisone reaching 120 mg daily. Recently a single-blind controlled trial of a single retrobulbar injection of triamcinolone in optic neuritis has been published (Gould, Bird, Leaver, and McDonald 1977). With treatment, vision tended to recover more rapidly, but conferred no long-term benefit when assessed by visual acuity, colour vision, or visual fields, though no patient was followed for more than six months.

Other forms of treatment

Following the acute episode of optic neuritis, residual impairment in visual function may be amenable to any form of treatment which modifies impulse conduction in the demyelinated optic nerve. Reduction in the ionized calcium concentration restores conduction in blocked demyelinated fibres and improves conduction velocity in fibres still conducting. In addition, the demyelinated fibres are rendered less sensitive to the blocking effects of increasing temperature (Davis and Schauf 1975). Lowering of calcium concentration by infusion of $NaHCO_3$ or EDTA decreases scotoma size in patients with multiple sclerosis (Fig. 10.1 a–f) (Davis, Becker, Michael, and Sorensen 1970), and a similar effect can be achieved by the oral intake of large doses of phosphate (Fig. 10.2) (Becker, Michael, and Davis 1974). Using the concept of a mathematical model to describe the properties of conduction in a demyelinated nerve fibre, Davis and Schauf (1975) have predicted that such conduction could be improved by any factor which increased the duration of the action potential. Agents which are capable of doing this, either by slowing the sodium inactivation process or reducing the maximum potassium permeability, exist but are not suitable for therapeutic trial. Despite this, it has been speculated that a non-toxic, clinically effective, agent might be developed which would be capable of achieving these effects, and hence of improving symptomatology (Davis and Schauf 1975).

Conclusions

There appear to be no clinical features of the original attack of optic neuritis which can be used to predict the likelihood of a poor visual outcome. As regards treatment, trials using fixed doses of intra-muscular corticotrophin or retro-ocular steroids have shown a lessening of ocular pain and a tendency to shorten the duration of visual symptoms, where patients have been treated relatively early after the onset of these symptoms. In our own trial, using fixed doses of subcutaneous corticotrophin in patients with a rather longer history, no benefit was conferred. No method of treatment, when assessed in a controlled manner, has been shown to influence the final visual outcome.

In patients with residual visual defects, temporary improvement can be achieved by reducing the ionized calcium concentration. On the basis of a mathematical model for conduction in demyelinated nerve, an agent capable of prolonging the action potential should lead to improvement in visual function.

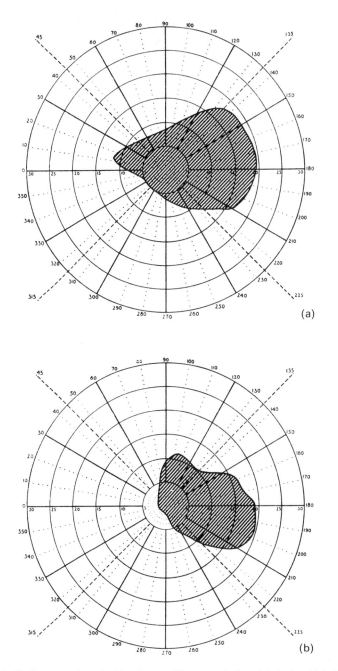

(a)

(b)

Fig. 10.1(a)–(f). Scotoma plotted with a 1 mm white target before (a), during ((b), (c)), and after ((d) (e) (f)) intravenous infusion of NaHCO$_3$. The scotoma slowly decreases in size during the infusion and then slowly increases, approaching control size after cessation of infusion (from Davis *et al.* 1970).

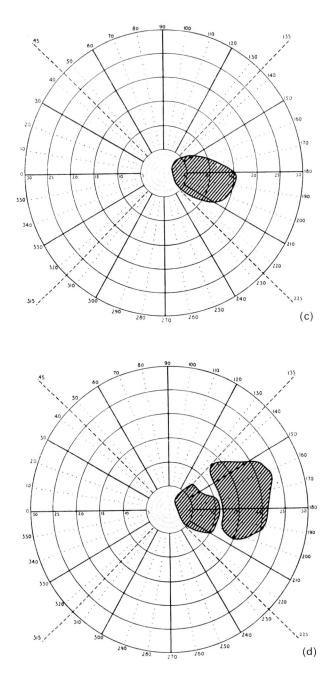

(c)

(d)

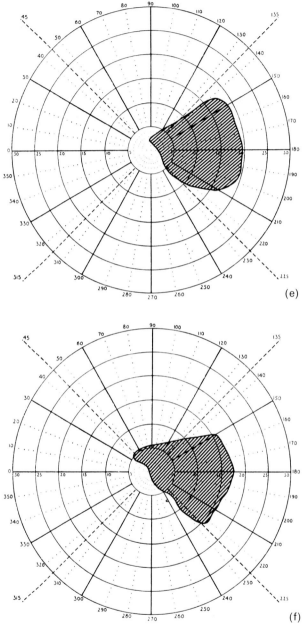

(e)

(f)

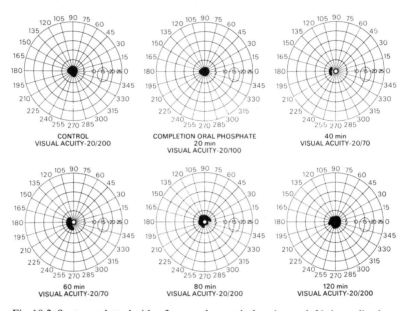

Fig. 10.2. Scotoma plotted with a 3 mm red target before (upper left), immediately on completion (upper middle), and after oral phosphate ingestion (upper right and lower row) in patient P.C. The scotoma slowly decreases in size following completion of oral phosphate and then slowly increases to control size after 120 minutes with improvement in visual acuity noted simultaneously (from Becker *et al.* 1974).

REFERENCES

Alexander, L. and Cass, L. J. (1963). The present status of A CT H therapy in multiple sclerosis. *Ann. intern. Med.* **58**, 454–71.

Becker, F. O., Michael, J. A., and Davis, F. A. (1974). Acute effects of oral phosphate on visual function in multiple sclerosis. *Neurology Minneap.* **24**, 601–7.

Benedict, W. L. (1933). Retrobulbar neuritis and disease of the nasal accessory sinuses. *Archs Ophthal., N.Y.* **9**, 893–906.

Bowden, A. N., Bowden, P. M. A., Friedmann, A. I., Perkin, G. D., and Rose, F. C. (1974). A trial of corticotrophin gelatin injection in acute optic neuritis. *J. Neurol. Neurosurg. Psychiat.* **37**, 869–73.

Bradley, W. G. and Whitty, C. W. M. (1967). Acute optic neuritis: its clinical features and their relation to prognosis for recovery of vision. *J. Neurol. Neurosurg. Psychiat.* **30**, 531–8.

Calvet, J., Calmettes, L., and Coll, L. (1967). Le rôle des sinusites dans l'étiologie des névrites optiques retro-bulbaires. *Revue Oto-Neuro-Ophtal.* **39**, 43–7.

Davis, F. A., Becker, F. O., Michael, J. A., and Sorensen, E. (1970). Effect of intravenous sodium bicarbonate, disodium edetate (Na_2EDTA), and hyperventilation on visual and oculomotor signs in multiple sclerosis. *J. Neurol. Neurosurg. Psychiat.* **33**, 723–32.

— and Schauf, C. L. (1975). Pathophysiology of multiple sclerosis. In *Multiple sclerosis research: Proceedings of a Joint Conference held by the Medical Research Council and the Multiple Sclerosis Society of Great Britain and Northern Ireland* (ed. A. N. Davison, J. H.

Humphrey, A. L. Liversedge, W. I. McDonald, and J. S. Porterfield), pp. 102–26. HMSO, London.

Dhir, B. K., Sofat, B. K., and Nahata, M. C. (1959). Optic neuritis: treatment by ACTH and cortisone. *J. Indian med. Ass.* **33**, 378–81.

Earl, C. J. and Martin, B. (1967). Prognosis in optic neuritis related to age. *Lancet* **1**, 74–6.

Giles, C. L. and Isaacson, J. D. (1961). The treatment of acute optic neuritis. *Archs Ophthal., N.Y.* **66**, 176–9.

Glaser, G. H. and Merritt, H. H. (1952). Effect of corticotrophin (ACTH) and cortisone on disorders of the nervous system. *J. Am. med. Ass.* **148**, 898–904.

Gould, E. S., Bird, A. C., Leaver, P. K., and McDonald, W. I. (1977). Treatment of optic neuritis by retrobulbar injection of triamcinolone. *Br. med. J.* **1**, 1495–7.

Gunn, M. (1904). Discussion on retro-ocular neuritis. *Br. med. J.* **2**, 1285.

Hutchinson, W. M. (1976). Acute optic neuritis and the prognosis for multiple sclerosis. *J. Neurol. Neurosurg. Psychiat.* **39**, 283–9.

Hyllested, K., Moller, P. M. (1961). Follow-up on patients with a history of optic neuritis. *Acta ophthal.* **39**, 655–62.

Kazdan, P. and Kennedy, R. J. (1955). Intravenous treatment of optic neuritis—comparison of corticotrophin and typhoid bacilli. *Archs Ophthal., N.Y.* **53**, 700–1.

Koch, F. L. P. (1946). The optic neuritides. *Conn. St. med. J.* **10**, 763–5.

Lawton Smith, J., McCrary, J. A., Bird, A. C., Kurstin, J., Kulvin, S. M., Skilling, F. D., Acers, T. E., and Coston, T. O. (1970). Sub-tenon steroid injection for optic neuritis. *Trans. Am. Acad. Ophthal. Oto-Lar.* **74**, 1249–53.

Leinfelder, P. J. (1950). Retrobulbar neuritis in multiple sclerosis. In *Multiple sclerosis and the demyelinating diseases.* Research Publications of the Association for Research in Nervous and Mental Diseases, Vol. 28, Chapter XXXIII, pp. 393–5. Williams and Wilkins, Baltimore.

Lillie, W. I. (1934). The clinical significance of retrobulbar and optic neuritis. *Am. J. Ophthal.* **17**, 110–19.

Lubow, M. and Adams, L. (1972). The changing management of acute optic neuritis. In *Neuro-ophthalmology,* Vol. 6 (Ed. J. Lawton Smith). C. V. Mosby Company, St. Louis.

Lynn, B. H. (1959). Retrobulbar neuritis. A survey of the present condition of cases occurring over the last fifty-six years. *Trans. ophthal. Soc. U.K.* **17**, 701–16.

Marshall, D. (1950). Ocular manifestations of multiple sclerosis and relationship to retrobulbar neuritis. *Trans. Am. ophthal. Soc.* **48**, 487–525.

Miller, H. (1961). Clinical applications of steroid therapy in neurology. *Proc. R. Soc. Med.* **54**, 571–5.

Miyazaki, S. (1952). Opening of the optic nerve canal via the nasal route in the treatment of acute retrobulbar optic neuritis. *Acta Soc. ophthal. jap.* **56**, 190–3.

Nettleship, E. (1884). On cases of retro-ocular neuritis. *Trans. ophthal. Soc. U.K.* **4**, 186–226.

Quinn, J. R. and Wolfson, W. Q. (1952). Improved results from individualized intensive hormonal treatment in certain eye diseases reported to respond poorly to ACTH or cortisone. *Univ. Mich. med. Bull.* **18**, 1–21.

Ravin, L. C. (1943). Treatment of acute optic neuritis with vasodilators. *Am. J. Ophthal.* **26**, 188–90.

Rawson, M. D. and Liversedge, L. A. (1969). Treatment of retrobulbar neuritis with corticotrophin. *Lancet* **2**, 222.

—— and Goldfarb, G. (1966). Treatment of acute retrobulbar neuritis with corticotrophin. *Lancet* **2**, 1044–6.

Rucker, C. W. (1956). The demyelinating diseases. *Trans. Am. Acad. Ophthal. Oto-lar.* **60**, 42–5.

Swanzy, H. R. (1897). In Discussion on retro-ocular neuritis. *Trans. ophthal. Soc. U.K.* **17**, 107–217.

Traquair, H. M. (1930). Toxic amblyopia, including retrobulbar neuritis. *Trans. ophthal. Soc. U.K.* **50**, 351–85.

White, L. E. (1924). An anatomic and X-ray study of the optic canal in cases of optic nerve involvement. *Ann. Otol. Rhinol. Lar.* **33**, 121–50.

— (1925). The optic canal in optic atrophy. *Ann. Otol. Rhinol. Lar.* **34**, 1210–23.
— (1928). The location of the focus in optic nerve disturbances from infection. *Ann. Otol. Rhinol. Lar.* **37**, 128–64.
Wray, S. H. (1972). The treatment of optic neuritis. *Sight Sav. Rev.* **42**, 5–13.
Young, G. A. and Bennett, A. E. (1927). Non-specific protein (typhoid vaccine) therapy of disseminated sclerosis. *Neb. St. med. J.* **12**, 401–6.

11 Uhthoff's syndrome

In letzter linie habe ich noch einer Erscheinung Erwahnung zu thun, die ich in
vier Fallen beobachten honnte, wo korperliche Anstrengung mit Ermudung
eine ausges prochene Verschlechterung des Sehens hervor brachte.*
(Uhthoff 1890).

Assumptions as to the pathogenesis of exacerbations of symptoms in
patients with multiple sclerosis need to be interpreted with caution. Symptoms appearing and disappearing within a few minutes, and possibly representing changes in nerve conductivity, should be distinguished from symptoms lasting for longer periods, more likely the result of fresh plaques of
demyelination. A consideration of precipitating factors may not help the
distinction, since some factors, for example emotional stress, appear capable
of producing either reaction. Even factors generally identified with short-
lived exacerbations, such as an increased temperature, may on occasion be
capable of producing a more prolonged deterioration. Kennedy (1914) for
example, described a patient who developed weakness and numbness of the
lower limbs within 20 minutes of taking a steam bath, but with progression of
symptoms thereafter for 2 days and recovery only after a further period of 2
weeks. In such cases, a fresh episode of demyelination seems a more likely
explanation than alteration of function in previously demyelinated nerve
fibres, despite the mode of onset.

Uhthoff was the first author to describe the phenomenon of exercise-
induced blurring of vision, often lasting only a few minutes, in patients with
multiple sclerosis, although he was aware of the description by Oppenheim
of the deleterious effect, in some patients, of exercise on walking ability.

Despite Uhthoff's description, it was not until 1947 that Franklin and
Brickner confirmed the observation, their patient developing visual blurring
whilst swimming. McAlpine and Compston (1952) subsequently found a
history of a deterioration of visual or other symptoms during exercise in
one-third of patients with multiple sclerosis.

In our follow-up of patients with optic neuritis, excluding those with a
history of visual symptoms exceeding 1 month before the original admission,
inquiry was made for the prevalence of transient visual blurring and any
precipitating factors (Perkin and Rose 1976). Of 125 patients questioned,
41 (32·8 per cent) described such episodes following recovery from the

* 'At last I have to mention a phenomenon which I could see in four cases, in which physical
exercise together with tiring caused a marked worsening of vision.'

original attack of optic neuritis. Table 11.1 gives details of the precipitating factors. Twenty-five patients were affected by one factor, 10 patients by two, 4 patients by three, and 2 patients by four factors.

Table 11.1 Factors producing transient visual blurring

Factor	Patients	
	No.	Percentage
Affective disturbance	20	16
Exercise	14	11
Temperature change	10	8
Menstruation	10	8
Unknown	4	3.2
Increased illumination	4	3.2
Eating	2	1.6
Smoking	1	0.8

Table 11.2 Clinical features of 125 patients at presentation

Feature at presentation	With subsequent transient blurring	Without subsequent transient blurring
Number of patients	41	84
Percentage of females	65.9	64.3
Age at presentation (mean) (years)	33.2	34.9
Eye affected (including multiple attacks)	Right 28 Left 28	Right 51 Left 50
Smokers (per cent) 20 cigarettes or more per day	65.9 24.4	54.3 24.4
Evidence of multiple sclerosis at onset (all criteria) (per cent)	53.7	39.5
Percentage* with visual acuity of 6/36 or better at onset	27.6	42.2
Duration of symptoms before admission (mean) (days)	15.2	16.0

* Excluding patients with previous attacks of optic neuritis in the same eye.

A comparison of the clinical features at presentation (Table 11.2) and follow-up (Table 11.3) between those with, and those without, subsequent transient blurring failed to reveal any significant difference.

J.R. (Male). In 1962, at the age of 24, this man had developed a left central scotoma with pain in the eye. Two weeks later numbness of the left face and weakness of the left limbs followed. The symptoms improved. In 1964 gradual visual impairment occurred on the right, with some pain, and he was found to have a right central scotoma. Further neurological episodes followed in 1965 and 1966 establishing the

Table 11.3 Clinical features of 125 patients at follow-up

Features at follow-up	With transient blurring	Without transient blurring
Attacks of optic neuritis (per cent)		
Single episode	75.6	87.5*
More than 1	24.4	12.5*
In originally affected eye	17.1	5*
More than 2	9.8	2.5*
Multiple (L=left R=right)	LL LL LL LR LR LR LLR RRL RRR LLRR	LL RR LR LR LR LR LR LR RRRL RRRRRLL
Evidence of multiple sclerosis at follow-up (all criteria) (per cent)	87.8	78.5
Mean follow-up for assessment of dissemination (months)	30.9	34.0
Percentage reaching visual acuity of 6/6†	77.4	75
Final macular threshold†	2.31	2.23
Time to measurement of stable macular threshold (weeks)	18	11
Colour vision: red/green abnormalities ± other defects (per cent)†	64.5 (unilateral 90)	44.4 (unilateral 81)
Percentage treated with steroids at onset	9.8	14.8

* These percentages were calculated on 80 patients. The possibility of multiple attacks had not been ascertained in the remaining four.
† Excluding patients with multiple attacks of optic neuritis in the same eye.

diagnosis of multiple sclerosis. From 1966, blurring of vision persisted and was made noticeably worse by exertion, hot baths, food, or emotional stress. The exacerbations would at times lead to almost complete loss of vision and might last from minutes up to 2 hours. His limb symptoms of weakness and heaviness of the legs would be similarly affected.

Fundal examination revealed bilateral temporal pallor, and the visual fields showed patchy central scotomata, more marked on the right. Friedmann fields were subsequently performed on the left eye before (Fig. 11.1), and shortly after (Fig. 11.2), a hot bath. The expected deterioration was confirmed, and found to be associated with a reduction in visual acuity from 6/18 to less than 6/60. Recovery occurred after approximately 1 hour.

In our series, the correlation between transient visual blurring and a history of more than one attack of optic neuritis in the originally affected eye only just fails to reach significance. Of seven patients with blurring of vision during exercise described by Thomson (1966), three had had two or more attacks of unilateral optic neuritis, as had two of the four patients with the same symptoms reported by Goldstein and Cogan (1964).

In a group of 185 patients with various types of optic neuritis, a decrease of visual acuity in relation to exercise or temperature was found in 20 per cent

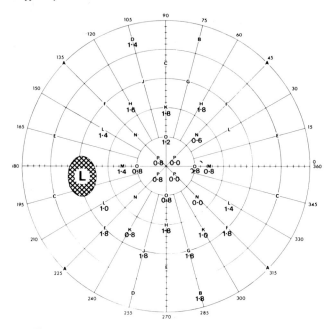

Fig. 11.1. Visual fields in subject J.R. before a hot bath.

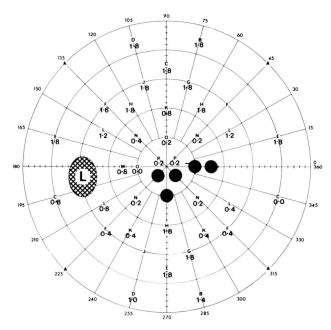

Fig. 11.2. Visual fields in subject J.R. after a hot bath.

(Nikoskelainen 1975) whilst McAlpine and Compston (1952) recorded a history of a short-lived deterioration of various symptoms in patients with definite multiple sclerosis, with exercise in 33·6 per cent, with emotional stimuli in 32·8 per cent, and with heat in 13·2 per cent.

Other provocative factors of transient exacerbations

Temperature change

The transient exacerbation of visual and other symptoms with increased temperature was probably first recorded in patients treated with typhoid vaccine therapy (Young and Bennett 1927). Subsequently, similar effects were reported in patients treated with hot baths (Lindemulder 1930; Collins 1938). Subjective worsening of motor function by heat was elicited in 62 per cent of a series of patients with multiple sclerosis (Simons 1937) and has since been recorded on numerous occasions (Franklin and Brickner 1947; Brickner 1950; Guthrie 1951; McAlpine and Compston 1952; Edmund and Fog 1955; Nelson, Jeffreys, and McDowell 1958; Nelson and McDowell 1959; Earl 1964; Goldstein and Cogan 1964; Thomson 1966; Namerow 1968). Watson (1959) observed the benefit of reduction in body temperature in eight patients with multiple sclerosis, and cast doubt on previous descriptions of exacerbation caused by cooling (Simons 1937; McAlpine and Compston 1952) suggesting that, in such cases, a paradoxical elevation of body temperature in response to cooling had occurred. Recently Geller (1974) has described the exacerbation of motor symptoms by cold in one patient, with the finding, on examination, of increased spasticity and cerebellar ataxia on cooling, with rapid reversal on rewarming. Body temperature was not recorded however.

The frequency with which hot baths produce symptomatic exacerbations becomes more impressive, when it is recalled that they also stimulate over breathing, leading to hypocapnia (Hill and Flack 1909) which is now known to cause improvement in certain manifestations of the disease—for example scotoma size (Davis, Becker, Michael, and Sorensen 1970).

Davis and his co-workers have recently studied the effect of temperature increase in greater detail (Davis, Michael, and Neer 1973; Michael and Davis 1973). Assessment of changes in oculomotor or optic nerve function in three patients showed that the responses to temperature increase were extremely variable (Fig. 11.3). The responses tended to be exaggerated immediately following a clinical relapse, but in other instances, spontaneous fluctuation occurred despite a stable clinical course. A discrepancy was found between the visual acuity of patients at a given temperature during

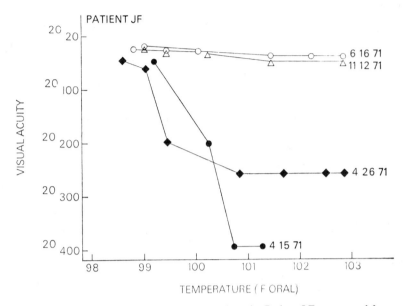

Fig. 11.3. Response of visual acuity to hyperthermia. Patient J.F. was tested four times over a 30-week period. The initial marked sensitivity to hyperthermia (15–71) was observed shortly following recovery from an exacerbation. It was less marked on 26.4.71 and by 16.6.71 was negligible. On the final test (12.11.71) the sensitivity was again minimal and appeared to have stabilized (from Davis *et al.* 1973).

heating compared with that at the same temperature during cooling, the latter being better. An analysis of the results obtained by Namerow (1968) produced a similar discrepancy, simulating the hysteresis curves obtained from various physical systems. In two patients, a temporary overshoot occurred after cooling, with a visual acuity better than had been obtained before heating commenced.

Emotion

Pratt (1951) found a significantly higher proportion of patients with multiple sclerosis had symptoms exacerbated by certain emotional stimuli, than did controls with other diseases of the nervous system.

Menstruation

Generally, menstruation leads to symptomatic improvement (McAlpine and Compston 1952). The pathogenesis of the exacerbations induced by menstruation in a patient described by McFarland (1969) remains uncertain, as their duration was generally several days.

Smoking

The ability of smoking to cause a short-lived deterioration of vision was first noted by Brickner (1950). Its adverse effect on other symptoms was later described by Courville, Maschmeyer, and Delay (1964). Although we have previously shown (Perkin, Bowden, and Rose 1975) that patients who are heavy smokers at the time of their attack of optic neuritis have, subsequently, a higher prevalence of colour vision defects, only one patient in this series noted visual deterioration while smoking, and smoking habits appeared to have no influence on the development of the symptom in relation to other precipitating factors.

Bright light

Gunn (1897) noted that patients with a previous history of optic neuritis tended to have worse vision in bright light, and suggested that 'some of the axis cylinders, though able to conduct momentarily, are soon exhausted, and the alternate action and loss of function of contiguous fibres, as they are earlier or later exhausted, lead to confused perception and confused movement from the irregularity of the stimulation forwarded and received'.

Conditions other than multiple sclerosis

Transient visual blurring with heat or exercise is not confined to multiple sclerosis. Using a hot bath, Nelson *et al*. (1958) described blurring of vision in patients with pituitary tumour, Friedreich's ataxia, and posterior cerebral artery insufficiency. The ability of exercise to cause a brief visual deterioration in patients with Leber's optic atrophy, first noted by Norris (1884), has recently been confirmed by Smith, Hoyt, and Susac (1973).

Pathogenesis

It has been suggested that heat, exercise, and eating, by inducing, respectively, cutaneous, muscular, and splanchnic vasodilatation, are capable of causing a reduction of blood flow in the region of the demyelinated nerve, thereby provoking a transient impairment of nerve function. The ability of increasing temperature to cause conduction block in demyelinated peripheral nerve fibres provides an alternative explanation for the effect of heating and indirectly exercise. In one patient, exercise produced a deterioration in visual acuity only when accompanied by a rise in body temperature (Namerow 1968), although in a similar case with visual blurring during exercise, body temperature remained stable (Goldstein and Cogan 1964).

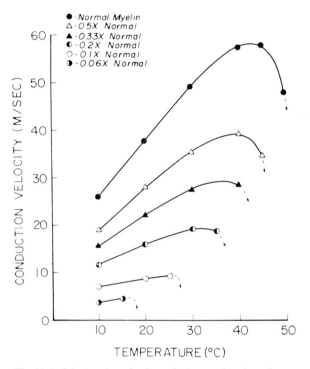

Fig. 11.4. Calculated conduction velocity as a function of temperature for a normal nerve fibre (upper curve) and fibres with increasing loss of myelin. For each curve the last datum point at the right is for the highest temperature at which continuous conduction is possible, the dashed lines and arrows simply being a convenient means of indicating block of conduction at a temperature 3 °C greater. The amount of demyelination is expressed in terms of the myelin resistance relative to normal (from Schauf and Davis 1974).

A rise in temperature of 0·5 °C can cause a reversible conduction block in severely demyelinated single peripheral nerve fibres, but enhances conduction in less affected fibres (Rasminsky 1973). It has been suggested, on this basis, that patients with multiple sclerosis developing symptoms with a slight increase in body temperature must have many fibres with severely demyelinated internodes, the conduction velocity of which would be significantly reduced (Figs. 11.4 and 11.5).

A number of authors (McDonald 1974; Heron, Regan, and Milner 1974; Asselman, Chadwick, and Marsden 1975) have suggested that the prolonged latencies of the visually evoked responses found in some patients with multiple sclerosis may not be entirely explicable on the basis of delayed

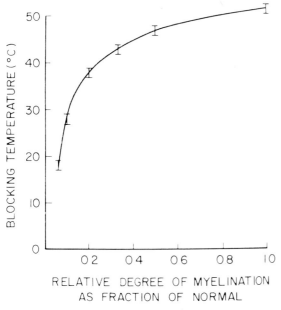

Fig. 11.5. Blocking temperature as a function of the amount of myelin loss. The error bars correspond to an uncertainty of 2 °C. The amount of demyelination is expressed in terms of the myelin resistance relative to normal (from Schauf and Davis 1974).

conduction in demyelinated internodes. Synaptic delay either within the retina or centrally has been considered as a possible factor (Halliday and McDonald 1977), as has the possibility that conduction in small demyelinated optic nerve fibres may be continuous. A study of continuous conduction in demyelinated segments of small peripheral myelinated fibres has shown a slowing by some 15 times compared with saltatory conduction in distal, normal segments (Bostock and Sears 1976). The effect of temperature increase on continuous conduction in demyelinated fibres is not known, though it may be similar to that on saltatory conduction (Bostock, personal communication).

If, however, the delay is related to a slowing of saltatory conduction in demyelinated internodes, then a number of predictions are possible. Firstly, those patients with the longest latencies would be the ones most likely to develop visual symptoms with rising body temperature, and, secondly, with elevation of body temperature the responses should be reduced in amplitude (due to conduction block in many of the fibres contributing to it) and possibly shortened in latency (due to enhanced conduction in unblocked fibres).

If visual blurring with rising temperature reflects a blockage of conduction in demyelinated optic nerve fibres, then the latter should be found in conditions other than multiple sclerosis where the phenomenon occurs. Two of the three diagnosed patients with visual blurring on heating described by

Nelson *et al*. (1958) had conditions (Friedreich's ataxia and pituitary tumour with supra-sellar extension) known to be associated with optic nerve demyelination, as, indeed, is Leber's optic atrophy (Wilson 1963).

Conclusions

A history of transient visual blurring is likely to be encountered in approximately one-third of patients with a previous episode of optic neuritis. Emotional disturbances and exercise are the commonest precipitating factors. The occurrence of the symptoms cannot be predicted from the characteristics of the original attack. The phenomenon has been described in other disorders of optic nerve function and may represent blockage of conduction in severely demyelinated nerve fibres. If the extent of the delay in the latencies of visually evoked responses in patients with optic neuritis reflects such demyelination, a correlation should exist between the delay and the occurrence of the symptom.

REFERENCES

Asselman, P., Chadwick, D. W., and Marsden, C. D. (1975). Visual evoked responses in the diagnosis and management of patients suspected of multiple sclerosis. *Brain* **98**, 261–82.
Bostock, H. and Sears, T. A. (1976). Continuous conduction in demyelinated mammalian nerve fibres. *Nature, Lond.* **263**, 786–7.
Brickner, R. M. (1950). The significance of localized vasoconstrictions in multiple sclerosis. In *Multiple sclerosis and the demyelinating diseases*. Research Publications of the Association for Research in Nervous and Mental Diseases, Vol. 28. Williams and Wilkins, Baltimore.
Collins, R. T. (1938). Transitory neurological changes during hyperthermia. *Bull. neurol. Inst. N.Y.* **7**, 291–6.
Courville, C. B., Maschmeyer, J. E., and Delay, C. P. (1964). Effect of smoking on the acute exacerbations of multiple sclerosis. *Bull. Los Ang. neurol. Soc.* **29**, 1–6.
Davis, F. A., Becker, F. O., Michael, J. A., and Sorensen, E. (1970). Effect of intravenous sodium bicarbonate, disodium edetate (Na_2 EDTA) and hyperventilation on visual and oculomotor signs in multiple sclerosis. *J. Neurol. Neurosurg. Psychiat.* **33**, 723–32.
— Michael, J. A., and Neer, D. (1973). Serial hyperthermia testing in multiple sclerosis: A method for monitoring subclinical fluctuations. *Acta Neurol. Scand.* **49**, 63–74.
Earl, C. J. (1964). Some aspects of optic atrophy. *Trans. ophthal. Soc. U.K.* **84**, 215–26.
Edmund, J. and Fog, T. (1955). Visual and motor instability in multiple sclerosis. *Archs Neurol. Psychiat., Chicago* **73**, 316–23.
Franklin, C. R. and Brickner, R. M. (1947). Vasospasm associated with multiple sclerosis. *Archs Neurol. Psychiat., Chicago* **58**, 125–62.
Geller, M. (1974). Appearance of signs and symptoms of multiple sclerosis in response to cold. *J. Mt. Sinai Hosp.* **41**, 127–30.
Goldstein, J. E. and Cogan, D. G. (1964). Exercise and the optic neuropathy of multiple sclerosis. *Archs Ophthal., N.Y.* **72**, 168–70.
Gunn, M. (1897). Discussion on retro-ocular neuritis. *Trans. ophthal. Soc. U.K.* **17**, 107–217.
Guthrie, T. C. (1951). Visual and motor changes in patients with multiple sclerosis. A result of induced changes in environmental temperature. *Archs Neurol. Psychiat., Chicago* **65**, 437–51.
Halliday, A. M. and McDonald, W. I. (1977). Pathophysiology of demyelinating disease. *Br. med. Bull.* **33**, 21–7.

Heron, J. R., Regan, D., and Milner, B. A. (1974). Delay in visual perception in unilateral optic atrophy after retrobulbar neuritis. *Brain* **97**, 69–78.

Hill, L. and Flack, M. (1909). The influence of hot bath on pulse frequency, blood pressure, body temperature, breathing volume and alveolar tension of man. *Proc. physiol. Soc. Camb.* **38**, 57–61.

Kennedy, F. (1914). Acute insular sclerosis and its concomitant visual disturbances. *J. Am. med. Ass.* **63**, 2001–5.

Lindemulder, F. G. (1930). The therapeutic value of high temperature baths in multiple sclerosis. *J. nerv. ment. Dis.* **72**, 154–8.

McAlpine, D. and Compston, N. (1952). Some aspects of the natural history of disseminated sclerosis. *Q. Jl. Med.* **21**, 135–67.

McDonald, W. I. (1974). Pathophysiology in multiple sclerosis. *Brain* **97**, 179–96.

McFarland, H. R. (1969). The management of multiple sclerosis. Apparent suppression of symptoms by an estrogen-progestin compound. *Missouri Med.* **66**, 209–11.

Michael, J. A. and Davis, F. A. (1973). Effects of induced hyperthermia in multiple sclerosis: differences in visual acuity during heating and recovery phases. *Acta Neurol. Scand.* **49**, 141–51.

Namerow, N. S. (1968). Circadian temperature rhythm and vision in multiple sclerosis. *Neurology Minneap.* **18**, 417–22.

Nelson, D. A., Jeffreys, W. H., and McDowell, F. (1958). Effect of induced hyperthermia on some neurological diseases. *Archs Neurol. Psychiat., Chicago* **79**, 31–9.

— and McDowell, F. (1959). The effects of induced hyperthermia on patients with multiple sclerosis. *J. Neurol. Neurosurg. Psychiat.* **22**, 113–16.

Nikoskelainen, E. (1975). Symptoms, signs and early course of optic neuritis. *Acta ophthal.* **53**, 254–72.

Norris, W. F. (1884). Hereditary atrophy of the optic nerves. *Trans. Am. ophthal. Soc.* **3**, 662–78.

Perkin, G. D., Bowden, P. M. A., and Rose, F. C. (1975). Smoking and optic neuritis. *Post-grad. med. J.* **51**, 22–5.

— and Rose, F. C. (1976). Uhthoff's syndrome. *Br. J. Ophthal.* **60**, 60–3.

Pratt, R. T. C. (1951). An investigation of the psychiatric aspects of disseminated sclerosis. *J. Neurol. Neurosurg. Psychiat.* **14**, 326–36.

Rasminsky, M. (1973). The effects of temperature on conduction in demyelinated single nerve fibres. *Archs Neurol., Chicago* **28**, 287–92.

Schauf, C. L. and Davis, F. A. (1974). Impulse conduction in multiple sclerosis: a theoretical basis for modification by temperature and pharmacological agents. *J. Neurol. Neurosurg. Psychiat.* **37**, 152–61.

Simons, D. J. (1937). A note on the effect of heat and of cold upon certain symptoms of multiple sclerosis. *Bull. neurol. Inst. N.Y.* **6**, 385–6.

Smith, J. L., Hoyt, W. F., and Susac, J. O. (1973). Ocular fundus in acute Leber optic neuropathy. *Archs Ophthal., N.Y.* **90**, 349–54.

Thomson, D. S. (1966). Blurring of vision on exercise. *Trans. ophthal. Soc. U.K.* **86**, 479–92.

Uhthoff, W. (1890). Untersuchungen uber die bei der Multiplen Herdsklerose vorkommenden Augenstorungen. *Arch. Psychiat. NervKrankh.* **21**, 55–116, 303–410.

Watson, C. W. (1959). Effect of lowering of body temperature on the symptoms and signs of multiple sclerosis. *New Engl. J. Med.* **261**, 1253–9.

Wilson, J. (1963). Leber's hereditary optic atrophy. Some clinical and aetiological considerations. *Brain* **86**, 347–62.

Young, G. A. and Bennett, A. E. (1927). Non-specific protein (typhoid vaccine) therapy of disseminated sclerosis. *Neb. St. med. J.* **12**, 401–6.

12 Subsequent visual signs

There was much more tendency to recovery, even in severe forms of retro-ocular neuritis, than would be expected judging from experience of other optic nerve lesions (Gunn 1904a).

Visual acuity during follow-up

The distribution of visual acuities (Fig. 12.1) during the first 6 months after the onset of optic neuritis indicates that 75 per cent of those examined at the end of that period had an acuity between 6/6 and 6/12 (Fig. 12.2). Patients with more than one attack in the same eye have been excluded. The distribution changes little for those patients followed for longer periods (Fig. 12.3), indeed such figures may be distorted by patients who have recovered failing

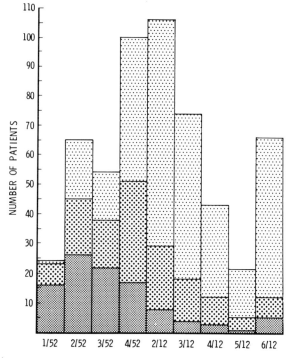

Fig. 12.1. Distribution of visual acuities during first 6 months after onset of optic neuritis. For this and subsequent figures, top band refers to visual acuity of 6/6–6/12, middle band to 6/18–6/60 and lower band to C.F. – no P.L.

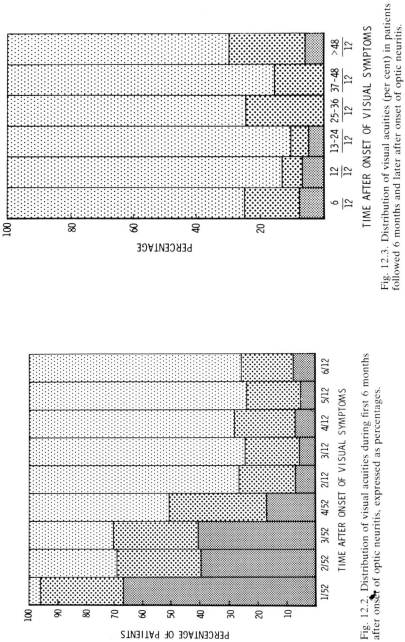

TIME AFTER ONSET OF VISUAL SYMPTOMS

Fig. 12.3. Distribution of visual acuities (per cent) in patients
followed 6 months and later after onset of optic neuritis.

TIME AFTER ONSET OF VISUAL SYMPTOMS

Fig. 12.2. Distribution of visual acuities during first 6 months
after onset of optic neuritis, expressed as percentages.

to attend for subsequent examination. Including those patients followed for at least 6 months, and using the final, stable, visual acuity, 85·7 per cent were between 6/6 and 6/12, 9·6 per cent between 6/18 and 6/60, and 4·7 per cent between CF and no PL. The mean period of recovery to 6/6 was 8·1 weeks (Table 12.1), the figure being not significantly affected by the severity of visual impairment at onset.

Table 12.1 Percentage of patients reaching 6/6 within first 6 months of onset of visual symptoms

Presenting V.A.	6/9	6/12	6/18	6/24	6/36	6/60	3/60	CF	HM	PL	No PL·	Mean
% recovering 6/6	88.9	84.6	55.6	63.6	80	92.3	71	66.7	86	66.7	50	69.7
Mean number of weeks to 6/6	6.3	7.4	7.8	7.6	7.9	9.6	7.2	9.3	8.9	7.5	6.0	8.1

Gunn (1904*b*) commented that occasional failure of recovery of vision was seen, without specifying its frequency. A number of authors have analysed the frequency of depressed vision in multiple sclerosis patients (Gipner 1925; Rosen 1965), some with a history of visual symptoms, whilst others (Rischbieth 1968; Kahana, Leibowitz, Fishback, and Alter 1973), though confining their study to optic neuritis, have failed to specify criteria for normal or decreased vision. In Table 12.2a, analogous visual angles have been used where possible to make comparison more valid. Where other forms of optic neuropathy have been included, for example Leber's disease, the percentage of cases with persistently poor vision is liable to be exaggerated (Hyllested and Moller 1961; Nikoskelainen 1975*a*).

The possible influence of the age at onset of visual symptoms on the final visual outcome has been considered previously (Table 12.2b). Müller (1949) found no differences between those above and below 25 years, the percentages achieving complete recovery being 51 and 61 respectively. Bradley and Whitty (1967) found no influence from age at onset except for a slower rate of recovery for those over 50 years. Lynn (1959) found recovery to be similar for those above and below the age of 30, but in two recent series, differences were encountered. Earl and Martin (1967) found patients over the age of 45 had a significantly greater chance of failing to recover good vision (6/9 or better), whilst Sandberg (1972) found a similar result in patients over 60 years. He considered many of the older patients had a vascular basis for their symptoms though Earl and Martin (1967) had taken some effort to exclude such cases. In this series (Fig. 12.4), the percentage of patients reaching an acuity between 6/6 and 6/12 at, and before, 6 months was unaffected by the age of onset.

A number of authors have considered the speed of recovery of optic

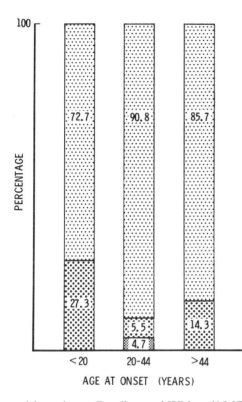

Fig. 12.4. Distribution of visual acuities up to six months after onset of optic neuritis, according to age at onset (no significant differences).

neuritis patients. Bradley and Whitty (1967) found 50 per cent of cases had recovered normal vision (6/6 or 6/9) by 1 month and 75 per cent by 6 months, figures very similar to our own. Those of our cases recovering to 6/6 did so in a mean period of 8·1 weeks, comparable to the 2 month period taken to optimal visual acuity reported by Earl and Martin (1967). Nikoskelainen (1975*a*) observed a slower rate of recovery, with 56 per cent having an acuity of above 0·8 at 6 months, though, as has been indicated, her material included cases with a worse prognosis.

The final outcome was unrelated to the appearance of the optic disc at presentation (Table 12.3), a conclusion shared by others (Bradley and Whitty 1967; Sandberg 1972).

Pupil asymmetry

Excluding patients with multiple attacks, pupil size was assessed in 138 cases at follow-up. Anisocoria was present in 15 (10·9 per cent), the dilated pupil being on the side previously affected by optic neuritis in all but one. Of these, 13 had had a dilated pupil at onset, though in one of them, on the

Table 12.2a Final visual acuity after optic neuritis (per cent)

Author	Number of eyes	Unilateral or bilateral	Aetiology	Follow-up period	Visual angle† 1.0–1.3	1.4–2.5	3.3 or more
Schlossman and Phillips (1954)	46	Both	MS	?	19.6	40	40.4
Bagley (1952)	60 (39 cases)	18 U / 21 B	?	Less than 6 months in 20	36.7	25	38.3
Marshall (1950)	164	Both	Mixed	?	L 39.0	27.5	33.4‡
Wybar (1952)	33	17 U / 8 B	MS	?	42.4	9.1	48.5
Marshall (1950)	164	Both	Mixed	?	R 44.5	24.4	30.4‡
Nikoskelainen (1975a)	194	U	Mixed	From 6 months to over 10 years	68.6	8.3	23.1
Hyllested et al. (1961)	52	Both	Mixed	From 2 to 15 years	71.1	11.5	17.4
Bradley and Whitty (1967)	78	Both	MS or ?	6 months	75 (spanning 1.0–1.3 and 1.4–2.5)		25
Hutchinson (1976)	121	71 U / 25 B	MS or ?	?	72§ / 72	15§ / 20	13§(U) / 8 (B)

† visual angle of 1.0–1.3 is equivalent to visual acuities of 6/6 or 5/6, 20/25 or above, 0.8 or above
  visual angle of 1.4–2.5 is equivalent to visual acuities of 5/12 to 6/9, 20/50 to 20/30, 0.4–0.7
  visual angle of 3.3 or more is equivalent to visual acuities of 6/18 or less, 20/70 or less, 0.3 or less
‡ These figures did not add up to 100 in the original publication.
§ these 3 columns correspond, not to the stated visual angles, but to acuities of 6/6–6/9, 6/12–6/36, and 6/60 or less respectively.

Table 12.2b Final visual acuity after optic neuritis (per cent) according to age at onset

Author	Number of eyes	Unilateral or bilateral	Aetiology	Follow-up period	Age at onset	Final visual acuity		
						6/6–6/9	6/12–6/36	6/60 or less
Lynn (1959)	200	Both	MS or ?	Less than 6 to over 21 years	Under 30	——46.5——		53.5
					Over 30	——40.9——		59.1
Earl and Martin (1967)	104	Both	MS or ?	Until acuity stable for 6 months	Under 45	——96——		4
					Over 45	——76——		24
Sandberg (1972)	58	Both	Mixed	3–7 years	Under 60	89.8†	2.0	8.2
					Over 60	37.5†	37.5	25

† In this series, the three categories of visual acuity were 6/6 to 6/8.5, 6/9 to 6/18, and 6/20 or less, respectively.

Table 12.3 Percentage of patients in three groups of visual acuities according to optic disc appearance at onset. Cases with multiple attacks excluded and minimum follow-up period of six months unless acuity of 6/6–6/12 achieved before that time

Eventual visual acuity	Disc appearance at presentation		
	Neuroretinitis	Papillitis	Normal
6/6–6/12	91.6	87.4	87.7
6/18–6/60	8.4	4.2	12.3
< 6/60	0	8.4	0

contralateral side. The final visual acuity was between 6/6 and 6/12 in 11, between 6/18 and 6/60 in three, and less than 6/60 in one.

In a group of 91 multiple sclerosis patients, Wybar (1952) found anisocoria in 11 (12·1 per cent), amounting to 0·5 mm in seven and 1·5 mm in four. Yaskin, Spaeth, and Vernlund (1951) reported the sign in 6 per cent of 100 cases. Following optic neuritis, anisocoria was found in 7 per cent of one series (Nikoskelainen 1975*a*) but in 20 per cent of 160 cases in another (Lynn 1959).

The pupillary reaction

This was assessed in 139 patients, excluding those with multiple attacks. An abnormal response (as defined in Chapter 4) was found in 54·7 per cent, coinciding in all cases with the affected eye.

Amongst multiple sclerosis patients, pupillary abnormalities have been reported in 1·1 (Savitsky and Rangell 1950), 4·5 (Gipner 1925), 6 (Yaskin *et al*. 1951) and 11·4 per cent of cases (Rosen 1965). In 160 patients with previous optic neuritis, Lynn (1959) elicited a pseudo-anisocoria by the 'modified Marcus Gunn test' in 16 (10 per cent) whilst Nikoskelainen (1975*a*) found a depressed or absent light response in 17 per cent of her cases. Wybar (1952) has analysed the pupillary reaction in some detail in 91 patients. An abnormality of the direct light reaction was found in 19, being bilateral in 12. In an attempt to overcome the difficulties in interpretation of minor pupillary abnormalities, the rate and amplitude of the pupillary oscillations induced by a fine light source applied to the pupil margin were studied. Of 177 eyes tested by this method, 70 were abnormal, including the 31 pupils found to have minor changes by conventional testing.

Thompson (1966) has used electronic pupillography to assess the light response. In the presence of an afferent defect, the reaction is of increased latency with reduced amplitude and duration (Fig. 12.5). With an alternating light source, pupillary escape occurs on the affected side, sometimes with a paradoxical dilatation (Fig. 12.6). The author concluded

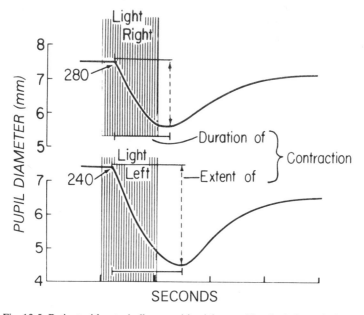

Fig. 12.5. Patient with retrobulbar neuritis, right eye. The shaded area indicates the duration of the light stimulus. Direct and consensual reactions of the right pupil are compared. When the right eye is stimulated, the latent period is longer (280 ms) and the reaction is less extensive and less sustained (from Thompson 1966).

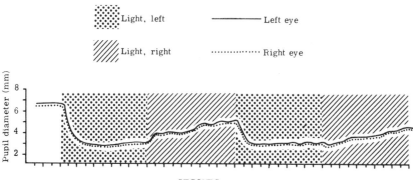

Fig. 12.6. Patient with retrobulbar neuritis, right eye. The stimulating light was shifted suddenly from one eye to the other. This swinging flashlight test made the afferent defect more apparent by contrasting the good and bad eyes (from Thompson 1966).

that an alternating stimulus was the best method for eliciting an afferent defect, an asymmetrical response implying a prechiasmal disturbance. In considering the phenomenon of amaurotic mydriasis, Thompson (1966) repeated Lowenstein's (1954) observation that no anisocoria occurred with one eye in darkness and the other illuminated, concluding that anisocoria, when present, implied some other defect in the pathway of pupillary control. If this is the case, this defect appears to be invariably ipsilateral to the side of the optic neuritis (at least in the patients studied in the acute stages), and, furthermore, shows a significant correlation with the degree of visual impairment.

Fundus appearance

The optic disc changes found at follow-up examination are summarized in Table 12.4. Patients followed for less than 6 months have been excluded, as have those with evidence of optic atrophy at presentation and those with a history of multiple attacks in the same eye. Neuro-retinitis was almost always followed by optic atrophy, whereas for those patients with a normal fundus initially, optic atrophy followed in only 48·1 per cent (Fig. 12.7).

Table 12.4 The final appearance of the optic disc according to presenting fundus examination

Disc appearance at follow-up	No.	Disc appearance at onset		
		Normal	Papillitis	Neuroretinitis
Normal	44	27 (61.4%)	16 (36.4%)	1 (2.2%)
Nasal pallor	1	1 (100%)		
Temporal pallor	44	18 (40.9%)	19 (43.2%)	7 (15.9%)
Generalized pallor	28	6 (21.4%)	17 (60.7%)	5 (17.9%)

The prevalence of optic atrophy in multiple sclerosis patients has been considered in Chapter 14 (Table 14.4). A number of authors have reported the frequency of optic atrophy after optic neuritis, some of the differences no doubt reflecting observer bias in interpreting this physical sign. Gunn (1904b) considered pallor of the disc to be almost inevitable, a view subsequently shared by Berliner (1935) and Benedict (1942), but in more recent series it has been reported less frequently (Table 12.5).

In this series, patients with optic atrophy were more likely to have a depressed visual acuity at follow-up (Table 12.6), though there are contradictory opinions regarding this correlation. Lynn (1959) found the degree of pallor was related to acuity, but Nikoskelainen (1975a) noted a frequent discrepancy between the two. Gipner (1925) reported good vision (6/10 or better) in 51 per cent of patients with optic atrophy compared with 92 per cent of those with normal fundi. Hyllested and Moller (1961) found an

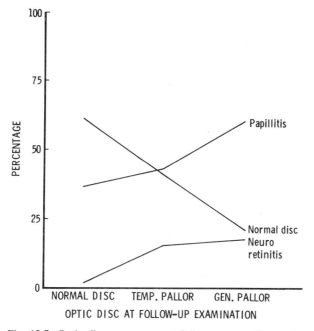

Fig. 12.7. Optic disc appearance at follow-up according to its appearance at presentation. The difference in distribution is significant (*P.*< 0·01).

Table 12.5 The frequency with which optic atrophy follows optic neuritis

Author	No. of patients	% with optic atrophy
Kahana *et al*. (1973)	91	49
Scott (1961)	20	50
Nikoskelainen (1975*a*)	194	58
Hyllested and Moller (1961)	52	60
Present series	117	62
Wybar (1952)	33	67
Lynn (1959)	160	80

Table 12.6 Distribution of final visual acuity according to optic disc appearance at follow-up

	6/6–6/12	6/18–6/60	< 6/60
Normal disc	45 (95.7%)	2 (4.3%)	0
Optic atrophy	78 (84.8%)	10 (10.9%)	4 (4.3%)

acuity of 6/6 in 55 per cent of patients with optic atrophy compared with 95 per cent of those without disc changes.

Colour vision

Colour vision, using Hardy–Rand–Rittler pseudoisochromatic plates, was tested in 112 patients, excluding those with a history of more than one attack in the affected eye. The findings are summarized in Table 12.7. Defects were found in 50 per cent of the patients, unilateral in 87·5 per cent of them. Of the 63 eyes with colour-vision abnormalities, 77·8 per cent had optic atrophy, compared with 46·4 per cent of those with normal colour vision.

Table 12.7 Colour vision abnormalities at follow-up

	Eyes affected
Colour vision abnormalities	63
Red/green—protan	7
Red/green—deutan	21
Red/green—unclassified	20
Red/green Blue/yellow	1
Red/green—⎫ Blue/yellow—⎬ unclassified	10
Red/green—deutan Blue/yellow—tritan	1
Red/green—protan Blue/yellow—tertaran	1
Red/green—deutan Blue/yellow—unclassified	1
Red/green—unclassified Blue/yellow—tritan	1

Nettleship (1884) reported colour-vision defects in some of his cases, using the test of Ole Bull (*sic*). Amongst 182 patients with multiple sclerosis, Kahana *et al*. (1973) found colour-vision loss (of unspecified type) in 7 per cent of those with a history of visual symptoms and in 4 per cent of those without. Rosen's (1965) comparable figures (using H-R-R plates) were 94·6 and 38·5 per cent. Wybar (1952) found abnormal colour vision (Ishihara) in 56 per cent of 25 cases with a history of optic neuritis. These, and the findings of Lynn (1959) and Nikoskelainen (1975*a*) are detailed in Table 12.8.

Table 12.8 Colour vision defects in patients with a history of optic neuritis

Author	Method	No. tested	% abnormal
Kahana *et al.* (1973)	?	107	7
Wybar (1952)	Ishihara	25	56
Nikoskalainen (1975*a*)	Ishihara+Farnsworth	23	65
Lynn (1959)	Ishihara	143	84
Rosen (1965)	H-R-R	111	95

The discrepancies are unexplained, though admittedly the methods used differed somewhat and the criteria for an abnormal response were not necessarily stated. In addition, in some cases, authors have failed to state whether their figures related to the number of patients, or to the number of eyes examined. Testing of the clinically unaffected eye was performed by Lynn (1959) who found, amongst 119 cases of unilateral optic neuritis, that 44·5 per cent had abnormal colour vision in the other eye. The figure is far higher than our own of 12·5 per cent, which incidentally included one patient who had subsequently had an episode in the second eye.

Excluding this patient, the percentage falls to 11. Lynn (1959) encountered recurrent attacks in 21 per cent of her patients and inclusion of these cases may well have inflated the number with colour-vision defects. Furthermore, the follow-up period exceeded 6 years in 75·5 per cent, whereas none of our patients had been followed for this length of time.

Intra-ocular tension

This was measured in 111 patients. Abnormal values (exceeding 24 mm) were found in two patients.

R.G., aged 40. In September 1964, developed painless visual blurring in the left eye. Visual acuity was 6/18 with temporal pallor of the optic disc and a centro-caecal defect. Intra-ocular tensions were not measured at this stage. Five years later, visual acuity was 6/12 with a left Marcus Gunn response and bilateral colour vision defects. The optic disc remained pale and the field defect had changed little. Tensions were 32 and 30 mm. The patient complained of paraesthesiae, but there was no evidence for multiple sclerosis on neurological examination.

M.M., aged 55. Developed blurring of vision in the left eye in March 1965 with pain below the eye. Visual acuity was counting fingers with a depressed light response. By 1969, the acuity had recovered to 6/6 with a Marcus Gunn pupillary response and abnormal colour vision. The optic disc was normal. Intra-ocular tensions were 26 and 26 mm. There was no evidence of multiple sclerosis.

Nikoskelainen (1975*a*) found high intraocular pressures in two of her cases and considered both to have chronic glaucoma. The nature of their original visual symptoms was not indicated.

Table 12.9 Distribution of visual fields at follow-up

Visual field at onset	Visual field at follow-up (number of patients)																			Totals
	Central				Central with periph. ext.				Arc.	Peripheral									Normal	
	5°	10°	15°	Unsp.	Gen.	Alt.	Sect.	Hem.		Diff.	Alt.	Sect.	5–15°	5–20°	5–25°	10–15°	10–20°	10–25°		
Central (total: 45)																				
5°														1		1			2	4
10°					1			1						1	1		1		4	10
15°		2	2											2	2	2	3		7	20
Unspecified		1	2		2									1		1	1		3	11
Central with peripheral extension to 25° (total: 33)																				
General		2	1		7	2	1							2	3	2			3	23
Altitudinal			1			1							1	1	1				2	7
Sectorial																	1		1	2
Hemianopic								1												1
Generalized depression to 25°			1	1	1											1			3	7
Arcuate									1				1				1			3
Peripheral defects with central sparing																				
Peripheral (diffuse)					1														2	3
Altitudinal											1						1			2
Sectorial																		1		1
No field possible					2									1	1			1		5
Unsatisfactory or unreliable			1		1	1		1							2	1	2	2	5	16
Normal		1	1													1		1	1	5
Totals	0	6	10	1	15	4	1	3	1	0	1	0	2	9	10	9	10	5	33	120
	17				23					1			45							

Visual fields

These have been analysed in those patients followed for a minimum period of 6 months, excluding cases with more than one attack in the originally affected eye. Details are given in Table 12.9 and summarized in Table 12.10,

Table 12.10 Visual fields after optic neuritis

Author	No. of cases	Normal	Central	Paracentral	Peripheral
Wybar (1952)	33	27.3	21.2	12.1	39.4
Present series	120	27.5	33.4	——39.1——	
Nikoskelainen (1975*a*)	194	41.0	27	——33.0——	
Hyllested and Moller (1961)	52	59.6	——21.1——		19.3

where a comparison is made with several other series. The designation of an arcuate defect at follow-up has been somewhat arbitrarily confined to a single patient, since, as we shall see, many of the patchy peripheral defects between 5° and 25° are probably arcuate in type.

Central defect to 15° (Fig. 12.8)

D.E., aged 24. Left papillitis, 1966. 3 years later, visual acuity was 6/6, with a left Marcus Gunn reaction, colour-vision defect and optic atrophy. Visual fields showed a patchy central defect extending to 15°. There had been a central scotoma at onset and neurological examination showed definite evidence of multiple sclerosis.

Central defect with peripheral extension (Fig. 12.9)

I.B., aged 41. Left retrobulbar neuritis, 1963, with evidence at that time of multiple sclerosis. Visual fields then showed a central scotoma to 15° with peripheral extension. Six years later, there was bilateral optic atrophy, bilateral colour-vision defects and acuities of 6/9 L and 1/60 R. The left visual field showed a central scotoma extending to the periphery.

Arcuate defect (Fig. 12.10)

R.G., aged 40. Left retrobulbar neuritis, 1964 with arcuate defect and evidence of optic atrophy. Five years later, left Marcus Gunn reaction with arcuate defect persisting, bilateral colour-vision defects, and left optic-atrophy. There was evidence by then of probable multiple sclerosis.

Peripheral defect (Fig. 12.11)

D.G., aged 19 (see also Chapter 4, Fig. 4.17). Right retrobulbar neuritis, 1963. Six years later, temporal pallor with normal pupillary reaction, normal colour vision, and an acuity of 6/12. A constricted field had been present at onset. By follow-up, there was evidence of definite multiple sclerosis.

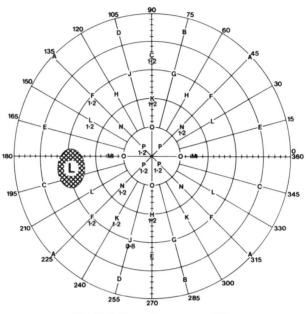

Fig. 12.8. Central scotoma to 15°.

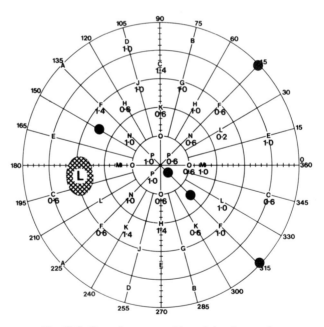

Fig. 12.9. Central scotoma with peripheral extension.

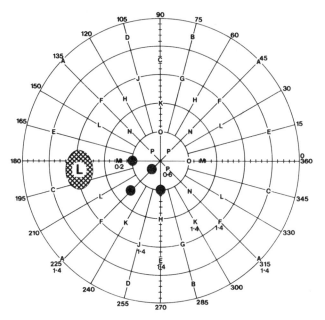

Fig. 12.10. Arcuate scotoma.

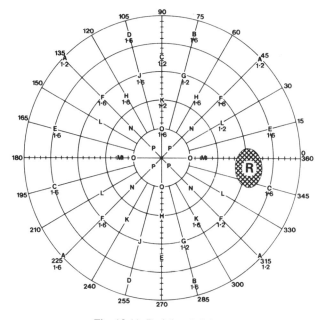

Fig. 12.11. Peripheral defect.

Scattered defect 5°–20° (Fig. 12.12)

J.C., aged 35. Right retrobulbar neuritis, 1964, with central 15° scotoma. Five years later, visual acuity was 6/4 with a Marcus Gunn response, abnormal colour vision and temporal pallor. There was no evidence of multiple sclerosis.

Scattered defect 5°–25° (Fig. 12.13)

M.S., aged 34. Left retrobulbar neuritis, 1964, with a central 5° scotoma. Five years later, visual acuity was 6/5 with a Marcus Gunn response, normal colour vision, and a normal optic disc. There was no evidence of multiple sclerosis.

Scattered defect 10°–15° (Fig. 12.14)

J.L., aged 24. Left retrobulbar neuritis, 1968, with central 10° scotoma extending to the periphery. Eight months later, visual acuity 6/12 with a Marcus Gunn response, colour-vision defect, and temporal pallor. Evidence by then of probable multiple sclerosis.

Scattered defect 10°–15° (Fig. 12.15)

M.S., aged 33. Right papillitis, 1966 with central 10° scotoma extending to the periphery. Three years later, visual acuity 6/9 with Marcus Gunn response, colour-vision defect, and temporal pallor. There was evidence of possible multiple sclerosis.

Scattered defect 10°–20° (Fig. 12.16)

S.S., aged 22. Left papillitis, 1968 with central scotoma extending to the periphery. Ten months later, acuity 6/4 with Marcus Gunn response, colour-vision defect, and optic atrophy. No evidence of multiple sclerosis.

Many descriptions of visual field defects in multiple sclerosis patients have emphasized central scotomata (Rosen 1965). Berliner (1935) considered central or paracentral scotomata to persist after an attack of optic neuritis, though often in association with enlargement of the blind spot and depression of the peripheral field. Lynn (1959) found residual field changes to fall into 4 groups, viz. central defects, scotoma with or without central depression, bizarre field defects (after multiple attacks), and incongruous hemianopic defects. Wybar (1952) found peripheral contraction in 39·4 per cent of his cases, with normal fields in only 27·3 per cent, though surprisingly the corresponding figure in Hyllested and Moller's series (1961) was 59·6 per cent.

Klingmann (1910) was perhaps the first to comment on paracentral field defects in multiple sclerosis patients, finding bilateral, predominantly temporal, paracentral scotomata in 10 of his 12 cases. Although he attributed these to chiasmatic lesions, inspection of the published fields shows similar, nasal, defects in some of them (Figs 12.17 and 12.18). Thirty-nine per cent

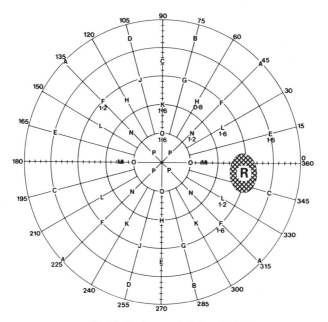

Fig. 12.12. Scattered defect 5°–20°.

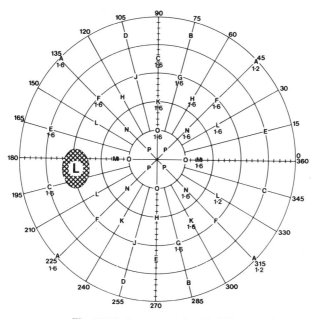

Fig. 12.13. Scattered defect 5°–25°.

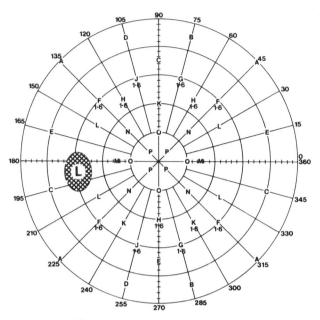

Fig. 12.14. Scattered defect 10°–15°.

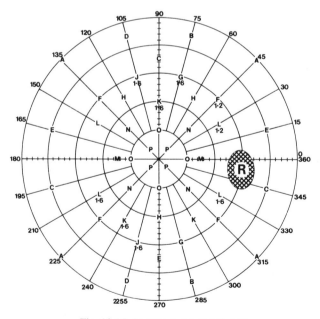

Fig. 12.15. Scattered defect 10°–15°.

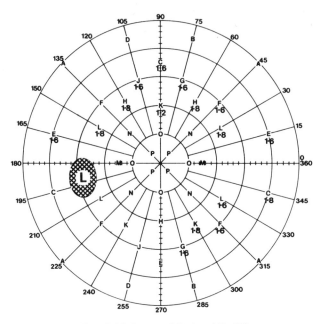

Fig. 12.16. Scattered Defect 10°–20°.

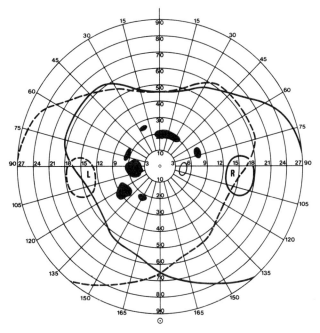

Fig. 12.17. Left eye. Visual acuity 20/40·5 mm white. 50-year-old
patient with numbness and weakness of the lower limbs, headache
and dizziness of 1 year's duration. Insidious visual failure for several
months.
Examination—bilateral optic atrophy, nystagmus and pyramidal
signs in the lower limbs.
(From Klingmann 1910.)

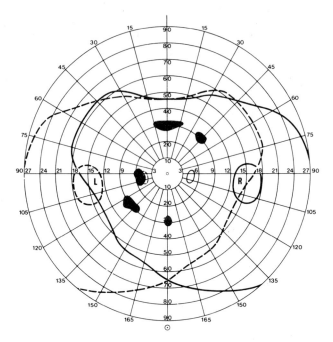

Fig. 12.18. Left eye. Visual Acuity 20/30. 5 mm white. 55-year-old patient. Stiffness when walking, dizziness and occasional visual blurring. Examination—nystagmus, intention tremor and a spastic gait with brisk reflexes and extensor plantar responses.
(From Klingmann 1910.)

of our patients, following optic neuritis, showed patchy depression of the field between 5° and 25° with preservation of central fields and acuity. Retinal nerve-fibre atrophy in patients with multiple sclerosis (Gartner 1953), most characteristically beginning in the upper arcuate bundles, is revealed not only by fundoscopy, but by related field defects, consisting of narrow, elongated scotomata between 10° and 25° from fixation (Frisen and Hoyt 1974 (Fig. 12.19). The patchy peripheral defects in many of our cases correspond to such scotomata, though a fundoscopic correlation with nerve-fibre atrophy was not attempted. Frisén and Hoyt (1974) suggested that the apparent tendency for this atrophy to be confined to the arcuate fibres might simply be due to their more ready identification on fundoscopy. The frequency of a corresponding field defect in this series, however, often in the presence of normal central fields, suggests that arcuate fibres, situated in the supero and infero temporal parts of the optic nerve (Hoyt 1962) may be more likely to degenerate after demyelination than corresponding fibres in the papillomacular bundle.

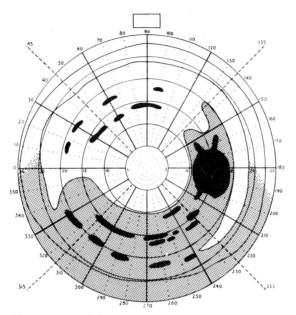

Fig. 12.19. Relative depression and multiple narrow scotomata in right visual field, corresponding with nerve fiber layer defects seen on fundoscopy. Patient with spinal cord disturbance and previous episode of slight dimness of vision in right eye (from Frisén and Hoyt 1974).

Recurrent optic neuritis

Thirty patients had experienced more than one episode of optic neuritis (Table 12.11). In two patients, bilateral involvement had occurred within the space of 4 weeks, although in one of them this had occurred several years

Table 12.11 Distribution (in chronological order) of recurrent attacks

Attacks	Distribution (No. of cases)
RR	3
LL	5
RL	5
LR	9
LRL	1
RLR	1
RRL	1
RRR	1
RLRLR	1
RRRLRL	1
RRRRLLRR	1
R and L within 1 month	1

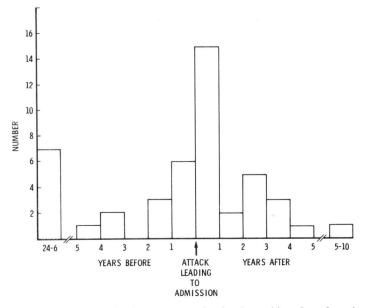

Fig. 12.20. Relationship of recurrent attacks of optic neuritis to time of attack leading to admission.

previously. The time relationship of these episodes to the attack leading to admission is summarized in Fig. 12.20. The final visual outcome where more than one attack had occurred in the same eye is shown in Table 12.12, excluding patients followed for less than 6 months after the final attack. It was found that 42·9 per cent had an acuity of less than 6/9, 83·3 per cent had an abnormal visual field (including those with sufficiently severely depressed vision to make field testing impossible), and 75 per cent had a colour-vision defect. Optic atrophy was present in 88·2 per cent. Twelve of these 13 patients had some evidence of multiple sclerosis at follow-up. It is apparent from this series that residual impairment of vision is more likely in those with a history of multiple attacks.

Recurrent attacks were reported in 11·3 per cent by Marshall (1950), in 14 per cent by Schlossman and Phillips (1954), in 20·6 per cent by Lynn (1959), and in 15 per cent by Scott (1961). Hutchinson (1976), defining recurrent attacks as those occurring after an interval of more than 2 weeks, found them in 24 per cent. Using the same definition, the analogous figure from this series is 16·7 per cent.

Benedict (1942) considered marked pallor of the optic disc to be usual after recurrent attacks. Schlossman and Phillips (1954) found poor recovery of vision in two of three patients with recurrent attacks in whom there was no

Table 12.12 Final visual outcome, and evidence of multiple sclerosis in patients with more than one attack in the same eye

Attacks	Final VA	Final field	Colour vision	Multiple sclerosis
RRRRRR	HM	Not poss.	Not poss.	Def.
LL	PL	Not poss.	Not poss.	
LL	6/7.5	Central + temporal	R/G D	Poss.
LL	6/9	General depression	R/G U	Poss.
LL	6/4	Patchy 10°–20°	?	Def.
RR	6/9	Altitudinal	Normal	Def.
LL	6/60	Paracentral	?	Def.
RR	6/6	Normal	R/G U	Prob.
RRRR	No PL	Not poss.	Not poss.	No
LL	No PL	Not poss.	Not poss.	
LL	6/6	?	?	Prob.
RR	6/4	Patchy 10°–20°	?	Prob.
RRR	6/6	Normal	?	Prob.
RRR	?	?	?	Prob.
LL	?	?	?	
RR	6/36	?	?	Poss.

HM = hand movements,   PL = perception of light,   No PL = no perception of light,
R/G = red green,   U = unclassified,   D = Deutan

evidence of multiple sclerosis, though Scott (1961) recorded good visual acuity in three patients after recurrent attacks. Recurrences occurred in 25 per cent of the patients reported by Nikoskelainen (1975*a*), though in 40 per cent of those with multiple sclerosis. Good or excellent vision (> 0·8) was found in 54 per cent of those with recurrent attacks compared with 69 per cent of the patients with single attacks. Similarly Hutchinson (1976) recorded good vision (6/6 to 6/9) in 72 per cent of unilateral attacks, but in 59 per cent of recurrent cases. Patients with recurrent attacks fared less well in Lynn's (1959) experience, only 24·2 per cent recovering to 6/9 or better.

Bilateral optic neuritis

Only one patient in this series had bilateral optic neuritis whilst under observation.

J.McG., aged 32. Admitted with a 2-week history of pain in the right eye followed, 4 days later, by blurring of vision. Two days before admission a similar pain had appeared in the left eye, followed by visual blurring in the left temporal field. On admission, visual acuities were HM right, and 6/6 left. There was a large right central scotoma and an altitudinal defect on the left (Fig. 12.21). The right pupil showed a Marcus Gunn reaction. The right disc was swollen uniformly, and the left showed blurring of the supero-nasal margin.

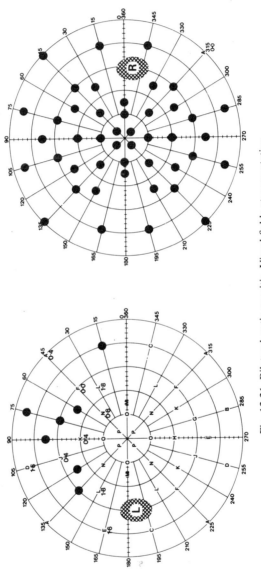

Fig. 12.21. Bilateral optic neuritis. Visual fields at presentation.

Vision deteriorated further on the left to 6/60. Six months later acuities were no PL right and PL left. The right pupil was fixed to the light, the left showed normal reactions. There was bilateral optic atrophy. Six years later, the patient had developed evidence of definite multiple sclerosis, with left-sided sensory symptoms, ataxia, and lower limb weakness.

Adie (1932) was unable to find a single case of simultaneous affection of both eyes in his material and considered both simultaneous and early consecutive cases to be very rare, suggesting other aetiological factors, such as disseminated encephalo-myelitis. Berliner (1935) concurred with this view, and McIntyre and McIntyre (1943) only found a single case in their own series. Although Kurland, Beebe, Kurtzke, Nagler, Auth, Lessell, and Nefzger (1966) recorded bilateral papillitis (the two eyes being affected within the space of 2 weeks) in 39 cases (representing 17·6 per cent of their total material) they excluded them on the assumption that a specific agent unrelated to multiple sclerosis was likely to be responsible. An examination of several other series indicates the relative frequency of these cases, in contradiction to Adie's (1932) assumption (Table 12.13). The variability is again considerable, although partly explicable, for some series, by the inclusion of disorders such as toxic amblyopia and Leber's disease which are generally bilateral.

Table 12.13 Percentage of bilateral cases

Author	No. of cases	% bilateral	Time relationship
Lynn (1959)	200	10.5	Within days
Hyllested and Moller (1961)	52	11.2	Not stated
Rischbieth (1968)	116	12.1	Within 2 weeks
Hutchinson (1976)	144	19	Within 2 weeks
Bradley and Whitty (1967)	73	19.2	Within 3 months
Nikoskelainen (1975*b*)	185	30	Within 1 month
Wybar (1952)	25	32	Not stated
Benedict (1942)	90	33.3	Not stated
Marshall (1950)	320	35	Not stated
Bagley (1952)	39	53.8	Not stated
Schlossman and Phillips (1954)	37	56.6	Not stated
White and Wheelan (1959)	33	75.7	Not stated

Several authors have considered the degree of visual recovery in bilateral as opposed to unilateral cases (Table 12.14). Bradley and Whitty (1967) found no significant differences in rate and degree of recovery in the two groups, and the other series have not shown a consistent difference. Although Kurland *et al.* (1966) excluded patients with bilateral papillitis, on the assumption that they were likely to have a 'toxic' basis, in one recent series (Hutchinson 1976), bilateral optic neuritis was more likely to progress

Table 12.14 Visual outcome in unilateral and bilateral cases

Author	% with good vision		% with poor vision	
	Unilateral	Bilateral	Unilateral	Bilateral
Rischbieth (1968)[1]	77.8	67.8	–	–
Nikoskelainen (1975a)[2]	–	–	23	34
Hutchinson (1976)[3]	72	72	13	8

[1] Not defined.
[2] Good vision: > 0.8; poor vision: < 0.3.
[3] Good vision: 6/6 or 6/9; poor vision: 6/60 or less.

to multiple sclerosis than unilateral cases. Hierons and Lyle (1959) analysed 34 adults with various types of bilateral optic neuritis. Of the cases with simultaneous or early consecutive involvement visual recovery occurred in approximately a half, but in none of them could a confident diagnosis of multiple sclerosis be made at follow-up.

Chronic optic neuritis

Many authors have used this term for cases with gradually progressive visual failure with or without an initial acute onset. None of our patients really fitted into this category, though in 7 an initially severely depressed vision showed little sign of subsequent recovery (Fig. 12.22). Lynn (1959) encountered two patients with gradual unilateral onset, without specifying the visual outcome. Scott's (1961) three similar cases all suffered severe impairment of vision which failed to recover.

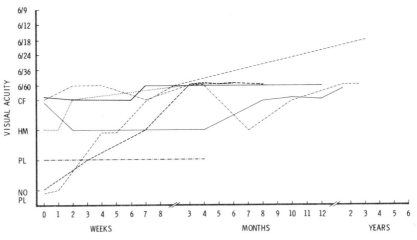

Fig. 12.22. Poor visual recovery in 7 patients.

Schlossman and Phillips (1954) considered chronic retrobulbar neuritis not to exist, reflecting in reality the result of repeated attacks on the optic nerve. Nikoskelainen (1975a) inclined to a similar conclusion, finding that of 24 eyes with chronic-progressive optic neuritis, half had had identifiable further attacks and, in the remainder, further assessment was thought to suggest recurrent episodes.

Ashworth (1967) published details of patients with various types of chronic retrobulbar neuritis, including acute cases initially recovering then subsequently deteriorating, acute cases with subsequent progression, and cases with insidious and progressive visual failure. Kahana *et al*. (1973) recorded progressive loss of vision in 25 patients. On the basis of an increase in signs of optic nerve damage with duration of illness, they concluded that the rate of optic nerve demyelination was more or less constant over the course of the disease, whether or not exacerbations had been identified.

A slowly progressive visual failure over several months may occasionally still recover. One such patient described by Hierons and Lyle (1959) had acuities of 1/60 in each eye at 6 months but recovered to 6/6, 2 years after onset. Nikoskelainen (1975a) recorded five cases with bilateral papillitis and poor vision at 6 months but subsequent recovery.

Uveitis and retinal vascular sheathing

One patient had evidence of healed choroiditis at both onset and follow-up, whilst another had cells in the vitreous on each occasion. Both had probable multiple sclerosis. Perivascular sheathing was noted in a third patient at the follow-up examination, when evidence of definite multiple sclerosis was obtained, and in a fourth, arteriolar sheathing was found, though this had not been noted at the initial presentation. This patient had probable multiple sclerosis.

Rucker (1972) considered retinal venous sheathing to occur in some 20 per cent of cases of multiple sclerosis, and believed the sign to be '90 per cent reliable for multiple sclerosis' if cases of choroiditis and syphilis were excluded. In addition, he described cloud-like patches overlying retinal veins, and small opacities in the vitreous close to the retina. In an extensive review of the literature similar descriptions were quoted, though in some reports observers had failed to find the abnormality. Some indication of the variability with which it has been reported in multiple sclerosis patients is given in Table 12.15.

Similar forms of periphlebitis occur in a number of ocular inflammatory diseases, though in such cases they are more likely to be associated with retinal haemorrhages or venous thromboses. Some of the reports in the literature of patients with retinal vasculitis and neurological disorders

Table 12.15 **Retinal venous sheathing in multiple sclerosis**

Author	No. of patients	% with 'periphlebitis'
Field and Foster (1962)	130	0
Marshall (1950)	322	0.3 (of R eyes)
Nikoskelainen (1975*b*)	240	1.3
Croll (1965)	140	2.8
Hyllested and Moller (1961)	52	7.7
Wybar (1952)	91	10
Scott (1961)	65	10.8

attributed to multiple sclerosis are probably in reality referring to disorders such as sarcoid with a known propensity to involve the nervous system.

Rucker (1972) has suggested that a localized phlebitis might be responsible for the plaques of multiple sclerosis, quoting Fog's (1965) post-mortem report of inflammatory changes in the wall of a retinal vein. Silfverskiöld (1951) described thickening of the retinal veins without cell infiltration in a single case, and Gartner (1953) considered the pathological correlate of sheathing to be 'a thickened sclerosis of the walls of blood vessels adjacent to the optic disc', though in Rucker's (1972) experience the sheathing is usually found between two and six disc diameters from the nerve-head. The description of variable arteriolar narrowing in patients with multiple sclerosis (Franklin and Brickner 1947) was not supported by our own observations, nor indeed does it appear to have been the experience of others.

Marshall (1950) found evidence of uveitis in some 5 per cent of his optic neuritis cases, Scott (1961) mentioned old iridocyclitis in one patient (representing 1·5 per cent of his material) and Nikoskelainen (1975*b*) reported cells in the vitreous in seven affected eyes (2·9 per cent). Again, in multiple sclerosis, signs of uveitis have been reported with extreme variability. Several studies from the Continent suggest the condition is more common in multiple sclerosis than in a control population. In Haarr's (1962) experience, uveitis when present was always accompanied by periphlebitis.

Conclusions

Some 75 per cent of the optic neuritis patients may be expected to recover to 6/12 or better within 6 months of onset, and eventually approximately 85 per cent will achieve this degree of recovery. For those reaching 6/6, the mean period to do so will be in the region of 8 weeks. Although some authors have found older patients to fare less well, this has not been the uniform view, nor was it our experience.

Anisocoria was encountered at follow-up in approximately 10 per cent, the dilated pupil nearly always corresponding to the eye previously affected.

An abnormality of the pupillary reaction was detected in 55 per cent, always appropriate to the side originally involved. Optic atrophy was found in 62 per cent, and was almost inevitable after neuro-retinitis. No consistent trend has been reported for the correlation of final visual acuity to the optic disc appearance, though generally residual impairment is more likely in those with optic atrophy.

Abnormalities of colour vision occurred in 50 per cent, and were more likely in those with optic atrophy. Changes in the other, clinically unaffected, eye were found in 11 per cent, compared with 45 per cent in one other series. Differences in the duration of follow-up were probably mainly responsible for the discrepancy.

Visual fields returned to normal in only 28 per cent of our patients, with approximately a third having central, and a third scattered, paracentral defects between 5° and 25°. A consideration of the field disturbances secondary to atrophy of arcuate fibres shows close correspondence with this third group, suggesting these fibres may be more prone to axonal degeneration after demyelination than those in the papillo-macular bundle.

With recurrent attacks of optic neuritis in the same eye, residual impairment of vision, as assessed by acuity, field defect, colour vision, or optic atrophy becomes more likely. Bilateral optic neuritis (as defined) was seldom seen in this series, though it has been reported frequently elsewhere. There is no consistent evidence that such cases fare less well in terms of visual outcome nor indeed that they should be considered a separate entity, apropos eventual multiple sclerosis, from unilateral cases.

A slowly progressive visual failure was not seen, though it is a recognized phenomenon in multiple sclerosis and may well give rise to diagnostic difficulty. Such cases show less tendency to recovery, though unexpected improvement even up to 2 years after onset has been encountered in some of them.

Periphlebitis, manifesting usually as perivenous sheathing seems more likely in multiple sclerosis than a control population, and the same conclusion probably applies to uveitis. Evidence for either was seldom seen in this study however.

REFERENCES

Adie, W. J. (1932). The aetiology and symptomatology of disseminated sclerosis. *Br. med. J.* **2**, 997–1000.
Ashworth, B. (1967). Chronic retrobulbar and chiasmal neuritis. *Br. J. Ophthal.* **51**, 698–702.
Bagley, C. H. (1952). An etiologic study of a series of optic neuropathies. *Am. J. Ophthal.* **35**, 761–72.
Benedict, W. L. (1942). Multiple sclerosis as an etiologic factor in retrobulbar neuritis. *Archs Ophthal. N.Y.* **28**, 988–95.

Berliner, M. L. (1935). Acute optic neuritis in demyelinating diseases of the nervous system. *Archs Ophthal., N.Y.* **13**, 83–98.

Bradley, W. G. and Whitty, C. W. M. (1967). Acute optic neuritis: its clinical features and their relation to prognosis for recovery of vision. *J. Neurol. Neurosurg. Psychiat.* **30**, 531–8.

Croll, M. (1965). The ocular manifestations of multiple sclerosis. *Am. J. Ophthal.* **60**, 822–9.

Earl, C. J. and Martin, B. (1967). Prognosis in optic neuritis related to age. *Lancet* **1**, 74–6.

Field, E. J. and Foster, J. B. (1962). Periphlebitis retinae and multiple sclerosis. *J. Neurol. Neurosurg. Psychiat.* **25**, 269–70.

Fog, T. (1965). The topography of plaques in multiple sclerosis with special reference to cerebral plaques. *Acta Neurol. Scand.* [Suppl] **15** (Vol. 41), 1–161.

Franklin, C. R. and Brickner, R. M. (1947). Vasospasm associated with multiple sclerosis. *Archs Neurol. Psychiat., Chicago* **58**, 125–62.

Frisén, L. and Hoyt, W. F. (1974). Insidious atrophy of retinal nerve fibers in multiple sclerosis. *Archs Ophthal., N.Y.* **92**, 91–7.

Gartner, S. (1953). Optic neuropathy in multiple sclerosis. *Archs Ophthal., N.Y.* **50**, 718–26.

Gipner, J. F. (1925). The ophthalmological findings in cases of multiple sclerosis. A study of 100 cases. *Med. Clins N. Am.* **8**, 1227–34.

Gunn, R. M. (1904a). Retro-ocular neuritis. *Lancet* **2**, 412–13.

— (1904b). Discussion on retro-ocular neuritis. *Br. med. J.* **2**, 1285.

Haarr, M. (1962). Uveitis with neurological symptoms. *Acta Neurol. Scand.* **38**, 171–87.

Hierons, R. and Lyle, T. K. (1959). Bilateral retrobulbar optic neuritis. *Brain* **82**, 56–67.

Hoyt, W. F. (1962). Anatomic considerations of arcuate scotomas associated with lesions of the optic nerve and chiasm. A nauta axon degeneration study in the monkey. *Bull. Johns Hopkins Hosp.* **111**, 57–71.

Hutchinson, W. M. (1976). Acute optic neuritis and the prognosis for multiple sclerosis. *J. Neurol. Neurosurg. Psychiat.* **39**, 283–9.

Hyllested, K. and Moller, P. M. (1961). Follow-up on patients with a history of optic neuritis. *Acta ophthal.* **39**, 655–62.

Kahana, E., Leibowitz, V., Fishback, N., and Alter, M. (1973). Slowly progressive and acute visual impairment in multiple sclerosis. *Neurology, Minneap.* **23**, 729–33.

Klingmann, T. (1910). Visual disturbances in multiple sclerosis. Their relations to changes in the visual field and ophthalmoscopic findings. Diagnostic significance. Report of twelve cases. *J. nerv. ment. Dis.* **37**, 734–48.

Kurland, L. T., Beebe, G. W., Kurtzke, J. F., Nagler, B., Auth, T. L., Lessel, S., and Nefzger, M. D. (1966). Studies on the natural history of multiple sclerosis. 2. The progression of optic neuritis to multiple sclerosis. *Acta Neurol. Scand.* [Suppl] **19** (Vol. 42), 157–76.

Lowenstein, O. (1954). Clinical pupillary symptoms in lesions of the optic nerve, optic chiasm and optic tract. *Archs Ophthal., N.Y.* **52**, 385–403.

Lynn, B. H. (1959). Retrobulbar neuritis. A survey of the present condition of cases occurring over the last fifty-six years. *Trans. ophthal. Soc. U.K.* **79**, 701–16.

McIntyre, H. D. and McIntyre, A. P. (1943). Prognosis of multiple sclerosis. *Archs Neurol. Psychiat., Chicago* **50**, 431–8.

Marshall, D. (1950). Ocular manifestations of multiple sclerosis and relationship to retrobulbar neuritis. *Trans. Am. ophthal. Soc.* **48**, 487–525.

Müller, R. (1949). Studies on disseminated sclerosis. *Acta med. scand. Suppl.* **222**, 1–214.

Nettleship, E. (1884). On cases of retro-ocular neuritis. *Trans. ophthal. Soc. U.K.* **4**, 186–226.

Nikoskelainen, E. (1975a). Later course and prognosis of optic neuritis. *Acta ophthal.* **53**, 273–91.

— (1975b). Symptoms, signs and early course of optic neuritis. *Acta ophthal.* **53**, 254–72.

Rischbieth, R. H. C. (1968). Retrobulbar neuritis in the State of South Australia. *Proc. Aust. Assoc. Neurol.* **5**, 573–5.

Rosen, J. A. (1965). Pseudoisochromatic visual testing in the diagnosis of disseminated sclerosis. *Trans. Am. neurol. Ass.* **90**, 283–4.

Rucker, C. W. (1972). Sheathing of the retinal veins in multiple sclerosis. *Proc. Staff Meet. Mayo Clin.* **47**, 335–40.

Sandberg, H. O. (1972). Acute retrobulbar neuritis—a retrospective study. *Acta ophthal.* **50**, 3–8.

Savitsky, N. and Rangell, L. (1950). The ocular findings in multiple sclerosis. In *Multiple sclerosis and the demyelinating diseases.* Research Publications of the Association for Research in Nervous and Mental Diseases, Vol. 28, pp. 403–13. Williams and Wilkins, Baltimore.

Schlossman, A. and Phillips, C. C. (1954). Optic neuritis in relation to demyelinating diseases. *Am. J. Ophthal.* **37**, 487–94.

Scott, G. I. (1961). Ophthalmic aspects of demyelinating diseases. *Proc. R. Soc. Med.* **54**, 38–42.

Silfverskiöld, B. P. (1951). Retinal periphlebitis and chronic disseminated encephalomyelitis. *Acta psychiat. scand. Suppl.* **74**, 55–7.

Thompson, H. S. (1966). Afferent pupillary defects. *Am. J. Ophthal.* **62**, 860–73.

White, D. N. and Wheelan, L. (1959). Disseminated sclerosis. A survey of patients in the Kingston, Ontario, area. *Neurology, Minneap.* **9**, 256–72.

Wybar, K. C. (1952). The ocular manifestations of disseminated sclerosis. *Proc. R. Soc. Med.* **45**, 315–20.

Yaskin, J. C., Spaeth, E. B., and Vernlund, R. J. (1951). Ocular manifestations of 100 consecutive cases of multiple sclerosis. *Am. J. Ophthal.* **3**, 687–97.

13 Prognosis for the development of multiple sclerosis

> I wish particularly to emphasise that in cases of unilateral acute optic neuritis one must always consider the possibility of disseminated sclerosis, even when no other signs of damage to the nervous system are demonstrable (Berliner 1935).

The frequency with which multiple sclerosis has been said to follow an attack of optic neuritis has varied from series to series (see Table 13.1). Information from several papers (see Table 13.1) on diagnostic criteria was sparse and further discussion on these pointless. Even when analysis is confined to those papers giving adequate clinical detail, considerable discrepancies remain. In this chapter we report the findings of an analysis which includes:

a the clinical material;
b the definition of optic neuritis;
c the definition of multiple sclerosis;
d The frequency of progression according to Kurland, Auth, Beebe, Kurtzke, Lessell, Nagler, and Nefzger (1963, 1966); Collis (1965); Bradley and Whitty (1968); Percy, Nobrega, and Kurland (1972); Nikoskelainen and Riekkinen (1974); Hutchinson (1976);
e the factors influencing progression;
f the rate of progression;
g the authors' clinical material;
h the relationship of optic neuritis to multiple sclerosis in children.
f the rate of progression;
g the authors' clinical material;
h the relationship of optic neuritis to multiple sclerosis in children.

The clinical material

The majority of authors have analysed retrospectively series of optic neuritis patients and then assessed them for evidence of multiple sclerosis. Although this has the advantage of a substantial period of follow-up in most instances, it relies on the accuracy of the original diagnosis and, more critically, on the assumption that a thorough neurological assessment was made at the original presentation with failure to find evidence of other lesions.

Series in which patients have been seen at the onset of visual symptoms and then followed personally are few, and suffer the disadvantage of a relatively short period of follow-up. For example, in the series of

Table 13.1 The frequency of multiple sclerosis following optic neuritis

	No of patients	% developing multiple sclerosis	Mean period, or range of follow-up (years)
Lenoire (1917)	11	0	
Heckford (1934)	10	0	9
Bagley (1952)	47	0	0–7
Friedinger (1925)	26	12	5
Kurland *et al*. (1966)	183	13‡	12–18
Percy *et al*. (1972)	24	17	18
Sandberg-Wollheim (1975)	56	19.6‡	2.6
Kennedy and Carter (1961)	30 (children)	27	8
Alter *et al*. (1973)		29*	10
Tatlow (1948)	26	31	
Taub & Rucker (1954)	87	32‡	10–15
Langenbeck (1914)		33	
Landy and Ohlrich (1970)	51	39	0.5–15
Marshall (1950)		36‡	4–20
Collis (1965)	75	36	7–20
Alter *et al*. (1973)		39†	10
Otradovec and Votockova (1962)	82	40‡	5–15
Sandberg (1972)	51	47	3–7
Hyllested and Moller (1961)	31	48	2–15
Nikoskelainen and Reikkinen (1974)		50	10.2
Lynn (1959)	97	50	
Bradley and Whitty (1968)	66	51‡	0.5–20
Hyllested (1966)	84	57	26–51
Rose *et al*. (1972)	78	58‡	0.5–5.5
Marburg (1920)	24	58	
Fleischer (1908)	42	62	
Behr (1924)		70	
Scheerer (1929)		71.5	
Hutchinson (1976)	132	78‡	1–15
McAlpine (1964)	67	85§	18
Rischbieth (1968)	100	85‡	4–54

* Patients of Caucasian origin. † Patients of Oriental origin. ‡ Represents a final value where figures indicated an increasing percentage with length of follow up. § McAlpine's series consists of those patients reported by Lynn and followed for at least 5 years.
The papers of Fleischer (1908), Langenbeck (1914), Lenoire (1917), Marburg (1920), Behr (1924), Friedinger (1925), Scheerer (1929), Heckford (1934) and Otradovec and Votockova (1962) have either not been consulted personally, or were never published in detailed form.

Sandberg-Wollheim (1975), the mean follow-up was 2·6 years and, with our own patients, only 11 had been followed for periods exceeding 54 months.

The definition of optic neuritis

In many instances, no adequate definition of optic neuritis has been stated (Marshall 1950; Bagley 1952; Taub and Rucker 1954; Hyllested and Moller

1961; Hyllested 1966; Rischbieth 1968). Those used in the series listed in Table 13.1 are given in Table 13.2.

Table 13.2 The definition of optic neuritis

	Bilateral cases included
Tatlow (1948): Sudden visual failure with or without disc swelling and usually recovering vision through a central scotoma	+
Lynn (1959)	
McAlpine (1964): Rapid deterioration of vision with minimal or no fundus change, and showing a tendency to recover	+
Collis (1965): Defective vision in one eye, not progressing for more than 3 days and with normal fundoscopy	−
Kurland *et al.* (1966)	
Percy *et al.* (1972): Rapid onset of blurring of vision, with or without pain, with demonstrable scotoma or reduced visual acuity, and temporal pallor, a normal disc, or swelling with or without haemorrhages or exudates	+ retrobulbar cases − papillitis
Bradley and Whitty (1968): Acute onset of blurred vision in one or both eyes without demonstrable cause	+
Landy and Ohlrich (1970): Sudden onset of blurred vision in one or both eyes, with central or centrocaecal scotoma, or total loss of vision or reduction to counting fingers. Patients over 55 years excluded	+
Sandberg (1972): Central scotoma of acute or sub-acute onset	+
Alter *et al.* (1973): Sudden onset of visual blurring with a central field defect, with or without disc swelling	+
Nikoskelainen and Riekkinen (1974): Involvement of the optic nerve by any inflammation, demyelination, or degeneration	+
Sandberg-Wollheim (1975): Acute monosymptomatic optic neuritis with exclusion of toxic, vascular, diabetic, or tumour cases	−
Hutchinson (1976): Acute or subacute onset of blurred vision in one or both eyes, associated with central, paracentral, or centro-caecal scotoma, excluding ischaemia, tumour, or retinal lesions.	+

An acute visual failure is usually stressed, though rarely is a specific time course stated. The presence of pain has been increasingly recognized as part of the symptomatology of optic neuritis, but it may be absent in otherwise typical cases, and its presence has no influence on the subsequent development of multiple sclerosis (Bradley and Whitty 1968). Not surprisingly, its presence has not been considered necessary in order to make the diagnosis.

Most definitions include the presence of a field defect, concentrating on central, paracentral, or centrocaecal scotomata. Atypical field defects, either quadrantic (Bradley and Whitty 1968), arcuate, altitudinal, or peripheral

(Lynn 1959), behave in a similar fashion, both in terms of the visual outcome and the subsequent incidence of multiple sclerosis.

The fundus changes thought to be compatible with the diagnosis have been variously stated. Generally, disc swelling has been accepted, although Collis (1965) excluded such cases and Lynn (1959) restricted her definition to discs showing minimal changes; her discussion on the problems of differential diagnosis between papilloedema and papillitis would suggest that more florid examples were included. Disc swelling in itself appears to have no significant effect on visual outcome (Bradley and Whitty 1968) or the progression to multiple sclerosis (Bradley and Whitty 1968; Hutchinson 1976).

The majority of series have included bilateral cases, though Kurland *et al.* (1966) excluded bilateral papillitis where the two eyes were involved within a period of 2 weeks, on the assumption, probably incorrect in adults, that a specific agent was more likely to be responsible.

The achievement of a homogeneous population of optic neuritis patients appears to chiefly depend on the careful search for other aetiological factors. The overlap of the syndrome with the symptoms produced by, for example, nerve compression (Chapter 5) is considerable, and a period of follow-up may be necessary before other aetiologies are established, e.g. in one series of 25 patients with optic neuritis one patient was subsequently shown to have a meningioma (Sandberg and Bynke 1973).

The criteria for the diagnosis of multiple sclerosis

In many reports, the criteria for the diagnosis of multiple sclerosis have been stated inadequately, if at all; for example 'evidence of a disseminated disease process' (Rischbieth 1968); 'abnormal neurological symptoms or signs' (Collis 1965); 'manifest or early (latent) disseminated sclerosis' (Hyllested and Moller 1961); 'abnormal neurological findings' (Tatlow 1948).

When more explicit criteria have been stated, emphasis has centred on a remitting and relapsing history, with the finding of at least two separate lesions known to be associated with multiple sclerosis (Table 13.3). The Schumacher committee (1965) definitions are similar to those of Nagler *et al.* (1966), explicable no doubt by the fact that several authors were involved in both publications. The slight changes between the criteria over a two-year period illustrate the difficulties in producing an acceptable definition of the disease on clinical criteria. Only Millar (1971) failed to insist on a remitting and relapsing history for a definite diagnosis, a fact which may help to explain the frequency with which multiple sclerosis was found to follow optic neuritis in Hutchinson's (1976) series. In some respects, these strict criteria, though unarguably valid, will exclude cases which, despite a relative lack of

Table 13.3 Diagnostic criteria for multiple sclerosis

Hyllested (1966)
Definite: dissemination in space and time with fluctuating course and signs of at least two lesions.
Possible: signs of involvement outside the optic nerves, but symptoms mild, non-progressive, or evanescent.

Kurland *et al.* (1966) used the criteria of Nagler *et al.* (1963)
Definite: 1. Dysfunction attributable to involvement of two or more parts of CNS white matter.
2. Two or more bouts of dysfunction 1 month or more apart or continuous over 6 months.
3. No other cause, including syphilis.
4. Especially critical assessment for onset outside the ages 15 to 45.
Possible: either 1. All definite criteria except either multiple bouts or progression.
or: 2. Single white matter lesion ? cause.
or: 3. Multiple lesions but other causes likely for all but one.

Bradley and Whitty (1968)
Definite: subsequently one or more neurological symptoms, relapsing and remitting in character, together with two or more signs (pyramidal and at least one other) of multiple lesions of the CNS.
Probable: development of a sign indicating a separate neurological lesion, without a history of relapsing symptoms.

Nikoskelainen and Riekkinen (1974) used criteria of Schumacher committee (1965)
Definite: 1. Objective signs of CNS dysfunction.
2. History or signs of at least two separate lesions of the CNS.
3. Signs suggesting white-matter disease.
4. Two or more relapses, separated by 1 month, or progression over at least 6 months.
5. Age at onset 10–50 yrs
6. No better explanation.
Possible: definite physical signs indicative of white-matter disease for which no other cause could be found, but not fulfilling all the first five criteria.

Hutchinson (1976) used the criteria of Millar (1971)
Probable: no reasonable doubt about diagnosis, physical disablement, clear-cut history of remission or relapses or undoubted evidence on examination of physical signs explicable only on the basis of multiple sclerosis.
Possible: no clear-cut evidence of multiplicity of lesions and history frequently one of slowly progressive disability, usually a spastic paraparesis.

neurological history, will show unequivocal evidence of multiple sclerosis at post-mortem. The more recent diagnostic criteria produced by the Medical Research Council Committee (1975) (Table 13.4) incorporating electrophysiological data, may go some way to resolve this problem when applied to cases with less overt neurological disease.

The frequency with which multiple sclerosis follows optic neuritis

The problems in interpretation of these figures is illustrated by the paper of Taub and Rucker (1954). Although, according to Kurland *et al.* (1966),

Table 13.4 Diagnostic classification criteria

Proven	Pathological proof
Clinically definite	Some physical disablement Remitting and relapsing ≥ 2 episodes
Early, probable, and latent	Signs of lesions at 2 or more sites Lesions predominantly white matter Age at onset 10–50 No better explanation Slight or no disability Remitting and relapsing ≥ 1 abnormal sign associated with MS Early single episode suggestive of MS with signs of multiple lesions
Progressive possible	Some physical disability Progressive history No definite evidence of > 1 lesion Other causes excluded
Progressive probable	As progressive possible but ≥ 2 lesions

these authors accepted 'the usual criteria' for the diagnosis of optic neuritis, these were never stated in the paper. The study was said to be confined to cases of retrobulbar neuritis, though it is quite clear that patients with papillitis were included. The inclusion or not of bilateral cases is never explicitly stated (Kurland *et al.* (1966) imply they were not), and the criteria for the diagnosis of multiple sclerosis were not given. From considering this study the time stated as the onset of multiple sclerosis needs to be interpreted with caution. There it was defined as the time when the patient was first seen for his neurological complaints (personal communication to Collis 1965), whereas other authors (for example Collis (1965)) have defined this as the time at which the patient recalled the onset of neurological symptoms.

An additional problem, already referred to and capable of exaggerating the apparent progression to multiple sclerosis, is how strictly patients presenting with optic neuritis are assessed for symptoms and signs referrable to lesions outside the visual pathway, and excluded if appropriate. Rischbieth (1968) included such patients, but in three the assumption of a more generalized neurological process was based on cerebrospinal fluid abnormalities alone. Similarly Tatlow (1948) and Hyllested and Moller (1961) included such patients, the latter observing that in some instances neurological abnormalities at the time of the attack of optic neuritis were not apparent at follow-up examination. Alter, Good, and Okihiro (1973) accepted those patients with retrobulbar neuritis who had other neurological symptoms, providing they were not accompanied by physical signs, or any such signs were not explicable on the basis of demyelination. When patients with previous symptoms or signs are excluded, the percentage appearing to progress to multiple sclerosis falls (Nikoskelainen and Riekkinen 1974).

It is also clear that some patients with neurological signs at follow-up, strongly suggestive of multiple sclerosis, may have had insufficient disability to warrant being under neurological review. Bradley and Whitty (1968) found that 33 per cent of patients personally examined had neurological signs unknown to their doctor. Similarly, of 12 patients examined by Tatlow (1948) and found to have neurological abnormalities, only five had previously stated the existence of a neurological problem in a written questionnaire. Nikoskelainen and Riekkinen (1974) commented that their multiple sclerosis patients included some whose symptoms were so mild that they would have been unlikely to seek a neurological examination unless specifically requested. Clearly, follow-up assessments which rely on anything other than personal examination are likely to under-estimate the presence of other neurological abnormalities.

Kurland *et al.* (1963, 1966)

These authors published their results in a brief précis in 1963, and in greater detail in 1966, though some discrepancies exist between the two papers United States Army World War Two personnel were studied, in whom a diagnosis of retrobulbar neuritis or papillitis had been made previously and, of necessity, only males were included. Bilateral cases were accepted, other than bilateral papillitis where the second eye had been affected within 2 weeks of the first. Of a total of 428 cases theoretically eligible, 245 were excluded, leaving 183. Of these, only 108 were personally examined by the authors for the possible presence of multiple sclerosis. Optic neuritis was defined strictly, with central or paracentral field defects predominating. Bilateral cases accounted for 27 per cent of the total.

Forty-five patients were encountered who had 'some evidence for possible neurologic dysfunction' but 21 were subsequently eliminated though the diagnoses in this group were never stated. The percentage of patients developing multiple sclerosis is extremely small in comparison with many other series. The criteria for the diagnosis (Nagler, Beebe, Kurtzke, Kurland, Auth, and Nefzger 1966) are clearly defined, and the authors considered the higher figures obtained by others to be partly explicable by the probable inclusion of cases already having evidence of disseminated lesions at the onset of optic neuritis, a conclusion supported to some extent by the results of Nikoskelainen and Riekkinen (1974). Their interpretation of Hyllested and Moller's (1961) paper is based on inaccurate figures, though it must be admitted that the paper itself gives a number of conflicting values. These criticisms could not be extended to series (Bradley and Whitty 1968; Hutchinson 1976; our own material) where a thorough neurological examination has been performed at onset. The timing of the subsequent neurological examination may be critical, since some patients with initial neurological abnormalities may not show them subsequently (Hyllested and Moller 1961). The decision to exclude patients with bilateral papillitis was based on an assumption that such cases were more likely to have a 'specific agent' responsible; 39 cases came under this category. Hutchinson (1976) has recently demonstrated that patients with bilateral optic neuritis (including papillitis) are more likely to develop multiple sclerosis over a ten-year period than unilateral cases.

The final problem in interpreting these results lies in the observer discrepancy in diagnosing multiple sclerosis, a difficulty referred to in the first publication (1963) but not the second (1966). Five diagnostic groups were defined: (1) definite multiple sclerosis, (2) possible multiple sclerosis, (3) not multiple sclerosis, (4) unknown, and (5) primary lateral sclerosis. Amongst three assessors, chief disagreement was showed between several categories including (1) and (3), a discrepancy difficult to understand considering the clear-cut diagnostic criteria. Disagreement within pairs of observers averaged 68 per cent, and it is impossible to assess how many patients were left in categories (3) and (4), what their diagnoses were, and how many patients were included in category (5). The combination of optic neuritis and a subsequent primary lateral sclerosis (presumably manifesting as a spastic paraplegia) would be categorized as progressive probable multiple sclerosis on more recent criteria (Davison *et al.* 1975).

Collis (1965)

This series covered patients with unilateral retrobulbar neuritis diagnosed at the Cleveland Clinic between 1942 and 1957. Multiple sclerosis was defined as 'the occurrence of abnormal neurological symptoms or signs, independent of the retrobulbar neuritis'. The symptoms had to be remissive in character but the diagnosis was still made in their absence if a patient presented with multiple neurological signs. Seventy-five of the 85 patients fulfilling the authors' criteria were available for examination, 41 being seen personally, 24 by other members of the Cleveland Neurology department, and 10 by other neurologists.

Bradley and Whitty (1968)

Sixty-six of a total of 85 patients were examined personally (63) or in the authors' department (3) in this survey. The mean follow-up period was 10·2 years, with a range of 6 months to 20 years. Twenty per cent were thought to have developed definite multiple sclerosis (including 2 with Devic's disease) and 31 per cent probable multiple sclerosis. All but one of the patients with definite multiple sclerosis had developed the disease within 4 years of the onset of optic neuritis. The time to onset of multiple sclerosis was taken as the time of neurological re-examination, irrespective of the presence or absence of symptoms in the intervening period, a necessary simplification adopted with our own material. Thus, in one patient, optic neuritis at the age of 46 was followed by an episode of vertigo 9 years later but neurological examination confirming multiple sclerosis, did not take place until the age of 64. The time taken for the establishment of multiple sclerosis, 18 years, may clearly represent an exaggeration in such cases.

Percy *et al.* (1972)

Kurland's presence as a co-author in this paper led to similar diagnostic criteria being used to those in his own study, though the definition of multiple sclerosis was never given. Over a mean follow-up period of 18 years only 17 per cent of 24 patients with optic neuritis developed multiple sclerosis, all within 4 years of the onset. The authors suggested that hospital series of optic neuritis patients might be distorted by a tendency to favour those with a more severe or persistent visual disturbance, though this criticism seems irrelevant when it is appreciated that the extent of vision loss has no influence on the subsequent incidence of multiple sclerosis (Bradley and Whitty 1968). They concluded 'the types of selection bias which would conceivably influence hospitalization for optic neuritis alone are not well established'. Patients with optic neuritis alone are probably not often admitted, and in our series, where they were, no selection operated since all patients with the diagnosis were admitted. As virtually all patients with established multiple sclerosis will have optic nerve demyelination histologically a considerable proportion of patients who develop such lesions will be asymptomatic, or have such minimal symptoms that they will not consult a neurologist.

The question of observer bias in the diagnosis of multiple sclerosis is raised by the fact that two series, reporting from the same hospital, produced widely differing figures. Percy *et al*. (1972) limited their Mayo Clinic cases to those resident in Rochester for at least 1 year before the onset of symptoms. Taub and Rucker (1954) included all Mayo Clinic cases seen between 1937 and 1942, irrespective of their residence, and found a subsequent incidence of multiple sclerosis approximately twice that of the other series. Neither group analysed the racial origins of their patients, though in one study from Israel (Leibowitz, Alter, and Halpern (1966) optic neuritis appeared more likely to arrest in the Afro-Asian population, whilst the likelihood of progression to multiple sclerosis from optic neuritis does not differ significantly between Oriental and Caucasian populations in Hawaii (Alter *et al*. 1973).

Nikoskelainen and Riekkinen (1974)

These authors reassessed 116 patients with an original diagnosis of optic neuritis; bilateral cases and those with papillitis were included. A hundred and four patients had had a neurological examination at the time of the initial attack, when seven had a definite diagnosis of multiple sclerosis made, and the diagnosis was suspected in a further 20, to be subsequently confirmed in 15. Optic neuritis was found to progress to multiple sclerosis in 63·3 per cent (69 of 109), though this figure includes 12 patients not examined initially and 20 patients in whom the diagnosis of multiple sclerosis was already suspected at the onset, presumably on the basis of other neurological symptoms. Since the authors included 15 patients with other causes of optic neuritis in their original material (for example polyneuropathy with uraemia, Leber's optic atrophy, and glaucoma), and also accepted in the idiopathic optic neuritis group some patients with subsequent neurological symptoms or signs, it is impossible to arrive at an accurate figure for the progression.

Hutchinson (1976)

A hundred and thirty-two patients were followed, of whom 67 (51 per cent) developed features suggesting multiple sclerosis; the mean follow-up period was 90·3 months. Probable multiple sclerosis accounted for 29·6 per cent and possible for 21·4 per cent. The author used a life-table method for assessing the long-term likelihood of developing multiple sclerosis, concluding that after 15 years the figure would have reached 77·8 per cent. The proportion of probable to possible cases in this final estimate is not given, though if it were similar to that of the total group, the respective percentages would be 45·1 and 32·7.

A total of 36 cases appear to have withdrawn during the first 10 years of follow-up, though the reasons for this are not stated. The figures indicate a progressive increase in the incidence of multiple sclerosis with time, though it is not possible to deduce whether this applies to both probable and possible cases or, as with Bradley and Whitty's (1968) study, to possible cases only.

Factors thought to influence the development of multiple sclerosis

Age at onset

The influence of this factor remains unsettled, although most authors have found that older patients are less likely to develop multiple sclerosis subsequently. In four series, the number progressing to multiple sclerosis were: over 44 years at onset 1/23 patients (Taub and Rucker 1954) and 0/17 patients (Collis 1965); over 46 years at onset 2/10 patients (Hyllested 1966); and over 50 years at onset 0/8 patients (Sandberg 1972). Forty per cent of Hutchinson's (1976) patients over 45 years developed multiple sclerosis, though it is not clear if this figure differed significantly from that for patients of other age groups. Bradley and Whitty (1968) found multiple sclerosis appeared in all their patients who developed optic neuritis over the age of 51, but the total was probably only five or six, and in three-quarters the diagnosis was 'possible' rather than 'probable' multiple sclerosis.

Sex
There is no significant difference in the likelihood of progression to multiple sclerosis between the sexes (Collis 1965; Bradley and Whitty 1968).

Unilateral or bilateral involvement
In most series, bilateral involvement has had no influence on the progression to multiple sclerosis (Kurland *et al.* 1966; Bradley and Whitty 1968). Otradovec and Votockova (1962) reported a higher incidence of multiple sclerosis where visual disturbances had affected the two eyes gradually after different time intervals, but these terms were never defined in detail. In a more recent study (Hutchinson 1976), bilateral optic neuritis affecting the two eyes together within the space of 2 weeks was more likely than unilateral optic neuritis to progress to multiple sclerosis over the first 10 years of follow-up. Bilateral cases in children appear to behave differently (*vide infra*). The side of involvement in unilateral cases has no significant effect on subsequent demyelination (Bradley and Whitty 1968, and our own series). In a recent series, recurrent attacks, whether unilateral, bilateral or both were associated with a higher risk of subsequent multiple sclerosis (Compston, Batchelor, Earl, and McDonald 1978).

The presence of pain
This appears to be without effect on prognosis (Collis 1965; Bradley and Whitty 1968).

The type of field defect
In some instances, cases with atypical field defects have been excluded on the assumption that they might represent a separate entity, though further experience has shown that they behave, both in terms of visual recovery and subsequent evidence of multiple sclerosis, like more typical cases (Bradley and Whitty 1968). In their first communication, Kurland *et al.* (1963) suggested that patients without a field defect at onset had a greater chance

of developing multiple sclerosis, but did not confirm this subsequently (Kurland *et al*. 1966).

The initial or subsequent appearance of the optic disc

Neither initial disc swelling (Kurland *et al*. 1966; Bradley and Whitty 1968) nor subsequent pallor (Collis 1965) have been found to influence progression.

Month of onset

In one series (Taub and Rucker 1954), 39·2 per cent of cases developing optic neuritis in April – October progressed to multiple sclerosis, compared to 16·7 per cent of those presenting in November – March. This discrepancy has not been confirmed by other studies (Kurland *et al*. 1966; Bradley and Whitty 1968). Patients possessing the determinant BT 101 who develop optic neuritis between October and March appear more likely to progress to multiple sclerosis than those with the same determinant whose attacks occur between April and September (Compston *et al*. 1978).

Progression of visual disturbance or visual outcome

Neither of these factors appears relevant (Kurland *et al*. 1966), nor indeed does the severity of vision loss, as measured by visual acuity (Bradley and Whitty 1968).

Race and birthplace

The evidence here is contradictory. In a series of U.S. servicemen, neither appeared significant (Kurland *et al*. 1966). It has been suggested (Leibowitz *et al*. 1966) that optic neuropathy is more likely to progress to multiple sclerosis in Europeans in Israel than in the Afro-Asian population. In a similar study comparing the Oriental and Caucasian populations in Hawaii (Alter *et al*. 1973), no significant differences were found.

Cerebrospinal fluid and histocompatibility status

These have already been discussed in Chapter 9. A raised cell count, protein concentration, and presence of colloidal gold curve abnormalities are of no prognostic significance (Bradley and Whitty 1968; Hutchinson 1976), although such changes have been considered to reflect evidence of multiple sclerosis (Rischbieth 1968). Over a limited follow-up period, the presence of oligoclonal IgG appears similarly without prognostic value (Sandberg-Wollheim 1975). Regarding histocompatibility status, the possession of certain determinants has been considered of predictive value for multiple sclerosis by some authors (Arnason 1975) but not by others (Sandberg-Wollheim, Platz, Ryder, Nielsen, and Thompson 1975). An analysis of B lymphocyte determinants in optic neuritis patients, and their effect on the subsequent development of multiple sclerosis has been published (Compston *et al*. 1978). Using an actuarial method of analysis, 73 per cent of those patients with BT 101 were likely to develop the disease over an 8-year follow-up, compared with 34 per cent of those without it.

Other factors

Kurland *et al*. (1966) assessed the possible influence of a large number of factors in optic neuritis patients on the subsequent incidence of demyelination elsewhere. Those found to be significant were:

a pupillary asymmetry;
b defective vision at entry to the Armed Service;
c twelve or more completed years of formal schooling prior to induction.

As these authors indicate, by considering the influence of a total of 42 factors, two significant associations would have been expected even with homogeneous material; the arbitrary quality of these associations would not seem to support the concept of their being influential.

The rate of progression

A study of the published series fails to resolve this question (Table 13.5 and Fig. 13.1). In many the impression is gained of a progressive increase with which multiple sclerosis is diagnosed according to the length of follow-up (Marshall 1950; Taub and Rucker 1954; Otradovec and Votockova 1962; Kurland *et al*. 1966; Bradley and Whitty 1968; Rischbieth 1968; Sandberg-Wollheim 1975; Hutchinson 1976). Periods of time between optic neuritis and subsequent multiple sclerosis amounting to 15 years (Adams 1927), 22 and 24 years (Adie 1930), and 29 years (Mackay 1953) have been used to further this argument. In other series, however, the cases

Table 13.5 Percentage of patients presenting with optic neuritis, who develop multiple sclerosis

	Years of follow-up									
	1	2	3	4	5	6	7	8	9	10
Kurland *et al*. (1966)		3.8	6.0		7.1		8.2		9.3	
Percy *et al*. (1972)	4.2	8.3		16.6						16.6
Taub and Rucker (1954)	4.6	6.9	9.2	10	14.9	17.2		21.7		
Otradovec and Votockova (1962)		8.8			32.9					
Sandberg-Wollheim (1975)	10.7	17.9	19.6							
Collis (1965)	14.7	24	31	32				32		
Bradley and Whitty (1968)	16	21		25		31		32		
Marshall (1950)				31.7						
* Hutchinson (1976)	18	23	33	36	41	41	48	52		59
Rischbieth (1968)	30	48								

* Refers to unilateral cases.

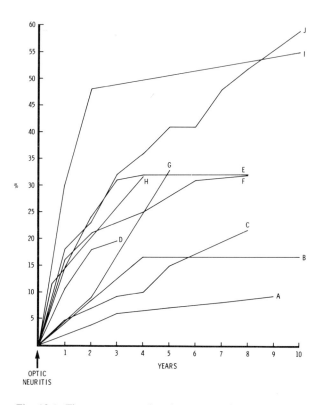

Fig. 13.1. The percentage of patients presenting with optic neuritis who develop evidence of multiple sclerosis during follow-up.
A, Kurland *et al.* (1966); B, Percy *et al.* (1972); C, Taub and Rucker (1954); D, Sandberg-Wollheim (1975); E, Collis (1965); F, Bradley and Whitty (1968); G, Otradovec and Votockova (1962); H, Marshall (1950); I, Rischbieth (1968); J, Hutchinson (1976).

progressing to multiple sclerosis have declared themselves within a relatively short time-interval. All the patients in two series (Collis 1965; Percy *et al.* 1972) had developed the disease within 4 years, despite a follow-up period overall of 7–20 years in the first, and 2–33 years in the second.

Where various diagnostic criteria have been applied for multiple sclerosis, it has been suggested that cases falling in the definite group may declare themselves relatively early, whilst more problematic examples are diagnosed with increasing frequency according to the length of follow-up. Thus with Bradley and Whitty's (1968) material, all but one of the cases with

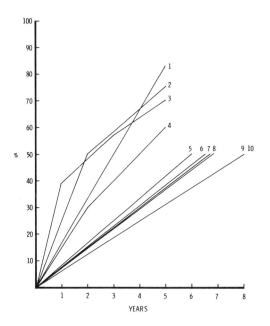

Fig. 13.2. Patients with multiple sclerosis whose initial symptom was optic neuritis. Time taken to establish the diagnosis (mean). 1. Nikoskelainen and Riekkinen (1974); 2. Symonds (1930); 3. Müller (1949); 4. White and Wheelan (1959); 5. Lazarte (1950); 6. Lynn (1959); 7. Leibowitz *et al.* (1966); 8. Adie (1932); 9. Wybar (1952); 10. Adie (1930).

definite multiple sclerosis were diagnosed within 4 years, but cases with probable multiple sclerosis continued to be diagnosed up to 20 years after the onset of optic neuritis. Hyllested (1966) concluded that all 'serious cases' of multiple sclerosis had declared themselves within 5 years of onset. None of the series referred to above, apart from that of Bradley and Whitty (1968) have attempted to divide their material according to the degree of certainty of diagnosis, in order to test this hypothesis. The question can be separately assessed by examining patients with definite multiple sclerosis and a past history of optic neuritis, to determine the time interval required to establish the diagnosis. The results of several series, however (Fig. 13.2), are at least as conflicting as the information from follow-up of optic neuritis cases. It seems probable that the quality of neurological review during the intervening period is the most variable factor, and thereby the one most likely to cause such marked differences.

The authors' material

Seventy-eight patients with optic neuritis alone were followed for a minimum of 6 months. The diagnostic criteria for optic neuritis were 'a condition causing a relatively rapid onset of visual failure, in which no evidence for a toxic, vascular, or compressive aetiology can be discovered, and where local retinal lesions have been excluded'.

All patients had a neurological examination at the onset of visual symptoms, the result of which, by definition, was normal. In addition, none gave a history of previous neurological symptoms. At follow-up, neurological examination, by two independent assessors, was only considered abnormal if agreed by both. The diagnostic criteria for multiple sclerosis were:

Definite (3)

A history of optic neuritis and of remitting and relapsing symptoms with physical signs of at least two separate neurological lesions outside the visual system.

Probable (2)

A history of optic neuritis and either
a remitting and relapsing symptoms but physical signs of only one lesion; or
b no history of remitting and relapsing symptoms but physical signs of two or more lesions.

Possible (1)

A history of optic neuritis and either
a remitting and relapsing symptoms without physical signs; or
b physical signs of one lesion without remitting and relapsing symptoms.

Overall, 57·7 per cent of patients showed some evidence of multiple sclerosis at follow-up examination, consisting of 20·5 per cent with possible, 24·4 per cent with probable, and 12·8 per cent with definite multiple sclerosis.

The factors influencing the progression

The following variables were studied: Age at onset, sex, unilateral v. bilateral, presence of pain, type of field defect, presence of disc swelling, subsequent optic atrophy, month of onset, worst visual acuity, degree of visual recovery, racial origin, abnormal CSF count, elevated CSF protein concentration, abnormal colloidal gold curve, and the presence of anisocoria at onset. Table 13.6 compares the findings in patients with and without any evidence of multiple sclerosis at follow-up. None of the apparent variations is significant. There is no evidence from this series that older patients developing optic neuritis are less likely to develop multiple sclerosis subsequently, though none of them were in the definite group, a result reminiscent

Table 13.6 Factors in optic neuritis patients relating to subsequent multiple sclerosis (authors' series) (figures in per cent)

	No evidence of subsequent MS	Any evidence of subsequent MS	Definite MS
* Over 45 years at onset	25	75	0
† Over 50 years at onset	28.5	71.5	0
Males	40	60	12
Females	42	58	14
Unilateral	All the cases in this series of 78 were unilateral		
Without pain	36	64	27
‡Atypical field defect	25	75	25
Disc swelling	50	50	2.5
Subsequent optic atrophy	41	59	12.2
Onset April–October	44	56	9.7
Visual acuity < 6/60	38	62	10.8
Recovery to < 6/6	30	70	20
§Non-caucasians	100	0	
Abnormal CSF cell count	20	80	10
Elevated CSF protein concentration	27	73	18
Abnormal colloidal gold curve	Only 1 patient without subsequent evidence of MS		
Anisocoria	38	62	9.5

* 14 patients
† 4 patients
‡ Refers to altitudinal, hemianopic, or peripheral field defects
§ 2 patients

of Bradley and Whitty's (1968) findings. The sexes developed multiple sclerosis with equal frequency, and in the absence of bilateral cases we are unable to confirm Hutchinson's (1976) impression. The absence of pain in the original attack is clearly irrelevant, and patients with atypical field defects at onset were somewhat more likely to develop disseminated lesions later. As with previous series, we have not found the initial or final disc appearance nor the severity of vision loss to be relevant. Anisocoria was detected relatively frequently (in 21 patients) but we could not confirm Kurland *et al.*'s (1966) impression that it was more often associated with multiple sclerosis. Abnormalities on the cerebrospinal fluid are clearly of no value in indicating subsequent prognosis.

The rate of progression in this series

This is summarized in Table 13.7 and Fig. 13.3. If all diagnostic groups are included, an impression of increasing frequency of the disease with length of follow-up is obtained. This impression, however, is not sustained when only the more definite cases (2 + 3) are considered; the marked increase in the number of definite cases diagnosed in patients followed between 54 and 65

Table 13.7 Frequency of multiple sclerosis (per cent) according to certainty of diagnosis, following presentation with isolated optic neuritis

	Period of follow-up (months)				
	6–17	18–29	30–41	42–53	54–65
Number of patients	26	9	13	19	11
Diagnostic criteria					
1	11.5	22.3	30.8	31.6	9.1
2	26.9	33.3	23.2	15.8	27.3
3	7.7	0	7.5	15.8	36.3
2+3	34.6	33.3	30.7	31.6	63.6
1+2+3	46.1	55.6	61.5	63.2	72.7

1, 2, 3, refer to diagnostic criteria for multiple sclerosis
1 = possible, 2 = probable, 3 = definite multiple sclerosis

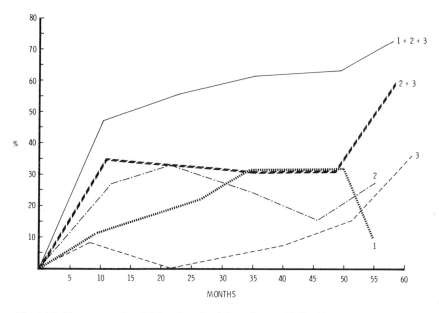

Fig. 13.3. Frequency of multiple sclerosis after optic neuritis in this series according to length of follow-up. 1. definite; 2. probable; 3. possible multiple sclerosis.

months is based on a total of only 11 patients and must be interpreted with caution. It would be premature to use these figures to support either of the hypotheses regarding the development of multiple sclerosis after optic neuritis.

The relationship of optic neuritis to multiple sclerosis in children (Table 13.7)

Kennedy and Carroll (1960) reviewed 41 cases of optic neuritis occurring in children under the age of 15, though adequate information was only obtainable in 37. Their mean age was 9·5 years and 12 had unilateral involvement. A specific diagnosis was made in 11, leaving 30 of unknown aetiology at the time of onset. Disc swelling was present in 22. No clinical features of the optic neuritis allowed subsequent prediction of multiple sclerosis. In a later paper (Kennedy and Carter 1961), the clinical details of the eight children subsequently developing multiple sclerosis were given in full; five had had unilateral and three bilateral optic neuritis. The mean follow-up period for the 30 children overall was 8 years. Meadows (1969) considered unilateral retrobulbar neuritis to be excessively rare in the first decade, but was able to collect nine cases presenting between the ages of 10 and 16. Only four of these were seen in the acute stage, the other five recalling an attack in retrospect when a diagnosis of multiple sclerosis had been established later. The four patients were followed for 2 to 8 years but none developed evidence of multiple sclerosis.

Bilateral optic neuritis

Hierons and Lyle (1959) collected 13 cases of bilateral optic neuritis in children under the age of 13, 10 of whom were females. All but one made a good visual recovery. Five had a history of specific exanthem or an indeterminate febrile illness prior to the onset of visual symptoms. One patient, who had developed diplopia and epilepsy during the acute illness, was found to have multiple sclerosis at follow-up 6 years later.

Meadows (1969) encountered 35 bilateral cases in childhood, the majority between the ages of 5 and 12. Seven followed specific infectious illnesses. Thirty-three of the 35 had disc swelling, with or without haemorrhages. The remainder of the neurological examination was usually normal, though of 24 cases seen in the acute stage, nine had extensor plantar responses, usually bilateral. Twelve patients were subsequently lost to follow-up, but none of the remainder developed evidence of multiple sclerosis over a period exceeding 3 years in 17.

Hutchinson (1976) had encountered six cases of bilateral optic neuritis in childhood who remained without evidence of further neurological involvement over a period of up to 14 years. Taub and Rucker (1954) described multiple sclerosis after optic neuritis in only one of seven children, and one child under 10 seen by Bradley and Whitty (1968) later developed the disease, but in neither case was it made apparent whether the visual disturbance had been unilateral or bilateral. We have already seen that bilateral

Table 13.8 The development of multiple sclerosis following optic neuritis in children

	Author	No. of cases	Age range	Length of follow-up	Percentage developing MS
Unilateral	Kennedy and Carroll (1960)	12	Up to 15 years	Mean 8 years	42
	Meadows (1969)	4	10–16 years	2–8 years	0
Bilateral	Hierons and Lyle (1959)	13	Up to 13 years	Mean 4 years	8
	Kennedy and Carter (1961)	18	Up to 15 years	Mean 8 years	17
	Meadows (1969)	23	Majority 5–12 years	Less than 3 to 18 years	0
	Hutchinson (1976)	6	?	Up to 14 years	8

optic neuritis in children is frequently related to a specific exanthematous illness (pp. 106–9) and a consideration of Table 13.8 suggests a much more benign long-term prognosis for these cases than for children with unilateral vision loss.

Conclusions

A consideration of the literature regarding the progression of optic neuritis to multiple sclerosis produces the inevitable conclusion that in the majority of series, inadequate diagnostic criteria and clinical information prohibit valid comparison. Although, in the remainder, a number of factors have been considered relevant for the subsequent development of multiple sclerosis, these have not been consistent between series, nor indeed have they been confirmed from a consideration of our own material. The frequency with which optic neuritis progresses to multiple sclerosis has been reported variously, and it is suggested that much of this variation represents differing diagnostic criteria, inadequate initial neurological examination, and a failure to specify the proportion of patients having definite as opposed to less certain signs of the disease. It is likely that a follow-up which does not rely on personal examination will miss cases which, despite a relative absence of symptoms, fulfil the most strict criteria in terms of multiple lesions. It can only be conjectured how frequently a 'benign' form of multiple sclerosis follows optic neuritis, though the introduction of electrophysiological techniques for the detection of demyelination may resolve this question.

The rate at which multiple sclerosis develops after optic neuritis remains unsettled. The alternative hypotheses appear to be a progressive increase with which the diagnosis is made according to length of follow-up, or the diagnosis being established, at least for 'definite' cases, within 4 or 5 years of onset.

Optic neuritis in children, when unilateral, probably behaves little differently, in terms of subsequent multiple sclerosis, from adult cases, but bilateral optic neuritis appears a much more benign condition, even where a specific preceding infectious illness cannot be identified.

REFERENCES

Adams, D. K. (1927). Disseminated sclerosis. Aetiology, symptomatology and occupational incidence. *Br. med. J.* **2**, 13–14.
Adie, W. J. (1930). Acute retrobulbar neuritis in disseminated sclerosis. *Trans. ophthal. Soc. U.K.* **50**, 262–7.
— (1932). The aetiology and symptomatology of disseminated sclerosis. *Br. med. J.* **2**, 997–1000.
Alter, M., Good, J., and Okihiro, M. (1973). Optic neuritis in Orientals and Caucasians. *Neurology, Minneap.* **23**, 631–9.
Arnason, B. G. W. (1975). In *Multiple sclerosis research: Proceedings of a Joint Conference held by the Medical Research Council and the Multiple Sclerosis Society of Great Britain and Northern Ireland* (ed. A. N. Davison, J. H. Humphrey, A. L. Liversedge, W. I. McDonald, and J. S. Porterfield), p. 84. HMSO, London.
Bagley, C. H. (1952). An etiologic study of a series of optic neuropathies. *Am. J. Ophthal.* **35**, 761–72.
*Behr, C. (1924). Zur entstehung der multiplen sklerose. *Münch. med. Wschr.* **71**, 633–6.
Berliner, M. L. (1935). Acute optic neuritis in demyelinating diseases of the nervous system. *Archs Ophthal., N.Y.* **13**, 83–98.
Bradley, W. G. and Whitty, C. W. M. (1968). Acute optic neuritis: prognosis for development of multiple sclerosis. *J. Neurol. Neurosurg. Psychiat.* **31**, 10–18.
Collis, W. J. (1965). Acute unilateral retrobulbar neuritis. *Archs Neurol., Chicago* **13**, 409–12.
Compston, D. A., Batchelor, J. R., Earl, C. J., and McDonald, W. I. (1978). Factors influencing the risk of multiple sclerosis developing in patients with optic neuritis. *Brain* **101**, 495–511.
Davison, A. N., Humphrey, J. H., Liversedge, A. L., McDonald, W. I., and Porterfield, J. S. (eds.) (1975). *Multiple sclerosis research: Proceedings of a Joint Conference held by the Medical Research Council and the Multiple Sclerosis Society of Great Britain and Northern Ireland*, p. 5. HMSO, London.
*Fleischer, B. (1908). Neuritis retrobulbaris acuta und multiple sklerose. *Klin. Mbl. Augenheilk.* **46/1**, 113–30.
*Friedinger, E. (1925). Klinische untersuchungen über die genese der neuritis neui optici mit besonderer berücksichtigung ihrer beziehungen zur multiplen sklerose. *Schweiz. med. Wschr.*, **55**, 1093–7.
Heckford, F. (1934). In Some varieties of acute optic and retrobulbar neuritis by W. R. Brain. *Trans. ophthal. Soc. U.K.* **54**, 230.
Hierons, R. and Lyle, T. K. (1959). Bilateral retrobulbar optic neuritis. *Brain* **82**, 56–67.
Hutchinson, W. M. (1976). Acute optic neuritis and the prognosis for multiple sclerosis. *J. Neurol. Neurosurg. Psychiat.* **39**, 283–9.
Hyllested, K. (1966). On the prognosis of retrobulbar neuritis. *Acta ophthal.* **44**, 246–52.
— and Moller, P. M. (1961). Follow-up on patients with a history of optic neuritis. *Acta ophthal.* **39**, 655–62.

Kennedy, C. and Carroll, F. D. (1960). Optic neuritis in children. *Archs Ophthal., N.Y.* **63**, 747–55.

— and Carter, S. (1961). Relation of optic neuritis to multiple sclerosis in children. *Pediatrics, Springfield* **28**, 377–87.

Kurland, L. T., Auth, T. L., Beebe, G. W., Kurtzke, J. F., Lessell, S., Nagler, B., and Nefzger, M. D. (1963). Studies on the natural history of multiple sclerosis. II. Progression from optic neuropathy to multiple sclerosis. *Trans. Am. neurol. Ass.* (ed. M. D. Yahr) Vol. 88, pp. 233–5. Springer Publishing Company Inc, New York.

— Beebe, G. W., Kurtzke, J. F., Nagler, B., Auth, T. L., Lessell, S., and Nefzger, M. D. (1966). Studies on the natural history of multiple sclerosis. *Acta Neurol. Scand.* [Suppl] **19** (Vol. 42), 157–76.

Landy, P. J. and Ohlrich, G. D. (1970). Optic neuritis and its relationship to disseminated sclerosis. *Proc. Aust. Assoc. Neurol.* **7**, 67–70.

*Langenbeck, K. (1914). Neuritis retrobulbaris und allgemeinerkrankungen. *Albrecht v. Graefes Arch. Ophthal.* **87**, 226–79.

Lazarte, J. A. (1950). Multiple sclerosis: prognosis for ambulatory and non-ambulatory patients. Research Publications of the Association for Research in Nervous and Mental Diseases, Vol. 28, Chapter 34, pp. 512–23. Williams and Wilkins, Baltimore.

Leibowitz, U., Alter, M., and Halpern, L. (1966). Clinical studies of multiple sclerosis in Israel. IV. Optic neuropathy and multiple sclerosis. *Archs Neurol. Chicago* **14**, 459–66.

*Lenoire, M. (1917). La neurite optique rétrobulbaire infectieuse aiguë, diagnostic étiologique et traitement. *Anns Oculist.* **154**, 411–26.

Lynn, B. H. (1959). Retrobulbar neuritis. A survey of the present condition of cases occurring over the last fifty-six years. *Trans. ophthal. Soc. U.K.* **79**, 701–16.

McAlpine, D. (1964). The benign form of multiple sclerosis: Results of a long-term study. *Br. med. J.* **2**, 1029–32.

Mackay, R. P. (1953). Multiple sclerosis: its onset and duration. A clinical study of 309 patients. *Med. Clins. N. Am.* **37**, 511–21.

*Marburg, O. (1920). Retrobulbäre neuritis optica und multiple sklerose. *Z. Augenheilk.* **44**, 125–31.

Marshall, D. (1950). Ocular manifestations of multiple sclerosis and relationship to retrobulbar neuritis. *Trans. Am. ophthal. Soc.* **48**, 487–525.

Meadows, S. P. (1969). Retrobulbar and optic neuritis in childhood and adolescence. *Trans. ophthal. Soc. U.K.* **89**, 603–38.

Millar, J. H. D. (1971). *Multiple sclerosis: a disease acquired in childhood*. Thomas, Springfield, Illinois.

Müller, R. (1949). Studies on disseminated sclerosis. *Acta med. scand. Supp.* **222**, 1–214.

Nagler, B., Beebe, G. W., Kurtzke, J. F., Kurland, L. T., Auth, T. L., and Nefzger, M. D. (1966). Studies on the natural history of multiple sclerosis. 1. Design and diagnosis. *Acta Neurol. Scand.* [Suppl] **19** (Vol. 42), 141–56.

Nikoskelainen, E. and Riekkinen, P. (1974). Optic neuritis—A sign of multiple sclerosis or other diseases of the central nervous system. A retrospective analysis of 116 patients. *Acta Neurol. Scand.* **50**, 690–718.

Otradovec, J. and Votockova, J. (1962). Etiologie akutnich neuritid optiku. *Mult. Scler. Abstr.* **7**, 264.

Percy, A. K., Nobrega, F. T., and Kurland, L. T. (1972). Optic neuritis and multiple sclerosis. *Archs Ophthal., N.Y.* **87**, 135–9.

Rischbieth, R. H. C. (1968). Retrobulbar neuritis in the state of Australia. *Proc. Aust. Assoc. Neurol.* **5**, 573–5.

Rose, F. C., Friedmann, A. I., Bowden, P. M. A., and Perkin, G. D. (1972). In *Multiple sclerosis. A reappraisal* (ed. D. McAlpine, C. E. Lumsden, and E. D. Acheson) (2nd edn.) pp. 151 *et seq*. Churchill Livingstone, Edinburgh.

Sandberg, H. O. (1972). Acute retrobulbar neuritis—A retrospective study. *Acta ophthal.* **50**, 3–8.

Sandberg, M. and Bynke, H. (1973). Cerebrospinal fluid in 25 cases of optic neuritis. *Acta Neurol. Scand.* **49**, 442–52.

Sandberg-Wollheim, M. (1975). Optic neuritis: studies on the cerebrospinal fluid in relation to clinical course in 61 patients. *Acta Neurol. Scand.* **52**, 167–78.
— Platz, P., Ryder, L. P., Nielsen, L. S., and Thomsen, M. (1975). HL-A histocompatibility antigens in optic neuritis. *Acta Neurol. Scand.* **52**, 161–6.
*Scheerer, R. (1929). Ueber die ursachen der neuritis retrobulbaris. *Klin. Mbl. Augenheilk.* **83**, 164–9.
Schumacher, G. A., Beebe, G., Kibler, R. F., Kurland, L. T., Kurtzke, J. F., McDowell, F., Nagler, B., Sibley, W. A., Tourtellotte, W. W., and Willmon, T. L. C. (1965). Problems of experimental trials of therapy in multiple sclerosis: Report by the panel on the evaluation of experimental trials of therapy in multiple sclerosis. *Ann. N.Y. Acad. Sci.* **122**, 552–68.
Symonds, C. P. (1930). Retrobulbar neuritis and disseminated sclerosis. *Lancet* **2**, 19–20.
Tatlow, W. F. T. (1948). The prognosis of retrobulbar neuritis. *Br. J. Ophthal.* **32**, 488–97.
Taub, R. G. and Rucker, C. W. (1954). The relationship of retrobulbar neuritis to multiple sclerosis. *Am. J. Ophthal.* **32**, 488–97.
White, D. N. and Wheelan, L. (1959). Disseminated sclerosis. A survey of patients in the Kingston, Ontario, area. *Neurology, Minneap.* **9**, 256–72.
Wybar, K. C. (1952). The ocular manifestations of disseminated sclerosis. *Proc. R. Soc. Med.* **45**, 315–20.

14 Methods for detecting optic nerve demyelination

> Since it is important to discover the early, minute, or latent symptoms, and thereby demonstrate the presence of multiple lesions, special methods of investigation may be needed (Lowenstein 1951).

The frequency of various ophthalmological abnormalities after optic neuritis has already been discussed (pp. 194–214). In this chapter, consideration will be given to abnormalities of optic nerve function detectable in the absence of such a history, but nevertheless of a degree sufficient to establish the likely diagnosis of optic nerve demyelination. On occasions, authors have failed, when describing ophthalmological findings, to indicate the presence or absence of previous visual symptoms. Where appropriate, such deficiencies have been recorded in the text.

The frequency of optic neuritis in patients with multiple sclerosis

Table 14.1 summarizes 17 series regarding the frequency of optic neuritis in multiple sclerosis, either as a presenting symptom or during the course of the

Table 14.1 The incidence of optic neuritis at the onset, or during, clinically definite multiple sclerosis (percentages have been rounded off to the nearest whole number)

Series	No. of Patients	% with optic neuritis at onset	% with optic neuritis at any stage
Lazarte (1950)	342	8	–
Marshall (1950)	822	13	47
Percy et al. (1972)	?	13	27
Leibowitz and Alter (1968)	266	14	–
Symonds (1930)	139	15	28
Lillie (1934)	>500	15	50–55
Brown and Putnam (1939)	133	15	39
White and Wheelan	47	15	45
Allison (1950)	40	18	–
Yaskin et al. (1951)	100	19	–
Müller (1949)	810	20	54
Croll (1965)	140	21	
Adie (1932)	80	25	36
Adie (1930)	84	33	50
Leinfelder (1950)	200	–	22
Wybar (1952)	91	–	27
Scott (1961)	65	–	31

disease. For the total of 3503 and 2971 patients, the respective percentages are 16 and 45.

Impaired visual acuity

Differing figures have been stated for the incidence of depressed acuity in patients with multiple sclerosis due, no doubt, to the extent to which patients with a history of optic neuritis have been excluded (Table 14.2), and also to the criteria used for normal vision. The percentage of patients with abnormal vision is higher in those with evidence of optic atrophy (Gipner 1925).

Table 14.2 The percentage of patients with multiple sclerosis who have normal visual acuity

	No. of patients	History of optic neuritis	Definition of normal vision	% with normal vision*
Rosen (1965)	272	111	?	66
Gipner (1925)	100 (197 eyes)	?	6/10 or better	73
Marshall (1950)	475	'Some'	20/30 or better	78.9 (Left) 79.6 (Right)
Yaskin *et al.* (1951)	100 (200 eyes)	'Some'	6/6	91

* It has generally not been possible to determine from individual figures whether these refer to observations on both eyes, and what proportion of the abnormalities have been bilateral.

Abnormal contrast sensitivity

As an alternative to visual acuity, which measures fine detail only, sine-wave gratings have been used to test visual sensitivity to coarse, medium, and fine detail (Regan, Silver, and Murray 1977*c*). In 11 of 42 multiple sclerosis patients, sensitivity to medium coarseness was severely impaired, though fine and coarse detail were unaffected and clinical evidence of visual impairment (measured by acuity, colour vision, and fundus examination) was lacking in many of them.

Impaired flight of colours

Following illumination of the eye by a bright light for 10 seconds, after dark adaptation, a large number of colour changes are seen subsequently with the eyes closed, of many different hues, and persisting for at least 1½ minutes. A disturbance of this phenomenon, producing few colour changes of brief duration, occurs with any lesion of the visual system. It has been found to be abnormal in 74 per cent of cases of multiple sclerosis (Mourik, van Donselaar, and Minderhoud 1978) in some of whom visual symptoms or signs were lacking. The abnormality is found bilaterally in approximately two-thirds of those cases where it is present.

Visual field defects

It is difficult to establish, regarding some of the reviews (Table 14.3) whether percentages refer to numbers of patients or to numbers of eyes tested. The frequency of peripheral constriction is surprising, but was not the experience of the two more recent series, nor indeed is it a common consequence of optic neuritis (p. 206–7).

Table 14.3 The incidence of visual field defects in patients with multiple sclerosis

Author	No. of patients	History of optic neuritis	% with field defects	Type of field defect (%)
Gipner (1925)	100	?	9	Central (5) Concentric constriction (3) Enlarged blind spot (1)
Savitsky and Rangell (1950)*	264	Some	10.2	Concentric constriction (6.8) Central (3.4)
Yaskin *et al.* (1951)	88	Some	20.5	Central/paracentral (9.1) Peripheral constriction (11.4)
Rosen (1965)	272	111	21.7	Central
Marshall (1950)	586	Some	32.8	Central/paracentral (18.5) Concentric constriction (10.4) Others (3.9)
White and Wheelan (1959)	68	33	56.2	Central/paracentral (46.1) Peripheral constriction (10.1)

* Includes cases from the literature.

Abnormal pupillary reactions

Pupillary abnormalities have been considered rare in multiple sclerosis (Gipner 1925; Savitsky and Rangell 1950) but may be expected in between 11·4 (Rosen 1965) and 12·8 per cent of patients (Marshall 1950). Pupillography may be capable of detecting more subtle changes (Lowenstein 1951).

Optic atrophy

In a total of 2118 patients, optic atrophy was encountered in 31 per cent (Table 14.4). The variability with which it has been reported probably reflects as much observer bias (Lynn 1959) as selection of material.

Colour-vision defects

Charcot emphasized (Buzzard 1893) the frequency with which dys-chromatopsy might be found in multiple sclerosis, whilst Sloan (1942) considered colour-vision testing of value in a variety of ophthalmological

Table 14.4 The incidence of optic atrophy (either unilateral or bilateral) in patients with multiple sclerosis (the figures have been rounded off to the nearest whole number)

Author	No. of patients	No. with optic atrophy	%
Leinfelder (1950)	200	21	11
Marshall (1950)			16
Croll (1965)	140	26	19
Rosen (1965)	272	72	26
Sachs and Friedman (1922)	141	46	33
Uhthoff (1890)	100	40	40
Müller (1949)	582	233	40
Savitsky and Rangell (1950)*	264	110	41
Buzzard (1893)	100	43	43
Gipner (1925)	100	47	47
Yaskin et al. (1951)	100	50	50
Halliday et al. (1973b)	51	28	55
White and Wheelan (1959)	68	48	71

* Includes cases from the literature.

disorders. Lynn (1959), using Ishihara plates, found bilateral colour-vision defects in 61 patients with a history of unilateral optic neuritis, of whom only eight had had visual symptoms in the second eye. It has been suggested (Rosen 1965) that errors on the Hardy–Rand–Rittler pseudoisochromatic plates, in the absence of ocular or retinal disease and congenital dyschromatopsia, reflect optic nerve dysfunction. In 272 cases of multiple sclerosis (diagnosed on classical clinical findings with or without CSF changes), 167 patients had abnormal colour vision (Rosen 1965) though it is impossible to say whether these were unilateral or bilateral findings, or a combination of the two. Of 111 patients with a history of retrobulbar neuritis, 105 had abnormal colour vision. All those with reduced visual acuity or central field defects had abnormal colour vision, as did 69 of 72 cases with optic atrophy or temporal pallor.

Retinal nerve-fibre atrophy

The development of axonal degeneration alongside demyelination in the optic nerve should lead to atrophy of nerve-fibre bundles within the retina. Such nerve-fibre bundle defects may be visible ophthalmoscopically and have an analogue in terms of visual field defects (Hoyt, Schlicke, and Eckelhoff 1972). The criteria for the recognition of these defects have been stated. They are usually initially noted amongst the upper arcuate fibres, irrespective of the cause of the optic neuropathy (Frisén and Hoyt 1974) between one and two disc-diameters from the nerve head. They are associated with narrow elongated scotomata, between 10 and 25° from fixation. The presence of such defects may allow a confident diagnosis of multiple sclerosis in patients with spinal cord or brain stem syndromes (Frisén and Hoyt 1974). In 25 patients with multiple sclerosis, 15 of whom had no visual symptoms or signs, an abnormality of the peripapillary nerve-fibre layer was detected in 17 (Feinsod and Hoyt 1975). Somewhat similar, multiple, peripheral scotomata were observed by Klingmann (1910) in 12 patients with multiple sclerosis, though they were predominantly temporal, whereas atrophy of arcuate fibres produces predominantly nasal defects.

Where there are medullated nerve fibres in the retina, atrophy of arcuate fibres may be associated with local loss of myelin (Sharpe and Sanders 1975; Gartner 1953).

Ultrasonography

Orbital ultrasonography has been performed in patients with optic neuropathies of various types, including cases due to multiple sclerosis and so-called idiopathic forms (Coleman and Carroll 1972). The method detected 90 per cent of the lesions, with two false positive results in a single patient with low-tension glaucoma. The findings included variable expansion of the nerve echo pattern with, in some instances, shadowing in the region of the fascii bulbi and enlargement, presumed oedematous, of the extraocular muscle outline. A study of optic neuritis patients has not been reported.

Computerized axial tomography

It has been suggested that computerized axial tomography may be capable of detecting demyelinating optic nerve lesions. Alternating high-density bulges and low-density constrictions have been reported (Eyerman, Archer, and Mayes, Jr. 1976) as have low-density areas (Mastaglia, Black, Cala, and Collins 1977), usually in the intra-orbital segment of the optic nerve close to the optic foramen (Cala and Mastaglia 1976). Correlation between these appearances and clinical or electrophysiological evidence of demyelination in the optic nerve has not yet been attempted.

Flicker fusion

Patients with multiple sclerosis have a depressed flicker fusion threshold compared with controls. In one series (Parsons and Miller 1957), the mean frequency at which subjective fusion of a flickering stimulus occurred was 29·8 Hz compared with 40·2 Hz for a control population. Abnormal thresholds have been found in 93 per cent of patients with, and in 52 per cent of those without, a history of optic neuritis (Titcombe and Willison 1961). Abnormal thresholds show a correlation with the presence of optic atrophy.

Flash-evoked potentials

It has been stated (Halliday, McDonald, and Mushin 1977) that flash-evoked potentials in patients with previous optic neuritis show either no delay or one of a few milliseconds only. Feinsod, Abramsky, and Auerbach (1973) however, found delays in seven of eight such patients, and in seven of nine without a history of visual symptoms. Subsequently (Feinsod, Hoyt, Wilson, and Spire 1977) using a flash stimulus at 1 Hz, abnormalities were demonstrated in all 20 of a group of patients with multiple sclerosis. In each case, the latency and shape of the initial negative wave were affected, with either prolongation of all components, or breakdown of the initial negative wave into 2–4 subcomponents with some normal, and others of prolonged latency. It was concluded that flash-evoked potentials were a sensitive and reliable index for optic nerve damage in multiple sclerosis.

Transient pattern evoked potentials (Fig. 14.1)

It has been established that stimulation of the optic nerve by an alternating pattern of light and dark squares produces a reproducible occipital potential with a well defined latency for normal individuals. The methodology has been recently discussed in detail (Sokol 1976). The amplitude of the poten-

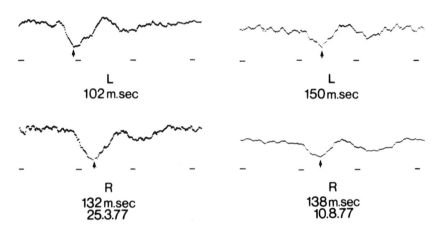

L
102 m.sec

L
150 m.sec

R
132 m.sec
25.3.77

R
138 m.sec
10.8.77

Fig. 14.1. C.N. aged 24

Onset January 1977, blurring vision R eye with slight pain on movement. Visual acuity 6/9 R, 6/6 L with mild arcuate field defect but normal pupil and fundus examination. Visual evoked responses (25.3.77) showed a significant delay for the R eye alone. Symptoms recovered and neurological examination was normal. Five months later a similar episode occurred in the L eye, and repeat evoked responses (10.8.77) showed now a marked delay in that eye, that on the right remaining essentially unaltered. By then, there was evidence of definite multiple sclerosis.

tial is dependent on the rate of alternation, luminance, check size, and retinal area stimulated. In addition, it is highly sensitive to refractive errors. Although the latency of the response is independent of acuity (Fig. 14.2), the amplitude falls to one third of normal when acuity reaches 6/60 or less (Fig. 14.3; Halliday, McDonald, and Mushin 1973*a*).

Halliday, McDonald, and Mushin (1973*b*) using a check size of 50' examined 51 patients with multiple sclerosis, divided into definite (34 cases), probable (five), and possible (12) according to the criteria of McAlpine, Lumsden, and Acheson (1972). A prolonged latency (defined as one exceeding the mean plus 2½ standard deviations) was found in over 90 per cent, unilaterally in 14 cases and bilaterally in 35. Other authors (using mean plus 3 standard deviations as their upper limit) have found delayed latencies less frequently. In a study of 51 patients (Asselman, Chadwick, and Marsden 1975) 67 per cent were abnormal (unilateral in 10 and bilateral in 24), the respective figures for definite, probable, and possible cases being 84, 83, and 21 per cent. Similar results have been reported by Hennerici, Wenzel, and Freund (1977), 61 per cent of their multiple sclerosis patients having abnormal values, with a breakdown of 81, 67, and 43 per cent for the same three diagnostic criteria.

Although Halliday, McDonald, and Mushin (1972) in an earlier study, found that one of 19 patients with acute unilateral optic neuritis had a

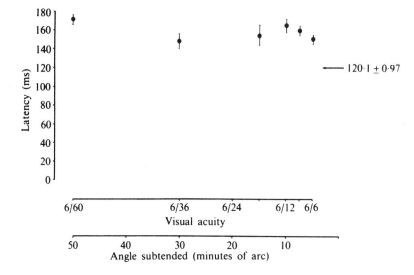

Fig. 14.2. Mean latency of visual evoked response ±S.E. from 69 records on 53 patients recovering from optic neuritis. The data at 6/60 includes those cases with a visual acuity of 6/60 or less. The mean latency ±S.E. in 17 healthy subjects is indicated by the arrow on the right (from Halliday *et al.* 1973*a*).

normal latency, subsequent reports (Halliday *et al.* 1973*b*; Cantor, Kurtzke, Schechter, Tsai, and Shirzadi 1974; Hennerici *et al.* 1977) suggested latencies were invariably prolonged in patients with previous optic neuritis. Further experience (Halliday *et al.* 1977) has indicated, however, that between five and six per cent of patients with a definite history will have normal latencies. Whether these represent patients in whom initially prolonged latencies have recovered (Asselman *et al.* 1975), or a group in whom latencies remain normal during a clinical attack remains to be established. The former hypothesis might be explained by remyelination of damaged optic nerve fibres (Halliday and McDonald 1977), the latter on the basis of an unusually short plaque within the optic nerve (Halliday *et al.* 1977).

Abnormal latencies may be found despite normal vision, fields, and colour discrimination (Halliday *et al.* 1973*b*; Asselman *et al.* 1975) and in the absence of evidence of retinal nerve-fibre atrophy (Hennerici *et al.* 1977). For multiple sclerosis patients with normal vision (6/9 or better), normal fundi and visual fields and intact colour discrimination (less than three mistakes with Ishihara colour plates) 28 per cent may still be expected to show prolonged latencies (Asselman *et al.* 1975).

The checkerboard stimulus in the studies quoted has been applied to the

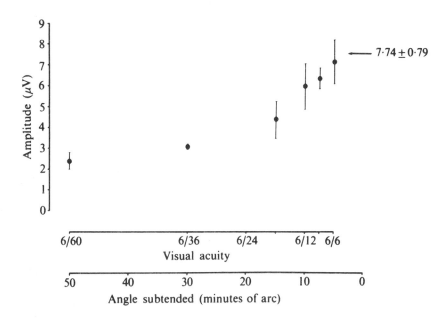

Fig. 14.3. Mean amplitude of response ±S.E. in the same group of patients as in Fig 14.1. The amplitude is significantly correlated with acuity (P<0·001). (From Halliday *et al.* 1973*a*.)

central 20–32° of vision, though the amplitude of the response probably changes little for stimulation beyond the central 12° (Sokol 1976). Small demyelinating lesions affecting foveal fibres might not be detected by such methods, since unaffected conducting axons from the peripheral retina would preserve the normal latency of the potential. Accordingly the responses to a single rectangular stimulus subtending 45′ of the central visual area have been studied (Hennerici *et al*. 1977), the latencies for which are prolonged, in normal individuals, in comparison with potentials from a checkerboard stimulating the central 20°. In 57 patients with multiple sclerosis, abnormal latencies were found in 88 per cent, with 94 per cent for definite, 94 per cent for probable, and 78 per cent for possible cases. The comparable overall figure for checkerboard stimulation was 61 per cent with, for the individual diagnostic groups, 81, 67, and 43 per cent abnormal respectively. All patients with a history of optic neuritis had delayed responses to both checkerboard and foveal stimulation.

Abnormal evoked responses may be of considerable value in establishing the presence of a second lesion in those patients manifesting isolated brain-stem syndromes or progressive spastic paraplegia. In the former category, Asselman *et al*. (1975) found six of 13 patients had delayed responses compared with one of 10 individuals with an undiagnosed spastic para-paresis. By contrast, Halliday, McDonald, and Mushin (1974) found delayed responses in 13 of 27 cases of spastic paraplegia, though in eight of these the diagnosis of multiple sclerosis was established on other grounds. Surprisingly, in two other patients with spastic paraplegia, though the diag-nosis of multiple sclerosis could be made on clinical grounds, visual evoked responses were normal. It has been postulated (Regan, Milner, and Heron 1976) that differing patterns of optic nerve damage occur in 'spinal' multiple sclerosis, distinguishable by their effects on various types of evoked poten-tial (see below).

Steady-state pattern evoked responses

These have been studied using a haphazardly changing checkerboard pattern, at between 4 and 14 Hz, with total light flux being kept constant. Large checks, of 50′ subtending a total field of 14°, and small checks, of 14′ subtending 4° overall were compared (Milner, Regan, and Heron 1974). Of 13 patients with optic neuritis who were examined, 11 had optic atrophy, three central field defects, and seven an acuity of less than J1 in the affected eye. Using larger checks, an abnormal latency was detected in seven of 10 eyes where a response could be elicited (two patients, with acuities of J20 and C.F., had no response) with, in the remainder, an abnormal latency difference between the two eyes, though individual values were within normal limits. For small checks, individual latencies were abnormal in four of eight affected eyes, with an abnormal inter-ocular difference in a further three. In a later communication (Regan *et al*. 1976) all 12 patients with a history of optic neuritis were found to have delayed potentials to a large check stimulus, though whether absolute or relative to the second eye was not stated. A residual depressed acuity after an episode of optic neuritis has no effect on the frequency with which delayed steady-state responses are elicited.

Latencies for either form of stimulation may be normal in the presence of depressed acuity or optic atrophy, but conversely may be abnormal despite preserved visual acuity. The contrast between the results of 4 and 14° stimulation is somewhat surprising, particularly as it represents the opposite of the experience of Hennerici *et al*. (1977). It must be presumed that the differing forms of central field stimulus used by these two groups of workers affect separate optic nerve pathways.

The latencies for large checks (50′ subtending a total of 14°) have been studied in patients with spinal multiple sclerosis (Regan *et al*. 1976). Clinical details in the patients is meagre, but they showed sensory or motor abnormalities, separately or in combination, with cerebellar signs in a small proportion. Using the criteria of McAlpine *et al*. (1972), seven were definite, four probable, and two possible examples of multiple sclerosis. Two patients had a history of oculomotor symptoms, one with blurring of the peripheral vision on sudden head movement, the other a previous sixth nerve palsy. Clinical evidence of optic nerve damage was accepted if visual acuity (presumably corrected) was less than J2, or if there was optic atrophy. Of the 13 patients studied, five had delayed potentials (bilateral in two) and one other had an abnormal inter-ocular difference. Of these six patients, five had a depressed visual acuity in one or other eye and three had optic atrophy. Amongst the seven patients with normal latencies, only one had a depressed acuity and none had optic atrophy.

It has been postulated that 'spinal' patients with visual signs have abnormal steady-state pattern responses but normal flicker responses (see below) whereas those without such signs have abnormal flicker but normal steady state pattern latencies. Some reservation needs to be expressed regarding this hypothesis, particularly when criteria for optic nerve damage have been confined to visual acuity and presence of optic atrophy.

Indeed, the curious finding from this work was that all three patients with bilateral optic atrophy had, in fact, only unilateral delay to pattern stimulation, making attempts to correlate certain visual signs with particular types of evoked potential abnormality even more tenuous. Halliday *et al*. (1977) found 80 per cent of their multiple sclerosis patients of 'spinal' type had abnormal transient pattern-evoked responses, though none of them, by definition, had either optic atrophy or a depressed visual acuity.

Steady-state flicker evoked potentials

Large evoked potentials can be elicited using an unpatterned light stimulus flickering at 13–25 Hz (medium-frequency) or 30–60 Hz (high-frequency). The properties of flicker, in terms of the resulting potential, differ according to the frequency. Medium-frequency flicker evoked potentials appear delayed for all patients with a history of optic neuritis, whereas values for high-frequency flicker are normal (Regan *et al.* 1976). Although responses were delayed for all 13 affected eyes in the patients with multiple sclerosis and a history of optic neuritis, only one of the unaffected eyes was abnormal (Milner *et al.* 1974). Testing of flicker responses is feasible in patients with poor visual acuity (even as low as counting fingers) and abnormalities appear to persist for at least 12 years after an attack of optic neuritis (Regan *et al.* 1977*a*).

The frequency with which the responses are abnormal in spinal multiple sclerosis has been made difficult to assess by errors in one of the tables in the paper on this subject by Regan *et al.* (1976). In six patients with normal visual acuity (J1 or 2) and no optic atrophy, responses were abnormal in all, with bilateral delays in three, unilateral delay in one, and an abnormal inter-ocular difference in the remainder. In seven patients with visual signs (defined as above), one had a bilateral delay and another an abnormal inter-ocular difference. In a recent communication (Regan *et al.* 1977*a*), the authors chose to emphasize the frequency of absolute delays in the two groups (four and one respectively). High-frequency flicker responses are more variable and were normal in all five 'spinal' cases studied (Regan *et al.* 1976).

The concept of differing evoked potential findings according to the presence or absence of visual signs is not sustained if optic atrophy alone is considered. For the three such patients in the group of 13 spinal multiple sclerosis cases, delayed pattern evoked potentials were found in all, but delayed flicker (either absolutely or between eyes) in two.

Perceptual delay

The delay in perception of a sudden increase in light intensity is increased in an eye previously affected by optic neuritis. The method involves stimulation of the, presumed, abnormal eye eccentrically between 0·6 and 8·6° from fixation whilst the reference eye is stimulated at the fovea. Delays for various retinal points can thus be assessed and plotted in the form of a 'delay field'. A reasonable visual acuity is necessary for the test.

Of 22 patients with a history of unilateral optic neuritis, all had a delay greater than two standard deviations above the mean of a control group, even in the absence of optic atrophy or depressed visual acuity, though with four patients, the delay was only found when a second retinal position was stimulated. Although the test uses the patient's other eye as a control, it may still reveal abnormalities in those with a history of bilateral optic neuritis, where the delay may change from one eye to the other according to the retinal site stimulated. The delay of perception of a sudden decrease in light intensity has also been measured. Although the delay for light increase and decrease may be comparable at a single retinal point, in some instances one or other alone may be affected.

Transretinal delay for a single eye can be measured by finding the time difference for perception of light falling on the fovea and on a point 5° eccentric to the fovea of the same eye. Both brightening and dimming stimuli have been used (Regan *et al*. 1976). Of nine patients with a history of optic neuritis, only one had a delay for a brightening stimulus and three for a dimming stimulus, though of the remaining six, four had a delayed perception for light increase or decrease when the affected eye was compared with its normal fellow.

In 'spinal' multiple sclerosis, an abnormal interocular delay has been detected in six of 19 cases (Regan *et al*. 1976) using a brightening stimulus, although for one of the six the delay was, in fact, at the upper limit of normal. Testing of a single retinal point (rather than two) would have produced a smaller yield of abnormal delays. Abnormal transretinal delay for a brightening stimulus using separate positions 5° from the fovea, was found in 10 of 19 patients, of whom four had been detected by an abnormal interocular difference. Combining the two measurements, 12 of 19 patients gave abnormal results and of these 12, seven had either optic atrophy or depressed acuity in one or both eyes. All three patients with optic atrophy had abnormal interocular and transretinal delays.

Perceptual delays in patients with 'spinal' multiple sclerosis appear to correlate with abnormalities of steady-state pattern-evoked responses. In some instances, however, they alone may be abnormal, possibly because the perceptual test can detect demyelination affecting retinal areas as small as 0·2° in diameter, whereas the pattern stimulation is applied to a much larger field.

Initial experience with this method suggested abnormalities were almost confined to those patients with visual signs (seven out of seven) compared with those without (one of six). In a further group of six patients, however, none of whom had visual signs, no fewer than three had abnormal perceptual delays by one or other method.

Combining the results of medium-frequency flicker, large-check pattern-evoked potentials and perceptual delay tests, 10 of 13 patients (77 per cent) with spinal multiple sclerosis were found to have abnormalities (Regan *et al*. 1976).

Delayed temporal resolution

Following optic neuritis, the ability to resolve two closely applied light stimuli becomes impaired. Twin light flashes of 10 ms duration separated by between 0 and 135 ms have been used (Galvin, Regan, and Heron 1976*a*). Using ascending and descending runs, thresholds at various retinal sites can be measured and compared with perceptual delay at the same site. Temporal resolution of stimuli between 0 and 6° eccentricity from fixation remains relatively stable but declines rapidly for more peripheral stimuli. Corresponding retinal points in the two eyes produce comparable resolution. Refractive errors do not influence the test and problems with fixation are seldom encountered.

In 14 patients with previous retrobulbar neuritis double flash threshold was impaired (using 99 per cent confidence limits) in 13. In six of these, the abnormality was confined to a single retinal area, but was found at all the tested sites in the remainder. 'Fields' of impaired temporal resolution and perceptual delay were not comparable in nine patients. The findings of an abnormal temporal resolution appears to be independent of any clinical sign of optic nerve dysfunction. In the 14 patients, three were found to have abnormalities in the clinically unaffected eye.

The method has been extended to patients with spinal forms of the disease (Galvin, Heron, and Regan 1977). Eleven patients without a history of optic neuritis, and with normal fundi, who presented with various combinations of spinal cord, brain stem, and cerebellar disturbances were studied. Of these 11, however, two had abnormal fields (Bjerrum screen), one other had a unilateral colour-vision defect (Ishihara), and three others had unilateral pupillary abnormalities (swinging light test). Of the remaining five patients, three (60 per cent) showed delayed temporal resolution, bilateral in all of them.

Pulfrich pendulum

In patients with a unilateral delay of visual perception, the orbit of a pendulum may be interpreted as an ellipse instead of a straight line (Pulfrich 1922). A similar effect in normal individuals can be achieved by placing a filter in front of one eye, the depth of the elliptical orbit being dependent on the speed of swing and the density of the filter (Frisén, Hoyt, Bird, and Weale 1973). This optical illusion has been reported by patients with normal vision, normal colour discrimination, and only minimal abnormality of the pupillary response.

Pupillary size must be equal for the test, since inequality can produce uneven retinal illumination and hence the same phenomenon, and successful testing necessitates normal stereoscopic vision.

Of 18 patients with definite multiple sclerosis, nine were shown to have the phenomenon (Rushton 1975), whilst 14 had delayed visual-evoked responses using the criteria of Asselman *et al*. (1975). Abnormal results were obtained in three of nine probable and two of eight possible cases. In patients with multiple sclerosis of all diagnostic types, but without visual signs (a total of 10 patients), an equal number (three) had optic nerve lesions detected with this method as by the use of evoked responses. No correlation has been found between inter-ocular latency differences of evoked responses and the latency detected by the Pulfrich pendulum.

Pathophysiological mechanisms

Experimental evidence suggests that large demyelinating lesions of fibres of the central nervous system produce complete conduction block, with the retained ability to conduct impulses in the nerve fibres distal to the block (McDonald 1977). With smaller lesions, the ability to conduct a train of impulses is impaired, resulting eventually, with prolonged stimulation, in periods of complete conduction failure. In addition, the conduction velocity of individual impulses is reduced. Slowing of conduction velocity to 1/6 of normal occurs with diphtheria toxin lesions of central myelin and up to 1/25 of normal with peripheral demyelinating lesions.

An attempt has been made (McDonald 1977) to calculate the delay expected from a lesion of mean size 1 cm, assuming an internodal length of 0·2 mm and a normal conduction velocity of 10 m/s. If delays by up to 25 times occurred, 25 ms would be required to traverse 1 cm, producing the degree of latency change encountered in optic neuritis; though experimentally conduction may fail completely through a series of internodes with such markedly prolonged conduction times. An alternative explanation may be that conduction in small demyelinated optic nerve fibres becomes continuous. Continuous conduction in demyelinated segments of small peripheral myelinated fibres is slowed by some fifteen times compared with saltatory conduction in distal, normal segments (Bostock and Sears 1976).

Delays in medium-frequency flicker or pattern reversal at 4–14 Hz are of similar degree (Regan *et al*. 1977a). Thus, 6 of 13 patients with retrobulbar neuritis had latencies exceeding 190 ms for flicker (upper normal 148 ms), and six of 10 patients had latencies exceeding 190 ms to large-check pattern stimulation (upper normal 148 ms).

A comparison in the same patients between pattern reversal latencies and those obtained by flash or estimation of simultaneity of two light sources indicated that the former were approximately twice as great (Cook and Arden 1977), suggesting the possibility that additional cortical delays might operate in the case of evoked pattern responses. Others (Regan *et al*. 1976), using different psychophysical methods, have however obtained latencies in some patients comparable to those occurring with pattern evoked stimulation. For example, in four patients with 'spinal' multiple sclerosis, the perceptual delay of one eye compared to the other was between 78 and 165 ms, the upper normal for interocular difference being 30 ms. It should be noted that Cook and Arden (1977) compared perceptual delay for foveal stimulation, whilst Regan *et al.* (1976) considered delay between foveal stimulation on one side and extra-foveal on the other. Indeed this particular discrepancy encapsulates in many ways the hazards of attempting comparison between series where differing methodologies have been used. However, in a more recent study (Regan *et al.* 1977*b*), the authors tested perceptual delay for one fovea against another, by a method very similar to that of Cook and Arden (1977), yet they found perceptual delays in eyes previously affected by retrobulbar neuritis, of 132, 35, 41, 194, 105, 23, and 94 ms respectively, comparable to the prolonged latencies associated with pattern stimulation.

Clearly, the perceptual tests used by Regan *et al.* (1976) are testing differing aspects of optic nerve function from those responding to pattern-evoked stimulation and, in some cases, only the former may reveal delays. The discrepant areas of retina stimulated by the two tests might be of relevance here. Similarly, perceptual delays may be abnormal for a sudden increase, but not decrease, in light intensity, suggesting such information is processed along different neural pathways, which can be selectively damaged in multiple sclerosis.

Double-flash thresholds after an attack of optic neuritis may be delayed to a degree (30 ms and more) comparable to that found with pattern stimulation. The results of this test are not comparable with those obtained from a perceptual test applied at the same retinal site (Galvin *et al.* 1976*a*).

Retinal delay has been suggested by some authors (Heron *et al.* 1974) as contributing to the latencies of evoked responses, but the evidence for a disturbance of retinal function in multiple sclerosis is conflicting.

It is considered that the perception of sudden light change and that of motion (as tested by the Pulfrich pendulum) depend on differing neural pathways. Opinions differ as to the retinal area involved in the perception of a moving pendulum. Whereas Regan *et al.* (1976) have considered the Pulfrich pendulum to test larger areas of retina than any perceptual test, Rushton (1975) concluded that tracking errors were generally of 1° or less, so that foveal latencies alone were being compared. In order to explain the large variation in perception of the phenomenon in individual multiple sclerosis patients, however, Rushton (1975) considered that small tracking errors might place the spot on areas of retina of widely differing latency.

Provocative tests

The exacerbation or appearance of symptoms in patients with multiple sclerosis during an increase in body temperature (Chapter 11) has led to the use of heating experiments as a test for sub-clinical involvement of the optic and other pathways.

Visual field defects

Elevation of body temperature may enlarge or cause the appearance of central scotomata (pp. 184–8; Davis, Michael, and Neer 1973). The precipitation of a field defect and nystagmus in a patient presenting with a right hemiparesis enabled the diagnosis of multiple sclerosis to be established (Davis 1966).

Critical flicker fusion

Namerow (1971) studied 18 multiple sclerosis patients, all of whom had a history of optic neuritis. Heating, in a hot-air cabinet, was continued until body temperature reached 38 °C or a marked change in flicker fusion frequency occurred. A marked sensitivity to temperature increase was noted, though individual responses were not recorded in detail. Patients without visual symptoms or signs were not examined.

Delayed temporal resolution

The effect of increasing and decreasing body temperature on double flash discrimination has been studied in four multiple sclerosis patients (Galvin, Regan, and Heron 1976*b*). All had experienced the development of symptoms with exercise or increased body temperature, either sensory (one patient), motor (two), or visual (one). Three of the four had had previous optic neuritis, whilst the fourth described visual blurring with exercise or heating. As body temperature increased, double-flash resolution deteriorated and visual acuity fell, with the reverse effects on cooling. Surprisingly, no recording of body temperature was made during the test. The depression of acuity on heating is explicable on the basis of blocking in severely demyelinated nerve fibres. Since heating increases conduction velocity in partially demyelinated peripheral nerve fibres (Rasminsky 1973), the impairment of double-flash resolution may represent increasing dispersal of the stimulus amongst optic nervefibres demyelinated by varying degrees.

Visual evoked responses

Regan *et al*. (1977*b*) have assessed the effects of cooling and heating in 10 patients with definite multiple sclerosis, one of whom had a previous history of optic neuritis. Four patients had optic atrophy, two of whom gave a history of temperature sensitivity. Measurements of evoked potentials to medium frequency flicker (13–25 Hz), perceptual delay and double flash threshold were made. In contrast to an earlier study (Regan *et al*. 1976) perceptual delay was measured for one fovea against another, rather than against a parafoveal site. Double flash resolution was assessed solely for foveal stimulation. The changes produced in body temperature were not measured.

In the cooling experiments, two of seven patients showed a reduction in flicker delay, whilst with heating, latencies were increased in two of four tests. A previous assessment of the effects of cooling (by a different method) on perceptual delay, had shown a lessening in all seven patients, not those, incidentally, studied in the later paper (Regan *et al*. 1977*b*). In one patient, the latency returned to its pre-cooling value two hours after the experiment was completed. In another, though heating produced a measurable deterioration in visual acuity, it was without effect on the evoked potential delay despite significantly prolonging visual perception. Paradoxically, heating actually improved double-flash resolution, though it had impaired resolution in six other patients tested.

Comparison of the effects of heating on flicker responses, perceptual delay, and temporal resolution was made in only a single patient, and since the change in body temperature was not measured, it is difficult to predict which type of response is more frequently affected. It has been suggested, however, that measurement of perceptual delay or double flash threshold will give a higher yield than that obtained from observing the effects on responses to medium-frequency flicker. The impairment of double-flash threshold with heating normally found may represent depression of maximum firing frequency in axons close to their blocking temperature, with the possible additional effect of dispersion of the stimulus due to heating affecting a population of axons to differing degree. The improvement in threshold in one patient was explained on the basis of blocking of conduction occurring in the fibres contributing to the major part of the dispersal of the stimulus. Where a patterned stimulus is presented at a lesser frequency, heating of a population of only mildly demyelinated fibres might reduce latency, from the known ability of heating to increase conduction velocity in partially demyelinated peripheral nerve fibres (Rasminsky 1973). Though this response might be less likely if the nerve contained axons demyelinated to markedly differing degrees, the recovery of the amplitude and wave form of the potential after optic neuritis argues that the fibres contributing to the potential have been affected to similar extents.

Evoked potentials and psychophysical tests in other conditions

Transient pattern responses

These are affected by a multiplicity of disorders other than multiple sclerosis. Halliday *et al*. (1973*b*) observed delays in patients with spino-cerebellar degeneration and optic atrophy and in some cases of optic nerve compression. Although delays have been reported in glaucoma, when all four quadrants of the visual field are stimulated simultaneously abnormal latencies are encountered only in the presence of large scotomata (Cappin and Nissim 1975). Earlier defects may be detectable by phase changes to quadrantic stimulation of the order of 10–20 ms. Delays have been seen in ischaemic optic neuropathy and tropical amblyopia (Asselman *et al*. 1975), and, rather surprisingly, with foveal stimulation in a case of medullary astrocytoma with mild papilloedema (Hennerici *et al*. 1977). The responses in patients with compression of the anterior visual pathways have been studied in detail (Halliday, A. M., Halliday, E., Kriss, McDonald, and Mushin, 1976). Abnormalities were found in 18 of 19 patients with proven compression of the optic nerve, though estimations of latencies was often difficult due to dispersion of the positive peak. Significant delays were found in only four patients and in none of them exceeded the upper limit of normal by more than 20 ms. In some instances a marked improvement in responses followed operation, but this did not extend to latencies, indeed they increased in three patients.

Steady-state evoked responses

These have not been found to be delayed in a group of patients with visual disturbances due to retinovascular lesions (Regan *et al*. 1976).

Psychophysical methods

Double-flash threshold is frequently abnormal in glaucoma, sometimes despite normal visual acuity or visual fields (Galvin *et al*. 1976*a*). Abnormalities are also seen in retinitis pigmentosa, retinal detachment and haemorrhage, but the extent of the delays has not been indicated, nor indeed have other optic nerve disorders been examined. Visual delays, as assessed by the Pulfrich pendulum, are occasionally abnormal in non-demyelinating disorders of the visual pathway (Rushton 1975).

Conclusions

It is an invidious task to summarize the material presented in this chapter. Seldom have the various types of evoked potential and psychophysical test been performed on the same patient, so that comparative evaluation is difficult.

In patients with previous optic neuritis, abnormal responses are the rule, whatever test is used. With transient pattern-evoked responses, some 5 per cent of patients will have normal latencies, but with steady-state stimulation by large checks (50′), medium-frequency flicker (13–25 Hz) or transient rectangular stimulation at the fovea, abnormalities are almost invariable provided prolonged interocular differences are included in the first two. A depressed critical flicker fusion frequency follows optic neuritis in some 90 per cent of patients but high-frequency flicker (30–60 Hz) produces delayed responses less often. The advantage of using medium-frequency flicker is that it does not require good visual acuity, though clearly these investigations are unlikely to be of diagnostic value when vision is severely impaired by a clinically recognizable optic nerve lesion.

Perceptual delay appears inevitable after optic neuritis (from testing of a small population), when parafoveal sites are compared with the other eye, though testing at more than one retinal site may be necessary. The delay in perception of a brightening or dimming stimulus between the fovea and an extra-foveal position is less often abnormal. Delayed temporal resolution of twin light flashes is nearly always found after optic neuritis, though some-times only at a single retinal site. In patients with unilateral optic neuritis, testing of the other eye gives abnormal results infrequently.

In patients with evidence of multiple sclerosis, but without a history of visual symptoms, the proportion with abnormal responses to these tests has varied (Table 14.5), though the small numbers studied by most authors hardly allows the findings to be compared with confidence. Bilateral delay of transient pattern evoked responses is more common in such cases, being reported approximately twice as often as unilateral delays in two studies.

It has been suggested that the type of visual damage sustained by patients with 'spinal' multiple sclerosis differs from that following optic neuritis, at least in terms of the responses to various electro-physiological and psychophysical tests. Stress has been laid on the association of abnormal steady-state pattern but normal flicker responses in 'spinal' patients with visual signs, but the reverse picture in those without such signs. The associa-tion does not extend to both eyes, even in the presence of bilateral optic atrophy, where delayed responses to steady-state pattern are just as likely to be unilateral. Furthermore delays to transient pattern responses are found in 80 per cent of patients with 'spinal' multiple sclerosis, despite the absence of visual signs. Considering the number of patients on which these conclusions have been based, it is clear that testing of a much larger population will be necessary before their validity can be accepted. In general, the use of perceptual tests for the detection of silent optic nerve lesions in patients

Table 14.5 The percentage of abnormal findings in patients with some evidence of multiple sclerosis but no history of visual symptoms

Method		Per cent				No. of patients
		Possible	Probable	Definite	Overall	
Steady-state pattern	Regan et al. (1976)†				0	6
Transient pattern	Asselman et al. (1975)				28	57 (eyes)
Medium-frequency flicker	Regan et al. (1976)‡				29	7
Pulfrich pendulum	Rushton (1975)	17	0	100	30	10
Perceptual delay (interocular + trans retinal)	Regan et al. (1976)†				42	19
Flicker fusion threshold	Titcombe and Willison (1961)				52	31
Transient pattern	Halliday et al. (1974)*				57	23
Abnormality of peripapillary nerve-fibre layer	Feinsod and Hoyt (1975)§				68	25
Delayed temporal resolution	Galvin et al. (1977)	80	——83——		82	11
Transient pattern	Halliday et al. (1973b)				86	14
Steady-state pattern	Regan et al. (1976)‡				86	7
Flash response	Feinsod et al. (1977)				100	15
Perceptual delay (interocular + trans retinal)	Regan et al. (1976)‡				100	7
Medium-frequency flicker	Regan et al. (1976)†				100	6

* Cases of spastic paraplegia
† Without visual signs
‡ With visual signs
§ Some had visual symptoms or signs

suspected of multiple sclerosis has been less valuable than the application of various electrophysiological techniques.

The delays revealed by evoked potential measurement have been explained on the basis of an experimental model, extrapolating from the conduction delays across demyelinated internodes in lesions of the central and peripheral nervous systems. Alternatively, some contribution may come from the conversion of conduction from saltatory to non-saltatory. Some authors have found less delay for various perceptual tests and argued that those associated with evoked potential stimulation may be partly explicable on delay at cortical levels. Other investigators, however, using similar psychophysical methods have found latencies of a comparable degree. Retinal delay has been considered as a possible further factor, but evidence for disturbed retinal function in multiple sclerosis is contradictory.

Artificial elevation of body temperature to reveal a higher proportion of abnormal findings has been used with a number of these methods. Heating may produce a measurable impairment of visual acuity or critical flicker fusion frequency, and in patients with previous optic neuritis, frequently impairs visual perception or double-flash resolution with a reversal of the effects on cooling. The depressant effect of increased temperature on the ability of partially demyelinated nerve fibres to conduct a rapid train of impulses has been considered the likeliest explanation. Responses to medium-frequency flicker are less often affected by these experiments.

Evoked potentials may be delayed in other disturbances of the optic nerve, including glaucoma, spino-cerebellar degeneration, ischaemic optic neuropathy, and compressive lesions. The degree of delay seldom extends to that encountered in patients with multiple sclerosis.

REFERENCES

Adie, W. J. (1930). Acute retrobulbar neuritis in disseminated sclerosis. *Trans. ophthal. Soc. U.K.* **50**, 262–7.
— (1932). The aetiology and symptomatology of disseminated sclerosis. *Br. med. J.* **2**, 997–1000.
Allison, R. S. (1950). Survival in disseminated sclerosis: A clinical study of a series of cases first seen twenty years ago. *Brain* **73**, 103–20.
Asselman, P., Chadwick, D. W., and Marsden, C. D. (1975). Visual evoked responses in the diagnosis and management of patients suspected of multiple sclerosis. *Brain* **98**, 261–82.
Bostock, H. and Sears, T. A. (1976). Continuous conduction in demyelinated mammalian nerve fibres. *Nature, Lond.* **263**, 786–7.
Brown, M. R. and Putnam, T. J. (1939). Remissions in multiple sclerosis. *Archs Neurol. Psychiat. Chicago* **41**, 913–20.
Buzzard, T. (1893). Atrophy of the optic nerve as a symptom of chronic disease of the central nervous system. *Br. med. J.* **2**, 779–84.
Cala, L. A. and Mastaglia, F. L. (1976). Computerized axial tomography in multiple sclerosis. *Lancet* **1**, 689.
Cantor, F. K., Kurtzke, J. F., Schechter, G., Tsai, S., and Shirzadi, M. G. (1974). Electrophysiologic evaluation of multiple sclerosis. *Neurology, Minneap.* **24**, 360.
Cappin, J. M. and Nissim, S. (1975). Visual evoked responses in the assessment of field defects in glaucoma. *Archs Ophthal. N.Y.* **93**, 9–18.
Coleman, D. J. and Carroll, F. D. (1972). A new technique for evaluation of optic neuropathy. *Trans. Am. ophthal. Soc.* **70**, 154–60.
Cook, J. H. and Arden, G. B. (1977). Unilateral retrobulbar neuritis: A comparison of evoked potentials and psychophysical measurements. In *Visual evoked potentials in man: New developments* (ed. J. E. Desmedt), Chap. 27, pp. 450–7. Clarendon Press, Oxford.
Croll, M. (1965). The ocular manifestations of multiple sclerosis. *Am. J. Ophthal.* **60**, 822–9.
Davis, F. A. (1966). The hot bath test in the diagnosis of multiple sclerosis. *J. Mt. Sinai Hosp.* **33**, 280–2.

— Michael, J. A., and Neer, D. (1973). Serial hyperthermia testing in multiple sclerosis: A method for monitoring subclinical fluctuations. *Acta Neurol. Scand.* **49**, 63–74.

Eyerman, E. L., Archer, C. R., and Mayes, Jr., B. (1976). Multiple sclerosis in brain and optic nerve as seen by standard and high-resolution C.T. (Artronix). *Neuroradiology* **12**, 52.

Feinsod, M., Abramsky, O., and Auerbach, E. (1973). Electrophysiological examinations of the visual systems in multiple sclerosis. *J. Neurol. Sci.* **20**, 161–75.

— and Hoyt, W. F. (1975). Subclinical optic neuropathy in multiple sclerosis. *J. Neurol. Neurosurg. Psychiat.* **38**, 1109–14.

— — Wilson, B. W., and Spire, J. P. (1977). The use of visual evoked potential in patients with multiple sclerosis. In *Visual evoked potentials in man: New developments* (ed. J. E. Desmedt), Chap. 28, pp.458–60. Clarendon Press, Oxford.

Frisén, L. and Hoyt, W. F. (1974). Insidious atrophy of retinal nerve fibers in multiple sclerosis. *Archs Ophthal. N.Y.* **92**, 91–7.

— — Bird, A. C., and Weale, R. A. (1973). Diagnostic use of the Pulfrich phenomenon. *Lancet* **2**, 385–6.

Galvin, R. J., Heron, J. R., and Regan, D. (1977). Subclinical optic neuropathy in multiple sclerosis. *Archs Neurol. Chicago* **34**, 666–70.

— Regan, D., and Heron, J. R. (1976*a*). Impaired temporal resolution of vision after acute retrobulbar neuritis. *Brain* **99**, 255–68.

— — — (1976*b*). A possible means of monitoring the progress of demyelination in multiple sclerosis: Effect of body temperature on visual perception of double light flashes. *J. Neurol. Neurosurg. Psychiat.* **39**, 861–5.

Gartner, S. (1953). Optic neuropathy in multiple sclerosis. Optic neuritis. *Archs Ophthal., N.Y.* **50**, 718–26.

Gipner, J. F. (1925). The ophthalmologic findings in cases of multiple sclerosis: A study of 100 cases. *Med. Clins. N. Am.* **8**, 1227–34.

Halliday, A. M., Halliday, E., Kriss, A., McDonald, W. I., and Mushin, J. (1976). The pattern-evoked potential in compression of the anterior visual pathways. *Brain* **99**, 357–74.

— and McDonald, W. I. (1977). Pathophysiology of demyelinating disease. *Br. med. Bull.* **33**, 21–7.

— — and Mushin, J. (1972). Delayed visual evoked responses in optic neuritis. *Lancet* **1**, 982–5.

— — — (1973*a*). Delayed pattern-evoked responses in optic neuritis in relation to visual acuity. *Trans. ophthal. Soc. U.K.* **93**, 315–22.

— — — (1973*b*). Visual evoked response in diagnosis of multiple sclerosis. *Br. med. J.* **4**, 661–4.

— — — (1974). Delayed visual evoked response in progressive spastic paraplegia. *Electroenceph. clin. Neurophysiol.* **37**, 328.

— — — (1977). Visual evoked potentials in patients with demyelinating disease. In *Visual evoked potentials in man: New developments* (ed. J. E. Desmedt), Chap. 26, pp.438–49. Clarendon Press, Oxford.

Hennerici, M., Wenzel, D., and Freund, H.-J. (1977). The comparison of small-size rectangle and checkerboard stimulation for the evaluation of delayed visual evoked responses in patients suspected of multiple sclerosis. *Brain* **100**, 119–36.

Heron, J. R., Regan, D., Milner, B. A. (1974). Delay in visual perception in unilateral optic atrophy after retrobulbar neuritis. *Brain* **97**, 69–78.

Hoyt, W. F., Schlicke, B., and Eckelhoff, R. J. (1972). Fundoscopic appearance of a nerve-fibre bundle defect. *Br. J. Ophthal.* **56**, 577–83.

Klingmann, T. (1910). Visual disturbances in multiple sclerosis. Their relations to changes in the visual field and ophthalmoscopic findings. Diagnostic significance. Report of twelve cases. *J. nerv. ment. Dis.* **37**, 734–48.

Lazarte, J. A. (1950). Multiple sclerosis: Prognosis for ambulatory and non-ambulatory patients. In *Multiple sclerosis and the demyelinating diseases*. Research Publications of the Association for Research in Nervous and Mental Diseases, Vol. 28, pp. 512–23. Williams and Wilkins, Baltimore.

Leibowitz, U. and Alter, M. (1968). Optic nerve involvement and diplopia as initial manifestations of multiple sclerosis. *Acta Neurol. Scand.* **44**, 70–80.

Leinfelder, P. J. (1950). Retrobulbar neuritis in multiple sclerosis. In *Multiple sclerosis and the demyelinating diseases*. Research Publications of the Association for Research in Nervous and Mental Diseases, Vol. 28, pp. 393–5. Williams and Wilkins, Baltimore.

Lillie, W. J. (1934) The clinical significance of retrobulbar and optic neuritis. *Am. J. Ophthal.* **17**, 110–19.

Lowenstein, O. (1951). Methods for the early diagnosis of multiple sclerosis. Observations with special reference to the so-called ocular type. *Archs Ophthal. N.Y.* **46**, 513–26.

Lynn, B. (1959). Retrobulbar neuritis. A survey of the present condition of cases occurring over the last fifty-six years. *Trans. ophthal. Soc. U.K.* **79**, 701–16.

McAlpine, D., Lumsden, C. E., and Acheson, E. C. (1972). In *Multiple Sclerosis. A reappraisal* (2nd edn), p. 202. Churchill Livingstone, Edinburgh.

McDonald, W. I. (1977). Pathophysiology of conduction in central nerve fibres. In *Visual evoked potentials in man: New developments* (ed. J. E. Desmedt), Chap. 25, pp.427–37. Clarendon Press, Oxford.

Marshall, D. (1950). Ocular manifestations of multiple sclerosis and relationship to retrobulbar neuritis. *Trans. Am. ophthal. Soc.* **48**, 487–525.

Mastaglia, F. L., Black, J. L., Cala, L. A., and Collins, D. W. K. (1977). Evoked potentials, saccadic velocities, and computerized tomography in diagnosis of multiple sclerosis. *Br. med. J.* **1**, 1315–17.

Milner, B. A., Regan, D., and Heron, J. R. (1974). Differential diagnosis of multiple sclerosis by visual evoked potential recording. *Brain* **97**, 755–72.

Müller, R. (1949). Studies on disseminated sclerosis. *Acta med. scand. Suppl.* **222**, (Vol. 133), 1–214.

Mourik, J., Van Donselaar, C. A., and Minderhoud, J. M. (1978). Disturbed 'flight of colours' in multiple sclerosis. *Lancet* **1**, 108.

Namerow, N. S. (1971). Temperature effect on critical flicker fusion in multiple sclerosis. *Archs Neurol. Chicago* **25**, 269–75.

Parsons, O. A. and Miller, P. N. (1957). Flicker fusion thresholds in multiple sclerosis. *Archs. Neurol. Psychiat., Chicago* **77**, 134–9.

Percy, A. K., Nobrega, F. T., and Kurland, L. T. (1972). Optic neuritis and multiple sclerosis. *Archs Ophthal. N.Y.* **87**, 135–9.

*Pulfrich, C. (1922). Die stereoskopie in dienste der isochromen und heterochromen photometrie. *Naturwissenschaften* **10**, 533–64, 569–74, 596–601, 714–22; 735–43, 751–61.

Rasminsky, M. (1973). The effects of temperature on conduction in demyelinated single nerve fibres. *Archs Neurol., Chicago* **25**, 269–75.

Regan, D., Milner, B. A., and Heron, J. R. (1976). Delayed visual perception and delayed visual evoked potentials in the spinal form of multiple sclerosis and in retrobulbar neuritis. *Brain* **99**, 43–66.

— — — (1977a) Slowing of visual signals in multiple sclerosis, measured psychophysically and by steady-state evoked potentials. In *Visual evoked potentials in man : new developments* (ed. J. E. Desmedt), Chap. 29, pp.461–9. Clarendon Press, Oxford.

—Murray, T. J., and Silver, R. (1977b). Effect of body temperature on visual evoked potential delay and visual perception in multiple sclerosis. *J. Neurol. Neurosurg. Psychiat.* **40**, 1083–91.

— Silver, R., and Murray, T. J. (1977c). Visual acuity and contrast sensitivity in multiple sclerosis—hidden visual loss. *Brain* **100**, 563–79.

Rosen, J. A. (1965). Pseudoisochromatic visual testing in the diagnosis of disseminated sclerosis. *Trans. Am. neurol. Ass.* **90**, 283–4.

Rushton, D. (1975). Use of the Pulfrich pendulum for detecting abnormal delay in the visual pathway in multiple sclerosis. *Brain* **98**, 283–93.

Sachs, B. and Friedman, E. D. (1922). *General and special symptomatology in multiple sclerosis. An investigation by the Association for Research in Nervous and Mental Diseases* (ed. C. L. Dana, S. E. Jelliffe, H. A. Riley, F. Tilney, and W. Timme), Chap. 11, pp. 49–131. New York, Paul B. Hoeber.

Savitsky, N. and Rangell, L. (1950). *The ocular findings in multiple sclerosis. In Multiple sclerosis and the demyelinating diseases.* Research Publications of the Association for Research in Nervous and Mental Diseases, Vol. 28, pp. 403–13. Williams and Wilkins, Baltimore.

Scott, G. I. (1961). Ophthalmic aspects of demyelinating diseases. *Proc. R. Soc. Med.* **54**, 38–42.

Sharpe, J. A. and Sanders, M. D. (1975). Atrophy of myelinated nerve fibres in the retina in optic neuritis. *Br. J. Ophthal.* **59**, 229–32.

Sloan, L. L. (1942). The use of pseudo-isochromatic charts in detecting central scotomas due to lesions in the conducting pathways. *Am. J. Ophthal.* **25**, 1352–6.

Sokol, S. (1976). Visually evoked potentials: theory, techniques and clinical applications. *Surv. Ophthal.* **21**, 18–44.

Symonds, C. P. (1930). Retrobulbar neuritis and disseminated sclerosis. *Lancet* **2**, 19–20.

Titcombe, A. F. and Willison, R. G. (1961). Flicker fusion in multiple sclerosis. *J. Neurol. Neurosurg. Psychiat.* **24**, 260–5.

Uhthoff, W. (1890). Untersuchungen über die bei der multiplen herdsklerose vorkommenden augenstörungen. *Arch. Psychiat. Nervkrankh.* **21**, 55–116, 303–410.

White, D. N. and Wheelan, L. (1959). Disseminated sclerosis. A survey of patients in the Kingston, Ontario, area. *Neurology, Minneap.* **9**, 256–72.

Wybar, K. C. (1952). The ocular manifestations of disseminated sclerosis. *Proc. R. Soc. Med.* **45**, 315–19.

Yaskin, J. C., Spaeth, E. B., and Vernlund, R. J. (1951). Ocular manifestations of 100 consecutive cases of multiple sclerosis. *Am. J. Ophthal.* **3**, 687–97.

15 The relationship of optic neuritis to multiple sclerosis

The main purpose of this communication is to keep alive the discussion that has been proceeding spasmodically for forty years or more on the relation of acute retrobulbar neuritis in general to disseminated sclerosis (Adie 1932).

Before considering the phenomenon of isolated optic neuritis, and the type of multiple sclerosis which sometimes follows it, it is appropriate to examine the form of optic nerve demyelination found in encephalitis periaxialis diffusa (Schilder's disease) and in neuromyelitis optica (Devic's disease).

Encephalitis periaxialis diffusa

This condition has been divided into diffuse sclerosis, where lesions are confined to the central white matter of the posterior hemispheres, and transitional sclerosis where more widespread demyelination is found in addition. The former condition is relatively rare, predominating in children and having a mean life expectancy of 3·2 years (Poser and Van Bogaert 1956). The latter disorder has an age of onset comparable to multiple sclerosis and may share many of its clinical characteristics, including a remitting and relapsing course.

Visual symptoms were stressed in early accounts, due to occipital lobe demyelination in diffuse sclerosis, but sometimes secondary to optic nerve demyelination in cases of transitional sclerosis. Shelden, Doyle, and Kernohan (1929) reported a woman of 27 with rapid visual failure followed by drowsiness, hemiparesis, and incontinence. Post-mortem examination revealed extensive optic nerve lesions. Similar cases have been described by Lillie (1934) and Paton (1936). Berliner (1935) considered the optic nerve lesions of multiple sclerosis, encephalomyelitis, neuromyelitis optica, and encephalitis periaxialis diffusa to share many pathological and clinical characteristics.

Whereas diffuse sclerosis produces a progressive course with combinations of deafness, blindness, pyramidal signs, psychiatric disturbances and, occasionally, seizures (Lhermitte 1950), transitional sclerosis is more often associated with a polysclerotic type showing sudden relapses and occasional remissions. The overlap with multiple sclerosis may extend to abnormalities of the cerebrospinal fluid, including an elevated cell count (Walsh and Ford 1940) and abnormalities of the colloidal gold curve (Poser 1957).

The myelin degeneration of the optic nerve seen with electron microscopy resembles that encountered in multiple sclerosis (de Preux and Mair 1974) though with a greater degree of axonal involvement (Suzuki and Grover 1970).

Neuromyelitis optica

Classically, the condition comprises bilateral optic neuritis and transverse myelitis, with lesions restricted to the optic nerves and spinal cord at post-mortem examination. It occurs in both sexes and though Stansbury (1949*a, b*) defined age limits between 9 and 60 years, cases developing outside this age range have been reported (Scott 1952, 1961). Beck (1927) found patients more commonly presented with visual symptoms, but further experience has indicated that onset with spinal cord symptoms is equally frequent. Unilateral visual failure, followed by involvement of the second eye within a few days, shows a characteristically rapid evolution and is sometimes associated with disc swelling. Central scotoma is usual but hemianopic defects may be found in one or both eyes. The cord lesion is usually in the upper dorsal region and may cause extensive destruction of grey matter in the dorsal and ventral horns. Rather than a transverse myelitis, it may manifest as a diffuse lesion, a Brown-Séquard syndrome, or with more focal symptomatology. Cerebrospinal fluid changes include a gross pleocytosis, often with polymorphonuclear cells and sometimes a substantial elevation of protein concentration. The colloidal gold curve is characteristically normal though one of Scott's (1952) cases had a slight mid-zone rise. The mortality of the condition was originally considered to approach 100 per cent, a view reinforced by Stansbury's (1949*a, b*) concentration on fatal cases, but recoveries, sometimes of a remarkable degree, are not uncommon.

The same clinical presentation may occur despite pathological evidence of demyelination in other parts of the central nervous system (Cestan, Riser, and Planques 1934; McKee and McNaughton 1938) or hemispheric lesions of the type seen in diffuse cerebral sclerosis (Van Bogaert 1932). In other patients, such lesions may be symptomatic, with ophthalmoplegia, epilepsy, confusional states, or dysphasia.

Besides death or varying degrees of recovery, patients may show subsequent neurological relapses. Though Miller and Evans (1953) suggested these reproduced the presenting symptoms, drawing an analogy with perivenous demyelinating encephalo-myelitis, it is clear that initially typical cases may progress to a condition indistinguishable from multiple sclerosis (Putnam and Forster 1942).

Neuromyelitis optica may thus be a self-limiting condition, with recovery or death, and pathological changes compatible with the clinical manifestations. There may be more widespread pathological abnormalities of the type seen in multiple sclerosis or diffuse sclerosis, despite the same confined clinical abnormalities, and finally typical cases sometimes progress to a remitting and relapsing neurological disorder indistinguishable from multiple sclerosis. It is perhaps not surprising that ultrastructural analysis of the optic-nerve pathology of this condition was thought to show quantitative rather than qualitative differences from those seen in multiple sclerosis (de Preux and Mair 1974).

Whether these differing clinical courses relate to distinguishable precipitating agents, or, perhaps, variations in the immunological status of the host is a matter of conjecture.

The type of multiple sclerosis following optic neuritis

It has often been suggested that a more benign multiple sclerosis follows presentation with optic neuritis compared with other symptomatology, both in terms of functional disability and mortality rates (McIntyre and McIntyre 1943; Lazarte 1950; Carter, Sciarra, and Houston Merritt 1950; Papac 1957). Other benign forms have been suggested, including onset with dorsal-column and brain-stem symptomatology (McAlpine 1961; Drake 1971).

MacLean and Berkson (1951) recorded disability and mortality rates in multiple sclerosis patients from the Mayo Clinic, finding 64 per cent to be working and walking at 5 years and 42 per cent at 10 years, with 79 per cent surviving at 10 years. Müller (1949) found 64 per cent of patients presenting with motor disability were invalids at 5 years and 72 per cent at 10 years. McAlpine (1961) reported 27 per cent of patients who had presented with non-visual symptoms to be completely unrestricted at 10 years. Bauer, Firnhaber, and Winkler (1965) found 50 per cent of 311 patients were independent 6 to 10 years after onset.

Müller's (1949) figures for invalidity at 5 and 10 years after onset with cranial nerve disturbances were 28 and 44 per cent respectively. Of those patients with optic neuritis followed by Bradley and Whitty (1968) who developed multiple sclerosis, 91 per cent were completely unrestricted at 10 years, the percentage falling to 64 per cent if only definite cases were included. Seventy-four per cent of the patients reviewed by Nikoskelainen and Riekkinen (1974), 11 to 20 years after the onset of multiple sclerosis with optic neuritis were independent. Although a comparison with Kurtzke's (1970) series of multiple sclerosis patients showed a similar type of system involvement, disability was less than in a series of patients with different presentation reported from the same area of Finland (Panelius 1969) using similar diagnostic and disability criteria. The mean follow-up period for 67 patients with optic neuritis progressing to multiple sclerosis was 93 months in Hutchinson's (1976) series, by when 73 per cent were independent and leading active lives.

An exception to these opinions has come from a study of multiple sclerosis in Israel. Leibowitz, Alter, and Halpern (1966), using Hyllested's (1961) disability scale, found 43 per cent of cases presenting with optic neuritis were severely disabled after a mean duration of illness of 11·5 years, compared with 49 per cent of those presenting with other symptoms, their duration of illness being similar. A remitting and relapsing course was more frequent in the optic neuritis patients. In further papers (Leibowitz and Alter 1968; Kahana, Leibowitz, Fishback, and Alter 1973) it was stated that cases of multiple sclerosis presenting with optic neuritis had similar mortality and disability rates to those cases presenting with other symptoms. Paradoxically these authors also concluded (Leibowitz, Kahana, and Alter 1969), from a consideration of the same material, that a higher death rate occurred in patients with initial combined motor-sensory, cerebello-vestibular, or mixed symptoms, compared with those with sensory or visual symptoms at the onset.

A more disabling form of multiple sclerosis was found to follow bilateral as opposed to unilateral optic neuritis in one series (Hutchinson 1976).

The phenomenon of isolated optic neuritis

In 1930, Adie wondered whether 'an attack of retrobulbar neuritis might be the only manifestation in a lifetime of the activity of the agent that causes disseminated sclerosis?' Support for this concept comes from their similar epidemiological characteristics, though Hutchinson (1976) has recently claimed a greater female predominance in optic neuritis (2·7 : 1) compared with multiple sclerosis (1·9 : 1) based on an analysis of 10 series by Acheson (1972). The female : male ratio in our own series was 1·84 : 1, and similar values have been recorded by others, for example Bradley and Whitty (1967)—1·70 : 1. The ratio in the cases described by Percy, Nobrega, and Kurland (1972) was comparable to a multiple sclerosis population from the same locality. Age-specific rates were also similar.

It has been suggested (Leibowitz and Alter 1968) that the female predominance lessens with increasing age at onset for cases presenting with non-visual but not visual symptoms. An epidemiological comparison between optic neuritis and multiple sclerosis was made in a Hawaian population by Alter, Good, and Okihiro (1973). They concluded that the two conditions had a similar age and sex incidence, a comparable geographical distribution, and essentially identical pathologies.

Most evidence therefore points to shared epidemiological characteristics, suggesting that the precipitating agent might be the same in the two conditions. If so, why should some patients progress to multiple sclerosis and others remain with apparently isolated lesions? Are such lesions really isolated, or do a proportion of patients with optic neuritis have more widespread areas of demyelination which remain asymptomatic?

The use of various electrophysiological techniques has begun to answer these questions, though it has been known for some time that discrepancies can occur between symptoms in life and the extent of the disease at post-mortem examination. So-called benign forms of the disease are described (McAlpine 1961, 1964; McAlpine, Lumsden, and Acheson 1972) and are the experience of all neurologists.

D.A. Presented at the age of 33 with a cervical cord lesion with a CSF cell count of 8 lymphocytes/cu mm. Two years later brief visual blurring occurred, confined to the right eye. Sixteen years later she developed weakness of the right leg. Examination showed a right afferent pupillary defect with temporal pallor of the optic disc and a slowing of saccadic eye movements. There was a mild spastic paraparesis. The patient remained unrestricted 18 years after the onset.

S.R. At the age of 27, developed transient diplopia. Four years later a right hemisensory disturbance occurred, again recovering. At the age of 44, she noticed a tendency to limp with increasing limb weakness. Examination revealed bilateral temporal pallor of the optic discs with mild pyramidal signs in the limbs. She was only mildly restricted in her activities, 18 years after the onset of her illness.

H.N. Developed vision loss in the right eye at the age of 16 with little recovery. Fifty-six years later, a progressive spastic paraparesis appeared with urgency of micturition and some clumsiness with paraesthesiae in the left hand. Visual acuity was less than N48 on the right and N5 on the left, with a right afferent pupillary defect. The right fundus showed myopic degeneration and there was temporal pallor of the left optic disc. The patient made 4 mistakes with 24 Ishihara colour plates, using the left eye alone. There was a mild spastic tetraparesis and some impairment of proprioception and vibration sense in the lower limbs. A myelogram was normal, though CSF protein concentration was 0·76 g/l. Computerized axial tomography showed mild ventricular dilatation. The latencies of visual evoked responses were 148 ms (right) and 144 ms (left), the upper limit of normal for the laboratory being 116 ms.

Many authors in following patients with optic neuritis have found some with unequivocal evidence of multiple lesions, despite an absence of appropriate symptoms (Tatlow 1948; Bradley and Whitty 1968; Nikoskelainen and Riekkinen 1974). Cases may fail to progress, sometimes soon after the onset of the disease, but in other instances after several years (Mackay and Hirano 1967). Autopsy evidence of multiple sclerosis may be found despite a lack of appropriate clinical history. In one series of 15 644 autopsies, of 64 cases of multiple sclerosis 12 had been unsuspected in life (Georgi 1961; quoted by Mackay and Hirano 1967). Mackay and Hirano (1967) described two such cases. The first patient had a history of possible poliomyelitis with consequent wasting of the right leg, but presented with late onset epilepsy in association with complete heart block. The neurological examination was compatible with the clinical history. Autopsy examination showed plaques in the cerebrum and brain stem but with sparing of optic chiasm, cerebellum, and spinal cord. The appearance of the optic nerves was not stated. The histological features were those of multiple sclerosis. The spinal cord examination did not show anterior horn cell changes consistent with the presumed diagnosis of poliomyelitis. The second case had a history of recurrent cerebrovascular accidents in association with hypertension and atrial fibrillation. On admission at the age of 71 years he had a left hemiparesis, hemisensory loss, and homonymous hemianopia. Autopsy examination revealed a right middle cerebral artery occlusion with multiple cerebral infarcts. In addition plaques were found in the right centrum semiovale and the restiform body of the medulla. Sections of the optic chiasm were unremarkable and the optic nerves apparently not examined. Fog, Hyllested, and Andersen (1972) reported a patient with a sensory disturbance followed by retrobulbar neuritis who remained well for 45 years, apart from occasional paraesthesiae. Autopsy examination showed demyelination of one optic nerve and numerous plaques throughout the central nervous system. Ghatak, Hirano, Lijtmaer, and Zimmerman (1974) described a man with skeletal metastases from a carcinoma of the bronchus who had a demyelinated lesion in the cervical cord at post-mortem examination undistinguishable from those occurring in multiple sclerosis. The intracranial contents were not examined. Thirty-three years before he had had an episode of diplopia with weakness of the lower limbs recovering after 12 months.

A number of techniques have been introduced which may establish the presence of multiple lesions in apparently monosymptomatic cases. The use of various visual evoked potentials and perceptual tests has been discussed in Chapter 14. Detection of silent lesions in the auditory pathway has been attempted by recording evoked responses to an auditory stimulus (Robinson and Rudge 1975). Early, middle, and late responses have been identified, but of the first, thought to arise from eighth nerve and brain stem nuclei, only component V appears to be reliably recorded in all normal individuals (Robinson and Rudge 1977). Abnormalities of this component were recorded in 65 per cent of 88 definite cases of multiple sclerosis, though these included disturbances of amplitude as well as latency. In patients with clinical evidence of a definite brain-stem lesion the figure rose to 82 per cent, compared to 51 per cent in those without such evidence.

Somatosensory potentials can be recorded over the spine and skull following stimulation of peripheral nerve in the upper or lower limb (Small, Beauchamp, and Matthews 1975). Abnormalities of cervical responses following median nerve stimulation, including both delayed and absent potentials, were detected in 58 per cent of 126 patients with multiple sclerosis (Small, D. G., Matthews, and Small, M. 1977). They may occur in the absence of sensory symptoms or signs, and have been found in 18 per cent of a small series of patients with isolated optic neuritis (Small, D. G., Matthews, and Small, M. 1978).

The blink reflex elicited by electrical stimulation of the supra-orbital nerve comprises early and late components (Kimura 1975). The early response, ipsilateral to the stimulus, is a simple pontine reflex, whilst the late, bilateral response is relayed through pons and lateral medulla. Afferent impulses for the late reflex enter the pons through the trigeminal root and, having descended in the ipsilateral spinal tract, ascend to connect with both ipsilateral and contralateral facial nuclei. The early response, a more specific test of brain-stem function, was abnormal in 145 of 260 patients tested, including 37 patients with either definite, probable, or possible multiple sclerosis, who had no clinical evidence of a brain-stem lesion. Abnormalities were more frequent in those patients with a longer history. In some cases, reduction of an initially prolonged latency is found during remission, in contrast to prolonged visual evoked responses which rarely change over many years of follow-up.

Measurement of saccadic and pursuit eye movements (Mastaglia, Black, and Collins 1977) has shown abnormalities of saccadic velocities in 50 per cent of multiple sclerosis patients, affecting abduction and adduction movements separately or together in one or both eyes. In half of these cases, no corresponding clinical disturbance was detectable.

Provocative tests, of the type already discussed in relation to visual evoked responses, have been used to elicit abnormalities in other fibre pathways. Electro-nystagmography detects nystagmus following an elevation of body temperature in many multiple sclerosis patients (Jestico and Ellis 1976).

These various tests serve to establish that in many patients with apparently isolated lesions, more widespread disturbances of neurological function exist. Their presence in some patients with optic neuritis, affecting pathways known to be frequently involved in multiple sclerosis, serves to further the concept, based partly on epidemiological evidence, that the two conditions have a common basis. Post-mortem examination of patients with isolated optic neuritis in life has not been reported, and it is likely that the application of these various electro-physiological techniques will be necessary to elicit how many such patients have more widespread lesions.

Accepting the hypothesis that optic neuritis, when strictly defined, is invariably due to the same agent that causes multiple sclerosis, one inevitably asks what factors determine the progression of one condition to the other. There is some evidence that a more rapidly progressive form of multiple sclerosis is associated with possession of certain histocompatibility determinants (Jersild, Dupont, Fog, Platz, and Svejgaard 1975), and that possession of the B lymphocyte determinant BT 101 in North European patients influences the progression from optic neuritis to multiple sclerosis (Compston, Batchelor, Earl, and McDonald 1978). It would seem more fruitful, in the light of the evidence available, to explore the immunological status of the host with optic neuritis in the hope that, if certain characteristics prove to be associated with a more favourable outcome, methods may be devised for altering the immune status in the remainder.

Conclusions

A similar form of optic nerve demyelination to that encountered in multiple sclerosis has been described in both encephalitis periaxialis diffusa and neuromyelitis optica. Though morphological differences exist, the pathological changes in the optic nerve in these three conditions are thought to be qualitatively similar.

The general experience is that the multiple sclerosis following optic neuritis pursues a more benign course, both in terms of mortality and disability, than that following other forms of presentation. Contradictory evidence, based on patients examined in Israel, has itself been open to differing interpretation.

Both epidemiological and morphological characteristics point to a common aetiological basis for optic neuritis and multiple sclerosis. Isolated optic neuritis is often found to be associated with more widespread demyelination when careful clinical assessment is available, and a number of reports suggest that a relatively benign form of the disease, with widespread lesions at post-mortem examination despite a paucity of clinical features, is more common than is usually appreciated.

A number of electro-physiological techniques have established the frequent occurrence of subclinical lesions in patients with isolated manifestation of the disease, including optic neuritis. Further experience will hopefully establish the factors, possibly based on the immunological status of the host, which determine both the progression of optic neuritis to multiple sclerosis and whether the development of more widespread demyelinating lesions becomes clinically manifest.

REFERENCES

Acheson, E. D. (1972). The epidemiology of multiple sclerosis. In *Multiple sclerosis: a reappraisal* (ed. D. McAlpine, C. E. Lumsden, and E. D. Acheson) (2nd edn.). Churchill Livingstone, Edinburgh.
Adie, W. J. (1930). Acute retrobulbar neuritis in disseminated sclerosis. *Trans. ophthal. Soc. U.K.* **50**, 262–7.
— (1932). Observations on the aetiology and symptomatology of disseminated sclerosis. *Br. med. J.* **2**, 997–1000.
Alter, M., Good, J., Okihiro, M. (1973). Optic neuritis in Orientals and Caucasians. *Neurology, Minneap.* **23**, 631–9.
Bauer, H. J., Firnhaber, W., and Winkler, W. (1965). Prognostic criteria in multiple sclerosis. *Ann. N.Y. Acad. Sci.* **122**, 542–51.
Beck, G. M. (1927). A case of diffuse myelitis associated with optic neuritis. *Brain* **50**, 687–702.

Berliner, M. L. (1935). Acute optic neuritis in demyelinating diseases of the nervous system. *Archs Ophthal., N.Y.* **13**, 83–98.

Bradley, W. G. and Whitty, C. W. M. (1967). Acute optic neuritis: its clinical features and their relation to prognosis for recovery of vision. *J. Neurol. Neurosurg. Psychiat.* **30**, 531–8.

—— (1968). Acute optic neuritis: prognosis for development of multiple sclerosis. *J. Neurol. Neurosurg. Psychiat.* **31**, 10–18.

Carter, S., Sciarra, D., and Houston Merritt, H. (1950). The course of multiple sclerosis as determined by autopsy proven cases. In *Multiple sclerosis and the demyelinating diseases.* Research Publications of the Association for Research in Nervous and Mental Diseases, Vol. 28, pp. 471–511. Williams and Wilkins, Baltimore.

Cestan, Riser, and Planques (1934). De la neuro-myélite optique. *Revue neurol.* **41**, (2), 741–62.

Compston, D. A., Batchelor, J. R., Earl, C. J., and McDonald, W. I. (1978). Factors influencing the risk of multiple sclerosis developing in patients with optic neuritis. *Brain* **101**, 495–511.

de Preux, J. and Mair, W. G. P. (1974). Ultra-structure of the optic nerve in Schilder's disease, Devic's disease and disseminated sclerosis. *Acta neuropathol., (Berl.)* **30**, 225–42.

Drake, R. L. (1971). Multiple sclerosis. The benign form of multiple sclerosis. *J. Kansas med. Soc.* **72**, 178–80.

Fog, T., Hyllested, K., and Andersen, S. R. (1972). A case of benign multiple sclerosis, with autopsy. *Acta Neurol. Scand.* [Suppl] **51** (Vol. 48), 369–70.

*Georgi, W. (1961). Multiple sklerose. Pathologisch-anatomische befunde multipler sklerose bei klinisch nicht diagnostizierten krankheiten. *Schweiz. med. Wschr.* **91**, 605–7.

Ghatak, N. R., Hirano, A., Lijtmaer, H., and Zimmerman, H. M. (1974). A symptomatic demyelinated plaque in the spinal cord. *Archs Neurol., Chicago* **30**, 484–6.

Hutchinson, W. M. (1976). Acute optic neuritis and the prognosis for multiple sclerosis. *J. Neurol. Neurosurg. Psychiat.,* **39**, 283–9.

Hyllested, K. (1961). Lethality, duration and mortality of disseminated sclerosis in Denmark. *Acta neurol. psychiat. scand.* **36**, 553–64.

Jersild, C., Dupont, B., Fog, T., Platz, P. J., and Svejgaard, A. (1975). Histocompatibility determinants in multiple sclerosis. *Transplant. Rev.* **22**, 148–63.

Jestico, J. V. and Ellis, P. D. M. (1976). Changes in nystagmus on raising body temperature in clinically suspected and proved multiple sclerosis. *Br. med. J.* **2**, 970–2.

Kahana, E., Leibowitz, U., Fishback, N., and Alter, M. (1973). Slowly progressive and acute visual impairment in multiple sclerosis. *Neurology, Minneap.* **23**, 729–33.

Kimura, J. (1975). Electrically elicited blink reflex in diagnosis of multiple sclerosis. Review of 260 patients over a seven-year period. *Brain* **98**, 413–26.

Kurtzke, J. F. (1970). Neurologic impairment in multiple sclerosis and the disability status scale. *Acta Neurol. Scand.* **46**, 493–512.

Lazarte, J. A. (1950). Multiple sclerosis: prognosis for ambulatory and non-ambulatory patients. In *Multiple sclerosis and the demyelinating diseases.* Research Publications of the Association for Research in Nervous and Mental Diseases, Vol. 28, pp. 512–23. Williams and Wilkins, Baltimore.

Leibowitz, U. and Alter, M. (1968). Optic nerve involvement and diplopia as initial manifestations of multiple sclerosis. *Acta Neurol. Scand.* **44**, 70–80.

—— and Halpern, L. (1966). Clinical studies of multiple sclerosis in Israel. IV. Optic neuropathy and multiple sclerosis. *Archs Neurol., Chicago* **14**, 459–66.

—Kahana, E., and Alter, M. (1969). Survival and death in multiple sclerosis. *Brain* **92**, 115–30.

*Lhermitte, F. (1950). *Les leuco-encephalites.* Flammarion, Paris.

Lillie, W. I. (1934). The clinical significance of retrobulbar and optic neuritis. *Am. J. Ophthal.* **17**, 110–19.

McAlpine, D. (1961). The benign form of multiple sclerosis. A study based on 241 cases seen within three years of onset and followed up until the tenth year or more of the disease. *Brain* **84**, 186–203.

—— (1964). The benign form of multiple sclerosis; result of a long-term study. *Br. med. J.* **2**, 1029–32.

— Lumsden, C. E., and Acheson, E. D. (1972). *Multiple sclerosis: a reappraisal* (2nd edn.), pp. 301–7. Churchill Livingstone, Edinburgh.

McIntyre, H. D. and McIntyre, A. P. (1943). Prognosis of multiple sclerosis. *Archs Neurol. Psychiat, Chicago* **50**, 431–8.

Mackay, R. P. and Hirano, A. (1967). Forms of benign multiple sclerosis. *Archs Neurol., Chicago* **17**, 588–600.

McKee, S. H. and McNaughton, F. L. (1938). Neuromyelitis optica. A report of two cases. *Am. J. Ophthal.* **21**, 130–7.

Maclean, A. R. and Berkson, J. (1951). Mortality and disability in multiple sclerosis. A statistical estimate of prognosis. *J. Am. med. Ass.* **146**, 1367–9.

Mastaglia, F. L., Black, J. L., and Collins, D. W. K. (1977). Saccadic and pursuit eye movements in patients with multiple sclerosis. *Electroenceph. clin. Neurophysiol.* **43**, 466–7.

Miller, H. G. and Evans, M. J. (1953). Prognosis in acute disseminated encephalomyelitis; with a note on neuromyelitis optica. *Q. Jl. Med.* **22**, 347–79.

Müller, R. (1949). Studies on disseminated sclerosis. *Acta med. scand.* [Suppl] **222** (Vol. 133), 1–214.

Nikoskelainen, N. and Riekkinen, P. (1974). Optic neuritis—a sign of multiple sclerosis or other diseases of the central nervous system. A retrospective analysis of 116 patients. *Acta Neurol. Scand.* **50**, 690–718.

Panelius, M. (1969). Studies on epidemiological, clinical and etiological aspects of multiple sclerosis. *Acta Neurol. Scand. Suppl.* **39**, 1–82.

Papac, R. (1957). Multiple sclerosis. A clinical review. *Stanford med. Bull.* **15**, 75–7.

Paton, L. (1936). Papilledema and optic neuritis. *Archs Ophthal., N.Y.* **15**, 1–20.

Percy, A. K., Nobrega, F. T., and Kurland, L. T. (1972). Optic neuritis and multiple sclerosis. *Archs Ophthal., N.Y.* **87**, 135–9.

Poser, C. M. (1957). Diffuse-disseminated sclerosis in the adult. *J. Neuropath. exp. Neurol.* **16**, 61–78.

— and Van Bogaert, L. (1956). Natural history and evolution of the concept of Schilder's diffuse sclerosis. *Acta neurol. psychiat. scand.* **31**, 285–331.

Putnam, T. J. and Forster, F. M. (1942). Neuromyelitis optica: its relation to multiple sclerosis. *Trans. Am. neurol. Ass.* **68**, 20–5.

Robinson, K. and Rudge, P. (1975). Auditory evoked responses in multiple sclerosis. *Lancet* **1**, 1164–9.

— — (1977). Abnormalities of the auditory evoked potentials in patients with multiple sclerosis. *Brain* **100**, 19–40.

Scott, G. I. (1952). Neuromyelitis optica. *Am. J. Ophthal.* **35**, 755–64.

— (1961). Ophthalmic aspects of demyelinating diseases. *Proc. R. Soc. Med.* **54**, 38–42.

Shelden, W. D., Doyle, J. B., and Kernohan, J. W. (1929). Encephalitis periaxialis diffusa. *Archs Neurol. Psychiat., Chicago* **21**, 1270–97.

Small, D. G., Beauchamp, M., and Matthews, W. B. (1975). Subcortical somatosensory evoked potentials in man. *Electroenceph. clin. Neurophysiol.* **38**, 215.

— Matthews, W. B., and Small, M. (1977). Subcortical somatosensory evoked potentials in multiple sclerosis. *Electroenceph. clin. Neurophysiol.* **43**, 536–7.

— — — (1978). The cervical somatosensory evoked potential (SEP) in the diagnosis of multiple sclerosis. *J. Neurol. Sci.* **35**, 211–24.

Stansbury, F. C. (1949a). Neuromyelitis optica. *Archs Ophthal., N.Y.* **42**, 292–335.

— (1949b). Neuromyelitis optica. *Archs Ophthal., N.Y.* **42**, 465–501.

Suzuki, K. and Grover, W. D. (1970). Ultrastructural and biochemical studies of Schilder's disease. 1. Ultrastructure. *J. Neuropath. exp. Neurol.* **29**, 392–404.

Tatlow, W. F. T. (1948). The prognosis of retrobulbar neuritis. *Br. J. Ophthal.* **32**, 488–97.

Van Bogaert, L. (1932). Erreur de diagnostic: neuromyelite optique aigue, premier stade d'une sclerose en plaques typique. *J. Neurol. Psychiat., Brux.* **32**, 234–9.

Walsh, F. B. and Ford, F. R. (1940). Central scotomas. Their importance in topical diagnosis. *Archs Ophthal., N.Y.* **24**, 500–32.

Index

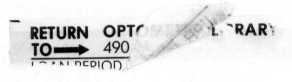